TMJ DISORDERS
MANAGEMENT of the CRANIOMANDIBULAR COMPLEX

CLINICS IN PHYSICAL THERAPY
VOLUME 18

TMJ DISORDERS
MANAGEMENT of the CRANIOMANDIBULAR COMPLEX

Edited by

Steven L. Kraus, P.T.

Clinical Assistant Professor
Orthodontic Residency Program
Part-time Faculty
TMJ/Facial Pain Clinic
Emory University School of Dentistry
Adjunct Faculty and Clinical Educator
Orthopedic Physical Therapy Master's Program
Emory University
Co-Director
Physical Therapy Associates of Metro Atlanta
Atlanta, Georgia

CHURCHILL LIVINGSTONE

NEW YORK, EDINBURGH, LONDON, MELBOURNE

1988

Library of Congress Cataloging-in-Publication Data

TMJ disorders.

 (Clinics in physical therapy ; v. 18)
 Includes bibliographies and index.
 1. Temporamandibular joint—Diseases.
2. Temporomandibular joint. I. Kraus, Steven L.
II. Series. [DNLM: 1. Temporomandibular Joint—
physiology. 2. Temporomandibular Joint Diseases—
therapy. W1 CL831CN v.18 / WU 140 T626]
RK470.T58 1988 617′.522 87-27742
ISBN 0-443-08484-X

© **Churchill Livingstone Inc. 1988**

Distributed in the United Kingdom by Churchill Livingstone,
Robert Stevenson House, 1-3 Baxter's Place, Leith Walk,
Edinburgh EH1 3AF, and by associated companies, branches,
and representatives throughout the world.

Acquisitions Editor: *Kim Loretucci*
Copy Editor: *Julia Muiño*
Production Designer: *Melanie Haber*
Production Supervisor: *Jocelyn Eckstein*

Printed in the United States of America

First published in 1988
Second printing in 1989

Dedicated to my parents Dottie and Kenneth L. Kraus, who have always given their time, energy, and love to their children. I would like to acknowledge my wife Pattie, for her patience and understanding during the editing of this book.

Contributors

Robert A. Bays, D.D.S.
Associate Professor and Chairman, and Graduate Program Director, Department of Oral and Maxillofacial Surgery, Emory University Post-Graduate School of Dentistry; Chief, Oral and Maxillofacial Surgery and Dentistry, Emory University Hospital; Consultant, Veterans Administration Medical Center, Atlanta, Georgia

Frank Benson, D.M.D.
Assistant Professor, Department of Periodontics, Emory University School of Dentistry; Private practice in periodontics, Atlanta, Georgia

Barbara M. Bourbon, Ph.D.
Adjunct Assistant Professor, Department of Physical Therapy, Philadelphia College of Pharmacy and Science, Philadelphia, Pennsylvania; Adjunct Assistant Professor, Graduate Program in Physical Therapy, Beaver College, Glenside, Pennsylvania; Co-Director, The Philadelphia Institute for Physical Therapy, Philadelphia, Pennsylvania

Barbara Connolly, Ed.D.
Associate Professor and Chairman, Department of Rehabilitation Sciences, University of Tennessee College of Allied Health Sciences, Memphis, Tennessee

David G. Gantt, Ph.D.
Associate Professor, Dental Research Center, Emory University School of Dentistry; Adjunct Associate Professor, Department of Anthropology, Emory University School of Arts and Sciences; Affiliate Research Scientist, Division of Reproductive Biology, Yerkes Regional Primate Center, Atlanta, Georgia

Duane Grummons, D.D.S., M.S.D.
Private Practice, Marina del Rey, California

Marty Kaput, M.S., P.T.
Clinical Faculty, Physical Therapy Master's Program, Georgia State University; Clinical Faculty, Physical Therapy Master's Program, Emory University; Co-Director, Physical Therapy Associates of Metro Atlanta, Atlanta, Georgia

Steven L. Kraus, P.T.
Clinical Assistant Professor, Orthodontic Residency Program, Part-time Faculty, TMJ/Facial Pain Clinic, Emory University School of Dentistry; Adjunct Faculty and Clinical Educator, Orthopedic Physical Therapy Master's Program, Emory University; Co-Director, Physical Therapy Associates of Metro Atlanta, Atlanta, Georgia

Eric S. Lawrence, D.D.S.
Private Practice in Orthodontics, Orofacial Orthopedics, and TMJ; Dental Staff in Orthodontics and TMJ, The Mount Sinai Medical Center, Cleveland, Ohio

Jeffrey S. Mannheimer, M.A., P.T.
Clinical Assistant Professor, Department of Orthopedic Surgery and Rehabilitation, Program in Physical Therapy, Hahnemann University School of Medicine, Philadelphia, Pennsylvania; Private Practice, Delaware Valley Physical Therapy Associates, Lawrenceville, New Jersey; Director, Physical Therapy Tract, Continuing Education Program in Diagnosis and Treatment of Orofacial Pain and TMJ Dysfunction (Craniomandibular Disorders), University of Medicine and Dentistry of New Jersey, New Jersey Dental School, Newark, New Jersey

Samuel J. Razook, D.D.S.
Prosthodontist; Oral and Maxillofacial Surgeon, Private Practice; Former Director, TMJ/Facial Pain Clinic, Emory University School of Dentistry; Consultant, Veterans Administration Medical Center, Atlanta, Georgia

Shirley A. Sahrmann, Ph.D.
Associate Director for Research; Associate Professor, Program in Physical Therapy; Associate Professor, Department of Neurology, Washington University School of Medicine; Consultant, Irene Johnson Institute of Rehabilitation, St. Louis, Missouri

Gerald S. Samson, D.D.S.
Assistant Professor, Department of Orthodontics, Emory University School of Dentistry; Private Practice in Orthodontics, Atlanta, Georgia

Charles G. Widmer, D.D.S., M.S.
Assistant Professor of Oral Biology, Dental Research Center; Director, TMJ/Facial Pain Clinic, Emory University School of Dentistry, Atlanta, Georgia

Foreword

The management of musculoskeletal disorders involving the temporomandibular joints or the neuromuscular components of the masticatory system is of common interest to physical therapists and dentists. Both are concerned with the relief of acute and chronic pain as well as with the restoration of normal function. Because the chief complaint of the majority of patients with temporomandibular disorders is pain, frequently accompanied by limited mobility or function of the mandible, an understanding of the etiology, diagnosis, and management of these disorders is important to physical therapists as well as to dentists.

Interest in temporomandibular disorders has increased enormously during the past 10 to 15 years. This interest is, to a large extent, reflected in the increasing number of health professionals who are seeing patients with these problems in their practices. Such clinicians are trying their best to deal with these problems, to help their patients, and to understand the underlying structural and behavioral factors involved. Unfortunately, the present state of our knowledge often places these clinicians in a difficult situation since they must contend with the problems, the patients, and the underlying factors in the presence of controversial and often conflicting ideas concerning etiology, diagnosis, and management.

It is within the context of increased professional interest, rapidly changing concepts, and lingering controversy that Steven Kraus and his colleagues have added this timely contribution to the physical therapy and dental literature. Such an undertaking entails some risk because, besides the current controversies, the results of subsequent research will almost certainly require revision of many prevailing ideas in this changing field. Nevertheless, patients have problems and are waiting to be treated, and one must deal with the perceived realities of the present. This volume is designed to inform and update the reader about the current role of physical therapy and its interface with dentistry in the management of temporomandibular disorders. It is unique because the physical therapy literature has not yet addressed this area in an organized manner. Thus, it is recommended reading for physical therapists and for those dentists interested in temporomandibular disorders.

In order to maintain a perspective between current management concepts and the likely prospect of future change, the reader is urged to remember that musculoskeletal disorders may involve various combinations of behavioral as well as structural factors and that the relative contribution of each is not always clear, that conditions may coexist in a given patient but not necessarily be directly related to each other, that signs and symptoms of these disorders are often naturally cyclic, that there is an overdependence on trial and error in much present clinical treatment, that proponents of diverse treatment regimens all claim clinical success, that there is an overdependence on anecdotal and often emotional lectures and reports of clinical success, and finally, that clinical success, however noteworthy, is not scientific proof of cause and effect.

How do we reconcile the issues of reported clinical success with those of cause and effect? The answer, simply stated, is research and the application of the scientific method to every proposed concept or hypothesis. Research has increased in this field but much more is required. For example, normative clinical data from groups of healthy asymptomatic subjects are needed in order to define ranges of normal variation. Comparison of such data with those from groups of temporomandibular disorder patients would help us to identify clinical relationships that may be truly associated with the disorders. We also need data from objective clinical efficacy studies of a variety of current or proposed treatment modalities. Many other examples of research needs may be cited. All health professionals must continue to find ways to separate conjecture from empiricism from scientifically derived data. These distinctions are important to our understanding of etiologic contributory factors, diagnostic criteria, and treatment efficacy. Thus, much more basic and clinical information is needed in areas that promise to enlighten us on the fundamental nature of these musculoskeletal disorders.

Norman D. Mohl, D.D.S., Ph.D.
Professor of Oral Medicine
State University of New York
at Buffalo

Preface

In developing this volume on TMJ disorders, I saw the goals as being threefold. The first objective is to provide the information necessary for understanding the biomechanical principles of the temporomandibular joint (TMJ). Once a knowledge base of the TMJ has been established, the clinician can better understand the process of evaluation and the management of non-surgical and surgical TMJ and myofascial disorders.

A second objective is to provide a clear picture of the cervical spine and its role in craniomandibular disorders (occlusion, TMJ, mandibular muscles). Different avenues relating the cervical spine to the craniomandibular region are explored; growth and development of the region, cervical spine influences on mandibular positioning and mobility, and utilization of intraoral appliances in the adult are covered. Cervical spine dysfunction is recognized as a common source of local and referred symptoms to the head, face, and jaw areas, and in order to understand the sequence and goals of treatment for TMJ and myofascial disorders, an understanding of the impact of the cervical spine is essential.

The final objective of this book is to stimulate research in the area of the craniomandibular and cervical spine regions and to serve as a catalyst in establishing the professional working-learning relationship between the physical therapy and dental professions.

Steven L. Kraus, P.T.

Contents

1 | Evolution of the Craniomandibular Region

David G. Gantt

Some 400 to 500 million years ago, chordate animals evolved in the sea and eventually gave rise to the group we know as vertebrates. The basic chordate stock was characterized by the possession of a notochord, a hollow dorsal nerve cord, and a pharynx with gill slits that formed a filter-feeding apparatus for collecting plankton. In general, plankton gathering is neither the quickest nor easiest way of obtaining food; therefore, it is not surprising that in the succeeding vertebrates a number of evolutionary experiments occurred, aimed at changing from a microphagous to a macrophagous habit. Such experiments included, for example, the development of a horny-toothed oral sucker and tongue for rasping away the flesh of other animals that still survives today in the lampreys.[1]

One of the greatest events in the history of the vertebrates was the appearance of the jaws. The importance of this evolutionary development can hardly be overestimated, for it opened to the vertebrates new lines of adaptation and new possibilities for evolutionary advancement that expanded immeasurably the potentialities of these animals. The jawless vertebrates were restricted as to their adaptations for different modes of life.

The appearance of the jaws in vertebrates was brought about by a transformation of anatomical elements that originally had performed a function quite different from that function of food gathering. The jaws were derived originally from gill arches. At an early stage in the history of vertebrates at least one and probably two of the original anterior gill "arches" were eliminated, while another arch, probably the third, was changed from gill support into a *pair of jaws*.

The one really successful experiment was the modification of the skeleton supporting the two anterior gill arches to form opposable jaws. Jaws themselves were derived from the first (mandibular) arch, and the attachment support was derived from the second (hyoid) arch. This change produced the true fishes, which can be claimed to be one of the most successful groups of vertebrates. As far as we can determine, teeth arose simultaneously with jaws by the simple modification of the dermal denticles surrounding the mouth and, in most fishes, teeth occur on all jaw bones as well as on several palatal bones and on the rod-like tongue. In cartilaginous and bony fish, both upper and lower jaws are movable, being suspended posteriorly from the hyoid apparatus. Jaw action consists of the approximation of upper and lower jaw elements with specialization of the teeth into cutting dentitions, as in sharks, or crushing dentitions with flattened teeth, as in rays and skates. Bony fishes evidence many variations on this basic theme, and in all fishes the teeth are replaced continuously throughout life.[1,2]

In crossopterygian fishes, which accomplished the evolutionary transition from water to land, the upper jaw, as in all succeeding groups of land vertebrates, was firmly attached to the skull, with the leverlike mandible pivoted posteriorly. This freed the hyoid skeleton to assume new functions, such as acting as the first ear bone, the stapes, and providing support to structures in the throat and pharynx. On land, the support once provided to both prey and predator by water disappeared; this necessitated firmer anchoring of the upper jaw and also development of a flexible neck. The range of mandibular movements remains limited, however, in the amphibians that succeeded the fishes and the reptiles that succeeded the amphibians.

Scrutiny of the jaw activities of amphibians and reptiles shows that they are all relatively simple up and down movements with little lateral displacement. Jaws are essentially grasping, restraining devices, and the simple, spike-like teeth are able to puncture the skin or cuticle of living prey and thereby facilitate the penetration of gastric juices. Tearing of food may occur but *never mastication*, and the living prey are usually seized head first and swallowed whole, facilitated by a tongue stiffened by a rodlike hyoid and by a large pharynx. Sometimes accessory devices are present, such as an anteriorly hinged, sticky tongue in frogs and toads to pick up insects and their larvae, and movable (kinetic) skull bones in lizards and snakes [a characteristic not found in mammals]. The mandible is compound, consisting of six separate bones (see Figures 1-1 and 1-2). Thus, the mouth and jaws gather food which begins to be digested in the stomach.

In mammals, the one great advantage of mastication is the breaking down of food at the beginning of the gut, that is, the mouth. This results in an enormous gain in digestive efficiency, necessary for the rapid metabolism associated with homoiothermy which evolved with the mammals. Furthermore, true salivary glands appeared for the first time in mammals, their secretions moistening and lubricating food and adding chemical degradation by enzymes to mechan-

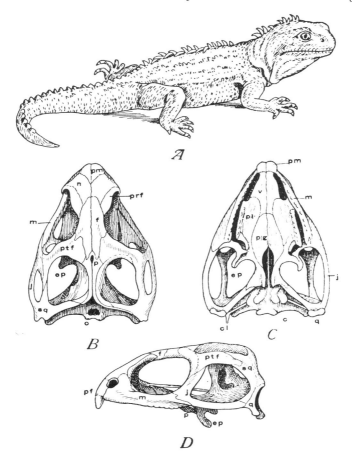

Fig. 1-1. *Sphenodon punctatum.* **(A)** Lateral view; **(B)** dorsal view of skull; **(C)** ventral view of skull; **(D)** lateral view of skull: *c,* condyle; *cl,* columella; *ep,* ectopterygoid; *f,* frontal; *j,* jugal; *m,* maxillary; *pm,* premaxillary; *n,* nasal; *p,* parietal; *pl,* palatine; *prf,* prefrontal; *ptf,* postfrontal and postorbital; *pg,* pterygoid; *Q,* quatrate or quadratojugal; *sq,* squamosal; *V,* vomer. (Newman H: Vertebrate Zoology. Macmillan, New York, 1920.)

ical degradation. Supersaturation with essential ions enabled buffering of natural and bacterial acidity to occur, as well as the restoration of the integrity of tooth surfaces by means of *remineralization*.

The teeth of mammals changed from being grasping and piercing devices with thin enamel to elements of a cutting and grinding machine with thick enamel. Wholesale modifications of the skull and mandible included the reduction of the mandible to a single bone, the *dentary*, and this occurred simultaneously with the rebuilding of the middle ear where all the ear ossicles have evolved from jaw bones. Also, profound restructuring of the cranio-

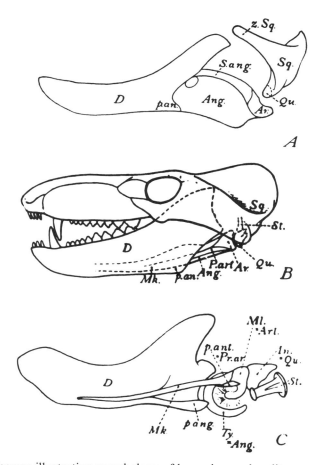

Fig. 1-2. Diagram illustrating morphology of lower jaw and auditory ossicles in mammallike reptiles and mammals. **(A)** Primitive therapsid condition: a jaw of reptilian type, in which the elements behind the dentary are not reduced. *D*, dentary; *p. an,* angular process of dentary, embracing the angular (*Ang*); *S. ang,* surangular; *Ar,* articular; *Qu,* quadrate, largely covered by *Sq,* squamosal; *s. Sq,* zygomatic process of squamosal. **(B)** Cynodont condition: jaw of submammalian type; the dentary the predominant element, with a very wide ascending ramus; postdentary elements reduced, the primary jaw (articular, Meckel's cartilage) and attached derm bones passing downward and forward and being received in the fossa on the inner side of the dentary; stapes in contact with quadrate, the latter small and largely covered by the squamosal. *Mk,* Meckel's cartilage; *P. art,* prearticular; *St,* stapes. **(C)** Condition in mammalian embryo (*Macropus*), seen from the inner side: the dentary is the sole functional element of the lower jaw; articulation with squamosal by means of a temporomandibular joint; elements behind dentary no longer functioning as jaw bones but as accessory auditory elements. *P. ang,* angular process; *Ty,* tympanic bone (probably derived from the angular of reptiles); *p. ant,* anterior process of malleus, a derm bone probably derived from the prearticular of reptiles; *Ml,* malleus, probably derived from the articular; *In,* incus, probably derived from the quadrate; *St,* stapes, probably derived from the stapes of reptiles. (Gregory WK: Origin and evolution of human dentition, Baltimore, Williams & Wilkins, 1922.)

mandibular musculature took place together with the emergence of new structures such as the lips and cheeks which, together with the tongue now powered entirely by intrinsic muscles, assist in positioning food between the teeth and in swallowing. The development of a secondary palate and an elaborate mechanism that safeguards the entrance to the pharynx, make it possible for breathing to continue during prolonged mastication.

The strengthening of the jaw joint, that is, an increase in the muscular and tendenous attachments, is usual where chewing consists of a unilateral, near-vertical shear. In the immediate ancestors of the mammals not only might chewing dislocate the jaw joint, but it could also dislocate the postdentary bones from the dentary. This may well be one the reasons for the development of the dentary-squamosal joint.

MAMMALIAN CHARACTERISTICS

The various diagnostic characteristics of the mammals as compared with mammal-like reptiles are that (1) mammals have a double occipital condyle forming the articulation for the skull on the first vertebra of the neck; (2) a secondary hard palate of bone which separates the nasal passage front from the mouth, with the external nasal opening as a single orifice in the front of the skull; (3) the joint between the skull and the lower jaw is formed by the squamosal and dentary bones, respectively; (4) the quadrate and articular bones (the articulating elements between the skull and jaw in the reptile) have in the mammal retreated into the middle ear to become transformed into two of the three ear ossicles, the incus and malleus, respectively, that together with the stapes make a chain to transmit vibrations from the eardrum to the inner ear. (This is one of the most remarkable transformations of anatomical structures from one function to another in the history of vertebrate evolution); (5) mammals have a differentiated dentition of incisors, canines, and molars of which the last has a crown of several cusps, held in the jaw by two or more roots; and (6) the enamel has increased in thickness in the form of prismatic enamel.

Mammals have the ability to maintain their temperature above that of their surroundings, which in turn requires a vastly increased food supply, especially in very small animals with a large surface area relative to volume, as is true of the recent shrews. Food is more efficiently used if it can be cut into smaller pieces (chewed) before ingestion. This involves the ability to shear the lower teeth against the upper, an ability that reptiles do not normally possess.

TMJ

The reptile jaw joint, where nearly all lateral movement is restricted, is formed between the quadrate bone attached to the cranium above and the articular bone attached by means of a suture to the back of the lower jaw. The

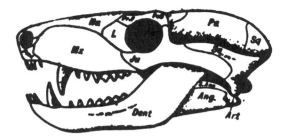

Fig. 1-3. Skull of cynodont reptile, *Nythosaurus larvalus,* Trias, South Africa. Note mammal-like tooth differentiation, but complex reptilian lower jaw. *Ang,* angulare; *Art,* articulare; *Dent,* dentary; *Ju,* jugal; *L,* lachrymal; *Mx,* maxillary; *Na,* nasal; *Pa,* parietal; *Pmx,* premaxillary; *PoO,* postorbital; *Pr. F,* prefrontal; *S. Ang,* surangulare; *sq,* squamosal. (Newman HH: Vetebrate Zoölogy. Macmillan, New York, 1920.)

lower jaw consists of several bones, with the dentary bone containing the teeth (see Fig. 1-2A).

Among recent vertebrates, the mammals from a well-defined class, differing from other classes in a number of ways, one of which is the possession of a dentary-squamosal jaw contact. This feature has been regarded as diagnostic of the mammals because it involves parts that are often preserved as fossils that evolved during the late Triassic, some 200 million years ago. Evidence of the development of this type of joint is a diagnostic feature found among the theridonts which link them to the mammals, especially among the cynodonts (small, mammalian-like reptiles) from the late Triassic (see Fig. 1-3). For millions of years, the mammal-like reptiles were evolving a new jaw joint between the dentary below, growing backward, and the squamosal above. Once the dentary had developed a joint with the squamosal, the quadrate and articular moved into the middle ear and joined the existing ear bones, the stapes; thus producing the three auditory ossicles (malleus, incus, and stapes).[3,4]

Until recently, it was generally accepted that the selective advantages of the backward growth of the dentary was a progressive strengthening of the lower jaw and ultimately of the jaw joint. Allen,[5] however, showed that if the lower jaw needed to be strengthened, it would have been a simple matter for the fibrous sutures between the bones to ossify as in birds. Allen argues that before the dentary began to grow backward the mammal-like reptiles picked up sound vibrations of the tympanum (eardrum) supported by and stretched between the bones at the back of the lower jaw. The vibrations of the tympanum caused the bones at the back of the lower jaw to vibrate. These vibrations were transmitted to the articular bone, across the jaw joint to the quadrate, and from here to the stapes and inner ear (see Fig. 1-2C). The selective advantage of the backward growth of the dentary was that it reduced the mass, and therefore the inertia of the bones behind the dentary, thereby improving hearing. Thus, the progressive increase in the size of the dentary and the formation of the new jaw joint may have had little or nothing to do with improving jaw function (these morphologic changes were designed to improve hearing). Having isolated hearing from jaw movement, the mammals were free to capitalize on the increased mobility allowed by the squamosal-dentary joint, now called the TMJ.[3-5]

The commonly accepted hypothesis that the mammalian jaw is functionally a lever implies that the jaw joint, the fulcrum of the lever system, is fixed with respect to the cranium.[6] In most reptiles, birds, and mammals, this is not true. The lower jaw is generally free to translate fore–aft with respect to the cranium by either of two mechanisms.[6,7] Translatory freedom is provided either by a sliding jaw joint (existing in most mammals, birds, and some reptiles, such as turtles) or by a two-jointed jaw suspension (streptostylic quadrate, existing in most lizards and snakes). An example of the sliding jaw joint is illustrated by the human skull.

THE SLIDING JAW JOINT

The jaw joint in humans consists of the articular fossa of the temporal bone above, an intermediate fibrocartilagenous articular disc, and the mandibular condyle below. The mandibular condyle and articular disc are separated by a synovial cavity permitting the condyle to rotate with respect to the articular disc. Both mandibular condyle and articular disc form the insertion for the external pterygoid muscle. The articular disc and temporal bone are also separated by a synovial cavity, permitting the articular disc–mandibular condyle assembly to translate forward when the external pterygoid muscle contracts. Mandibular depression–elevation is accompanied by simultaneous fore–aft translation of the mandible.[6-9] The chief muscle adducting the human jaw is the temporalis; it originates from the side of the cranium and inserts on the coronoid process of the mandible.[10-12]

JAW ARTICULATION AND MIDDLE EAR APPARATUS OF MAMMALS AND REPTILES

In all mammals, the lower jaw consists of a single element, the dentary. Anteriorly, it bears the teeth; posteriorly, it develops an ascending ramus with a coronoid, angular, and articular process (the mandibular condyle). These three processes of the dentary have the same names as the separate individual bones that occupied the equivalent positions in the reptile jaw. Of the reptile postdentary bones, the splenial, coronoid, and surangular have disappeared (they have no homologue in mammals); although the positions and functions of the articular (plus prearticular) and angular have been changed, just like those of the quadrate of the upper jaw.

In non-mammals, the lower jaw articulates with the upper jaw by the quadrate-articular joint, the concave surface of the articular bone fitting around a convexity of the quadrate. The quadrate lies at the posterior corner of the skull at the end of a series of bones (premaxilla, maxilla, pterygoid jugal, quadratojugal, quadrate) along the upper jaw. A single auditory ossicle, the stapes (known as the columella auris in reptiles), has two outwardly directed processes: one braced against the quadrate, the other being attached to the tympanum (see Figs 1-1 and 1-2). The inner end of the stapes fits into the fenestra ovalis of the otic capsule.[3,5,9]

In mammals, the condyle of the lower jaw articulates with a fossa in the squamosal bone (the squamous temporal of humans). The stapes has a single outwardly directed process articulating with the incus (quadrate), which in turn articulates with the malleus (articular). The malleus is attached to the tympanum by a lever arm, the manubrium mallei. The incus and malleus are separate from the jaw and skull but remain articulated with each other, being intercalated between the stapes and the tympanic membrane as a part of the vibration-transmission mechanism of the middle ear. A third bone, the angular bone of a reptile, has also lost its connection with the lower jaw and is instead fused with the skull in mammals. It supports the membranous tympanum, and in most mammals is known as the tympanic bone. In humans, it has become a part of the (composite) temporal bone, although it still develops from separate dermal ossification centers.

The articulating chain consisting of three bones—stapes, incus, malleus— exists in both recent reptiles and mammals, but the function is entirely different. In the former, it is a jaw joint; in the latter it is a "hearing aid."[5]

EVOLUTION OF THE TMJ AND MIDDLE EAR

To understand the evolution of the mammalian middle ear, it is important to understand that the middle ear of recent amphibians, reptiles and mammals are not homologous. Each type has evolved independently and in a different position in each line. The common ancestor of diapsid reptiles (the basal stock of modern reptiles) and synapsid reptiles (the basal stock of mammals) either had no tympanum or had developed a simple middle ear apparatus that subsequently became improved in two very different ways.[5,9]

In the diapsid reptiles and their descendants, the birds, the tympanum developed behind and was supported by the quadrate. In mammal-like reptiles, however, the tympanum formed on the lower jaw, lateral to the articular, and was supported in this position by the angular and hyoid bones (see Fig. 1-2C). The reasons for this difference of strategy probably had to do with the relative sizes and postures of the two types of reptiles; the mammal-like reptiles, being small, had a selective advantage in improving their hearing.[9] Initially, in the earlier mammal-like reptiles, the hyoid bone would have transmitted tympanic vibrations directly to the stapes and inner ear; in later forms, however, the hyoid bone transmission route decreased in importance as tympanic vibrations were transmitted through the jaw joint bones to the stapes. The small quadrate was streptostylic (attached movably to the skull), and the articular–angular complex was only loosely attached to the adjacent postdentary bones; quadrate and articular could both articulate the jaw and transmit vibrations of the tympanum to the inner ear.[3,5,9] The evolutionary advantage of subsequent separation of the quadrate, articular, and angular ossicles from the jaws was the reduction in ligamentous and muscular impedance that previously limited the sensitivity or frequency response of the middle ear.[9] The progressive diminution of the postdentary bones in mammal-like reptiles was an essential prerequisite of this separation. The selective advantage for each increment of size reduction must have been the improved hearing that resulted from decreased mass and inertia of the transmission elements.[3,5,9] As the postdentary bones decreased in size and loosened their attachment to the tooth-bearing dentary bone, the jaw joint became increasingly weakened, although the dentary had increased in size proportional to the diminution of the postdentary bones and had taken over the attachment areas of the jaw musculature.

Differentiation of the single reptilian adductor muscle into separate units (temporals, masseters, and pterygoids) with different directions of pull effectively reduced the masticatory loading of this weakened jaw joint.[3,8,10,11]

The evolutionary changes to these structures are clearly the result of selection for improved hearing. Further advantages were gained from the reorganization of the bones and musculature: (1) There was a great increase in bite force across the postcanine teeth; (2) more important still, the varied musculature could produce side-to-side movements of the lower jaw; and (3) mastication was finally possible.[3,9,12]

EVOLUTION OF JAWS IN PRIMATES AND HUMANS

The evidence of the earliest primates comes from the Cretaceous period, approximately 70 million years ago. These tiny primates, *Purgatorius*, are represented by isolated jaws and teeth. The following primates of the Paleocene and Eocene time periods (65 to 38 million years) document the transition of the primates from a generalized primitive mammal, to the highly specialized order we are today. The first evidence of higher primates leading to the genus *Homo* appears in the late Oligocene, about 30 million years ago, with the appearance of *Aegyptopithecus*, from the Fayum of Egypt. This evidence is represented by a nearly complete skull, including the jaw joint. This evidence, and associated skeletal remains, indicates that *Aegyptopithecus* was a quadrupedal primate with an enlarged brain, yet prognathic face. The jaws are characterized by large anterior incisors and canines and large, relatively rounded molars with five cusps.

The next major clue comes from the Miocene, approximately 20 million years ago, with the discovery of *Proconsul*. This fossil ape consists of a nearly complete skull and most of a skeleton. The remains document a monkeylike skeleton with an apelike skull.

The evidence from the Miocene (25 to 6 million years) of Africa, Europe, and Asia reveals that during the late Miocene, the hominoids appear to have migrated out of Africa and into Europe and Asia. The fossil evidence from Asia clearly documents that our earliest ancestors were orangutanlike, with powerful jaws and teeth.[13] Some genera, such as *Gigantopithecus*, had massive jaws and teeth several times the size of human teeth.

The jaws, TMJ, and craniofacial morphology architecture resemble that of most herbivores (plant-eating animals). The hominoid dentition indicates heavy crushing and grinding, with little lateral excursion. Little exists of the postcranial remains of the later Miocene hominoids, however, specifically, *Sivapithecus* (15 to 10 million years), which most closely resembles extant hominids (humanlike forms) and apes.

EVOLUTIONARY CHANGES IN THE CRANIUM

The evidence for the evolution of the cranium and brain in primates is derived from two sources: the fossil record and comparisons between the brains of living primates. The fossil record consists of two types, the endocast (a cast of the inside of the cranium that reflects the size and shape of the brain as well as certain external morphologies) and the fossil remains of the cranium itself.

One of the more distinctive traits of the primates is the tendency toward development of a brain that is larger in proportion to total body weight and that is particularly characterized by a relatively extensive and often richly convoluted cerebral cortex. Brain size relates to behavior, learning performance and the rate of behavioral development. Species with larger than average brains in relation to body size show a greater ability to process and use complex information. Furthermore, increase in brain size need not be confined to only one area of the brain. Those areas that do increase in size are often related to some specialization in certain areas or sense organs.

The primate brain shows certain features of its intrinsic organization that also distinguish it from that of other mammals (e.g., the neural apparatus of vision becomes highly developed, and the olfactory regions are reduced). The result of these changes is the forward rotation of the orbits with subsequent development of enclosed orbits. The significantly expanded occipital lobe of the primates reflects the expansion of the primary visual cortex. The increasing dominance of vision over the other sense organs played a major role in the evolution of the primates, especially in the hominoids.

One of the earliest hominoid fossil species comes from the late Oligocene (38 to 25 million years) of East Africa. Analysis of *Aegyptopithecus* indicates that this species was advanced with respect to the amount of visual cortex as compared with the lower primates, the Strepsirhine (lemurs, etc.). A number of hominoid forms from the Miocene (25 to 6 million years), of Africa, Europe, and Asia are now known. These hominoids document an increase in brain size.[14]

During the Plio/Pleistocene (6 to 2 million years), the ancestors of *Homo* arose, in the form of a small-bodied, but large-brained hominid known as *Australopithecus*. Analysis of endocasts from these fossils documents that the australopithecine brains do not appear to have been reorganized along human lines at a gross external neuroanatomic level, but were similar to the brain of a chimpanzee brain.[14] Evidence of dramatic increases in brain size is found in the East African forms from 3.5 to 1.75 million years, however. This size range expands from as small as 250 cc to nearly 800 cc during this period, with a reduction in facial prognathism. The evolution of the brain has a direct impact of the expansion of the upper face (the orbits, and frontal bone) and strong influence on the midface (nasal region, maxilla, and zygomatic region).

EVOLUTION OF POSTURE AND *HOMO*

One of the most important characteristics that separates humans from apes is human adaptation to a primarily bipedal form of locomotion and stance. Although many primates can walk bipedally, only humans use this form of locomotion on a regular and habitual basis. Morphologic changes in the muscular and skeletal systems of the hominids involved changes in both the upper and lower appendages. The most dramatic changes, however, were centered in the lower limbs.

The major changes in the lower limb involved modifications in the lumbar vertebrae, pelvis, and especially the hindlimb. The most radical alterations occurred in the ilium, femur, and foot. These changes first occur in the hominid known as *Australopithecus*.

The first evidence of *Australopithecus* comes from the limestone fissures of South Africa. The remains are of a small hominid known as *Australopithecus africanusor,* the Taung baby found in 1924 by Raymond Dart. Evidence of the locomotor behavior of *Australopithecus*, until recently, indicated an upright, possibly bipedal creature, living about 2 to 3 million years ago. Recent discoveries from East Africa in the form of skeletal remains and fossilized footprints, especially from Laetolil, Afar and Lake Turkana, now clearly document that *Australopithecus* was totally bipedal some 3.5 million years ago. The craniofacial morphology, however, is very primitive. The overall morphology resembles that of a chimp with a slightly larger brain.

Based on the evidence from *Homo erectus*, which was discovered in the 1890s in Java and in the early 1920s in China, it was proposed that the final and decisive changes in the human skull are related to the acquisition of upright posture.[1,2] Until recently, evolutionary changes in the craniofacial morphology of hominids leading to the genus *Homo* were generally believed to be the result of selective pressures of upright posture, that is, bipedality.[1,2] The discoveries in East Africa, however, clearly negate this hypothesis. Furthermore, the recently discovery of the first, nearly totally complete *Homo erectus* skeleton (KNM-WT 15K), also from Lake Turkana in East Africa, dating back about 1.5 million years, provides us with a much clearer understanding of the skeletal anatomy of *Homo erectus* than ever before. This evidence is of a young boy aged about 12 years, totally erect, with a large brain of about 900 cc. *Australopithecus* is estimated to have an average brain size of 450 cc, with *Homo* ranging from 650 to more than 1,600 cc in the Neanderthals. The most surprising evidence is that the thoracic cavity is chimplike, the spinous processes of the lumbar vertebrae are horizontal and not inclined as in humans, there are six lumbar vertebrae, and the neural foramen is much reduced in size (about one-half the size of that of modern humans). This point is of much interest because it indicates neurological input and output to the brain (A. Walker, personal communication).

Therefore, what does this evidence provide us? What is evident from the recent discoveries in East Africa, which span some 2 to 3 million years of fossil hominid evolution, is that the acquisition of bipedality did not mandate the craniofacial morphology of modern humans. These earliest hominids had massive jaws and teeth with powerful masticatory muscles.[14] The face was very prognathic, with heavy anterior loading. With the acquisition of culture (tool-using and the development of social groups), brain size increased correspondingly and masticatory loading reduced. As brain size increases, there was concomitant reduction in facial prognathism and in tooth and jaw size. This trend continued from *Australopithecus* through *Homo sapiens* until the development of a "chin" appeared about 65,000 years ago in the early representatives of *Homo sapiens sapiens* (modern humans).[14]

SUMMARY

The evolutionary adaptations resulting in the existing morphology and physiology of the craniomandibular region are the consequence of many factors. Most important have been the evolution of (1) the ear region in mammals and primate; (2) the development of the binocular, stereoscopic, and color vision in the hominoids; (3) the dietary adaptations of the hominoids; and (4) the acquisition of culture in the hominids.

These data present more questions than answers, since new evidence and recent discoveries have disproven and/or questioned long-standing assumptions concerning the evolution and development of the TMJ and related craniomandibular regions in humans. What is clear is that we actually do not fully understand the effects of posture on the TMJ region. The effects are complicated by the radical departure in our dietary habits from the adaptions of our ancestors. Therefore, I believe that attempts to use animal models to interpret clinical problems concerning the TMJ may prove fruitless.

Malocclusion and TMJ problems are commonplace among modern populations; however, analysis of American Indian skeletal remains documents large jaws and teeth with very little to no evidence of malocclusion or TMJ problems. The problems faced by modern populations are the result of present-day behavioral and dietary habits as well as the continued selective pressures resulting in facial flattening and dental reduction (both tooth and jaw size).

REFERENCES

1. Du Brul EL: Origin and evolution of the oral apparatus. p. 1. In Kawamura Y (ed): Physiology of Mastication. Frontiers of Oral Physiology. Vol. 1. Karger, Basel, 1974

2. Du Brul EL: Origin and adaptations of the hominid jaw joint. p. 5. In Sarnat BG, Laskin DM (eds): The Temporomandibular Joint. 3rd Ed. Charles C Thomas, Springfield, IL, 1979

3. Crompton AW: Origin of the mammalian temporomandibular joint. p. 1. In Carlson DS (ed): Developmental Aspects of Temporomandibular Joint Disorders, Monograph No. 16, Craniofacial Growth Series. Center for Human Growth and Development, The University of Michigan, Ann Arbor, MI, 1985

4. Bramble DM: Origin of the mammalian feeding complex: models and mechanisms. Paleobiology 4:271, 1978

5. Allin EF: Evolution of the mammalian middle ear. J Morphol 147:403, 1975

6. Lumsden AGS, Osborn JW: The evolution of chewing: a dentist's view of palaeontology. J Dent 5:269, 1977

7. Gingerich PD: Functional significance of mandibular translation in vertebrate jaw mechanics. Postilla 152:1, 1971

8. Roberts D, Tattersall I: Skull form and the mechanics of mandibular elevation in mammals. American Museum Novitates 2436:1, 9, 1972

9. Lumsden AGS: Evolution and adaptation of the vertebrate mouth. p. 88. In Osborn JW (ed): Dental Anatomy and Embryology. Vol. 1, Blackwell Scientific Publications, Oxford, 1981

10. Noble HW: Comparative functional anatomy. p. 35. In Sarnat BG, Laskin DM (eds): The Temporomandibular Joint, 3rd Ed. Charles C Thomas, Springfield, IL 1979

11. Noble HW: Comparative functional anatomy of the temporomandibular joint. p. 15. In Zarb GA, Carlsson GE (eds): Temporomandibular Joint Function and Dysfunction. CV Mosby, St. Louis, 1976

12. Hylander WL: Functional anatomy. p. 85. In Sarnat BG, Laskin DM (eds): The Temporomandibular Joint. 3rd Ed. Charles C Thomas, Springfield, IL, 1979

13. Gantt, DG: Enamel thickness and ultrastructure in hominoids: with reference to form, function, and phylogeny. p. 453. In D. Swindler and J. Erwin (ed): Comparative Primate Biology, Volume 1: Systematics, Evolution, and Anatomy, Alan R. Liss, Inc. New York, 1986

14. Falk D: Hominid brain evolution: the approach from paleoneurology. Yearbook Phys Anthropol 23:93, 1980

15. Wolpoff MH: Some aspects of human mandibular evolution. p. 1. In McNamara JA (ed): Determinants of Mandibular Form and Growth. Monograph No. 4, Craniofacial Growth Series. Center for Human Growth and Development, The University of Michigan, Ann Arbor, MI, 1975

Cartilage is a fundamental biological material that forms the model from which most bone develops. Throughout life, cartilage also provides a covering for bones that withstand compression loads, yet enables these bones to move smoothly against one another. Cartilage is a tissue whose properties are established not by the properties of its cells but by what the cells secrete. Chondroblasts, or cartilage-producing cells, produce an elaborate network of giant molecules that form an extracellular matrix. This matrix includes some of the largest proteins made by any cell in nature. It also includes great volumes of water. The water-binding properties of the large molecules yield the tissues' properties of strength and smoothness.

Body cartilage exists in three forms: elastic, hyaline, and fibrocartilage.

Elastic cartilage is a very specialized connective tissue primarily found in the symphysis pubis and the larynx.

Hyaline cartilage covers the ends of long bones and, along with the synovial fluid which bathes it, provides a smoothly articulating, slippery friction-free surface when two bones move against each other.

Fibrocartilage basically acts as a shock absorber in both weightbearing and nonweightbearing joints. This fibrocartilage provides space between bones, allowing freedom of movement. Its large fiber content makes it ideal for bearing large stresses in all directions. It covers the articulating surfaces of the mandible as well as the articular eminence of the temporal bone.[5,6] It also exists in the form of a disc interposed between the mandibular condyle and the temporal bone. Therefore, the TMJ is unique among synovial joints because its articular cartilage is fibrocartilage rather than hyaline cartilage. The presence of fibro, rather than hyaline cartilage implies that the TMJ is specialized to withstand large and repeated stresses.[7] On the other hand, the fibrocartilaginous covering is thinnest where it lines the roof of the glenoid fossa. The thinness of the cartilage at the roof of the fossa has helped researchers determine that the fossa itself bears little or no load even during chewing. The load-bearing surface of the joint is the eminence where the fibrocartilage is the thickest.

The fibrous covering of the articulating surfaces consists of heavy and densely packed bundles of collagenous fibers. These fiber bundles are arranged into two fairly distinct layers. In the deep layer adjacent to the remnants of the growth cartilage, the fibers are arranged radially, at approximately right angles to the surface. In the superficial layers, the fibers are parallel to the surface. The deeper layers appear to be adapted to withstand large pressures while the superficial layers appear to enhance gliding under pressure.[8]

Fibrocartilagenous Disc

Interposed between the under surface of the temporal bone and the mandibular condyle and dividing the TMJ into an upper and lower compartment is a fibrocartilaginous disc. The upper, or superior compartment, is bordered by the mandibular fossa and the superior surface of the articular disc. The lower, or inferior compartment, is bordered by the mandibular condyle and the inferior surface of the articular disc. The attachment of the articular disc to the capsular ligament anteriorly and posteriorly, and the attachment of the disc to the medial and lateral poles of condyle, divides the TMJ into two distinct cavities. The coarse bundles of collagenous fibers that constitute this disc interlace to form a three-dimensional network. Blood vessels and nerves are found only in the thickened periphery of this disc; the thinner center is avascular and aneural.

This fibrocartilaginous disc exhibits three clearly defined transverse, ellipsoidal zones that are divided into three regions: posterior band, intermediate zone, and anterior band.[9] The intermediate zone is considerably thinner (1 mm) than the posterior and anterior bands, and the posterior band is generally thicker (3 mm) than the anterior band (2 mm).[10] The intermediate zone comes into contact with the articular surface of the condyle. The upper surface of the disc adapts to the contours of the fossa and eminence of the temporal bone. The significance of the varying thicknesses of the disc is not entirely understood, but the interposition of a thin zone between two thicker zones may allow the intermediate zone to alter its shape from concave below to convex above as it slides forward from the articular fossa onto the articular eminence. In addition, the disc, with its varying thicknesses, seems to smooth the course of the mandible as it glides along the temporal surface.

Posteriorly, the disc is contiguous with the bilaminar retrodiscal pad, which in turn fuses with the posterior wall of the articular capsule. As its name implies, this loosely organized tissue is composed of two laminae. The superior lamina is composed of connective tissue containing many elastic fibers.[11] This superior lamina is attached to the tympanic plate of the temporal bone posterosuperiorly.

The inferior retrodiscal lamina is attached posteroinferiorly to the neck of the condyle and anteriorly to the disc. This lamina is composed chiefly of collagenous fibers, making it nonelastic.[12]

This retrodiscal tissue is highly vascular and neural loose connective tissue. A synovial membrane covers both the superior and inferior laminae. The retrodiscal tissue, therefore, ensures free metabolic exchange, nutrition, and lubrication of the articulating surfaces in both upper and lower joints. The morphology of the bilaminar zone also appears suited to fill the vacated glenoid fossa when the condyle assumes the protruded posture. The great vascularity of the bilaminar zone may allow a venous engorgement to occupy the glenoid fossa more completely.

Medially and laterally, the fibrocartilaginous disc is firmly attached to the medial and lateral poles of the condyle. Attachment of the articular disc to the medial and lateral condylar poles is performed by collateral, discal ligaments (Fig. 2-3). These ligaments permit anterior and posterior rotation of the disc on the condyle. They function to restrict movement of the disc from the condyle, either from an anterior or posterior dislocation. Therefore, they are responsible for the hingelike movement that occurs between the condyle and the articular disc. Innervation of the discal ligaments provide proprioceptive feedback relative to harmonious interplay between disc–condylar relationships. The disc is not directly attached to the temporal bone; therefore, the disc has

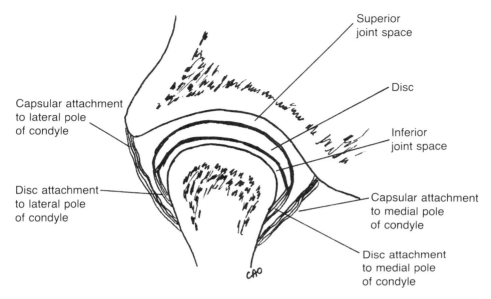

Fig. 2-3. Frontal view of the right TMJ.

liberty to move with the condyle as the condyle translates in relation to the articular eminence.

SYNOVIAL MEMBRANE

A synovial membrane is characterized by a rich supply of blood vessels, a prerequisite for the function of a synovial membrane, namely to manufacture lubricating and nutritional synovial fluid. The synovial membrane of the TMJ is a highly vascularized layer of connective tissue that lines the fibrous capsule and covers the loose connective tissue between it and the posterior border of the disc. The synovial membrane inserts inferior from the articulating surface of the mandible and reflects on, and covers, the bone to the boundaries of the articulating surfaces. Therefore, part of the mandibular neck is covered by the synovial membrane and is intracapsular. The largest area of synovial lining covers the superior and inferior surfaces of the retrodiscal pad where the synovial capsule forms small folds and villi that permit freedom of forward translation of the disc–condyle complex without injury to the membrane. The passive volume of synovial fluid in the upper joint averages about 1.2 ml,[13] whereas that of the inferior cavity averages 0.9 ml.[14]

The interposition of the fibrocartilaginous disc between the temporal bone and the mandibular condyle divides the potential articular space into an upper and lower compartment (Fig. 2-4). Each compartment is enclosed and lined with its own synovial membrane. The synovial cavity above the disc, the su-

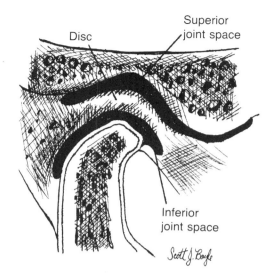

Fig. 2-4.   Sagittal view of the right TMJ.

perior, larger, and looser of the two, is continuous from the margin of the cartilage covering the mandibular fossa and articular tubercle to the superior surface of the disc. It generally extends to the greatest curvature of the articular eminence. The upper joint space always extends farther anteriorly than the lower joint space.[10]

The separate inferior cavity below the disc passes from the under surface of the disc to the neck of the condyle and extends a little posteriorly. The lower joint is contiguous with the condyle and extends only slightly anterior to the condyle along the superior aspect of the superior head of the lateral pterygoid muscle. The articulating surfaces of the temporal bone, the mandible, and the disc are free of any synovial membrane.

This synovial membrane produces synovial fluid which fills both joint cavities. This synovial fluid provides the metabolic requirements of the avascular articular surfaces of the joints. There is a rapid exchange of nutrients and waste products between the vessels of the capsule, the synovial fluid, and the articular tissues. The synovial fluid also serves as a lubricant between articular surfaces during function, thus minimizing friction.

In any synovial joint, there exists a potential position in which the articular surfaces are maximally congruent and cannot accomplish any further movement in that direction and in which the ligaments surrounding that joint are taut. These positions are known as border positions. Border positions, although attainable, are not functional positions.[15] Movements within the temporomandibular articulations are referred to as interborder movements.

ARTICULAR RECEPTORS

Static and dynamic changes of the condyle will be recognized by the receptor system due to stimulation of mechanoreceptors I, II, and III or the nociceptive receptor system if sufficient mechanical or chemical stimulation exists around the periarticular connective tissue of the joint. All synovial joints of the body are provided with a quadruple array of corpuscular (mechanoreceptors) and noncorpuscular (nociceptors) receptor endings with varying characteristic behaviors and distributions depending on articular tissue.

Type I receptors consist of small, thinly incapsulated globular corpuscles located in the peripheral layers of the fibrous joint capsule, each cluster being innervated by a small myelinated afferent fiber that enters the related articular nerve. These are low-threshold, slowly adapting mechanoreceptors whose frequency of discharge is a continuous function of the prevailing tension in the region of the joint capsule where they are located. They have an inhibitory effect on the trans-synaptic centripetal form of nociceptive activity from the type IV articular receptor system. Their activity exerts powerful tonic reflexogenic influences on the motor neuronal pool of the muscles of mastication.

Type I receptors are most numerous in the posterior region of the joint capsule; therefore, the contribution to the reflex regulation of postural tone in the mandibular musculature appears to be greater from this region. Variations in applied load produce differences in the rate of change in capsular tension. Type I mechanoreceptors contribute to reflex regulation of postural muscle tone, to coordination of muscle activity, and to preceptional awareness of mandibular position.

Type II receptors are large, thickly encapsulated conical corpuscles imbedded in the deeper parasynovial layers of the posterior fibrous joint capsule. They are innervated by thicker myelinated afferent fibers in the articular nerves. These receptors operate as low-threshold, rapidly adapting mechanoreceptors that fire off brief bursts of impulses only at the onset of changes in tension in the joint capsule. At the onset of mandibular movements, type II mechanoreceptors in the stressed region of the joint capsule are stimulated simultaneously. Their behavior suggests their role as a control mechanism to regulate motor-unit activity of the prime movers of the TMJ.

Type III mechanoreceptors are found in the superficial layers of the capsular ligament. They may be regarded as high threshold; therefore, only during strong capsular tension will the type III mechanoreceptors evoke discharges.

The type IV nociceptive receptor system is a plexiform array of unmyelinated nerve fibers distributed three-dimensionally throughout the fibrous joint capsule. No nerve endings of this or any other kind exist in the articular cartilage, synovial tissues, or central portion of the disc; this suggests that these structures cannot be the source of pain in the TMJ. The type IV receptor system is activated when its nerve fibers are depolarized by the generation of high mechanical or chemical stresses in the joint capsule.

SUPPORTING STRUCTURES OF THE TMJ

The ligaments of the TMJ are composed of nonelastic collagenous connective tissue whose role is that of protecting and supporting joint structures. These ligaments act as passive restraints designed to limit and restrict joint movement. Two strong ligaments that provide joint stability are (1) the joint capsule, and (2) the temporomandibular ligament. Three lesser ligaments may contribute to the integrity of the joint are (1) stylomandibular, (2) sphenomandibular, and (3) malleomandibular, or Pintos ligament.

Capsular Ligament

The capsular ligament is compsed of fibrous connective tissue that is well vascularized and innervated. It is a thin, loose envelope that surrounds and encompasses the entire joint and is attached to the circumference of the mandibular fossa and the articular tubercle and to the neck of the mandibular condyle. Although the capsule is quite thin anteriorly, medially, and posteriorly, it is strongly reinforced laterally as the temporomandibular ligament. Anteriorly, the capsule fuses with the articular disc. Posteriorly, it attaches to the retrodiscal pad in loose folds that permit disc-condyle freedom anteriorly. The capsule is also attached posteriorly to the postglenoid spine and to the neck of the condylar process.

The capsule tends to restrain the extremes of medial, lateral, or inferior forces that tend to separate the articular surfaces. As in all synovial joints, the capsule retains the synovial fluid. In the closed mouth position, the synovial fluid in both upper and lower joint cavities appears to be distributed evenly from an anterior and posterior relationship to the disc. During translation, much of the synovial fluid is located posteriorly as the fluid conforms to the shape of the capsule.[16]

The joint capsule is highly innervated and provides proprioceptive feedback regarding joint posture and movement. Afferent nerve fibers for proprioception and nociception are branches of the auriculotemporal, masseteric, and posterior deep temporal nerves.[17] Nourishment is provided by the superficial temporal artery, whereas the anterior tympanic artery supplies the well-vascularized retrodiscal tissue.[3]

Temporomandibular Ligament

The capsule of the TMJ is reinforced laterally by strong fibers that make up the temporomandibular ligament. This ligament consists of two parts, an outer oblique portion that extends down and back to insert onto the outer surface of the condylar neck, and an inner horizontal portion that arises from the outer surface of the articular tubercle, along with the oblique portion, and runs backward to insert onto the lateral pole of the condyle and posterior part of the articular disc (Fig. 2-5). These ligaments are the suspensory mechanism of the mandible, resisting downward and posterior displacement.

The outer portion limits normal rotational opening movements; the inner portion limits posterior movement of the disc–condyle complex. This ligament

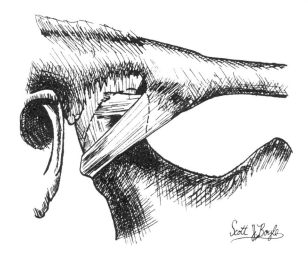

Fig. 2-5. Two parts of the temporomandibular ligament of the right TMJ.

prevents excessive posterior gliding of the condyle and thereby protects the sensitive retrodiscal tissue from encroachment by the condyle.

Stylomandibular Ligament

The stylomandibular ligament is a specialized band of deep cervical fascia that splits away from the superficial lamina of the deep cervical fascia to run deep to both pterygoid muscles. This ligament attaches to the posterior border of the mandibular ramus between the masseter and medial pterygoid muscles. It then runs deep to both pterygoid muscles to reach the styloid process of the temporal bone.[18] This ligament becomes taut when the mandible is protruded, but is most relaxed when the mandible is opened. It acts as a brake for the mandible, preventing excessive anterior drift of the mandible during extreme opening.

Sphenomandibular Ligament

The sphenomandibular ligament is a thin band that runs from the spine of the sphenoid bone and the tympanosquamous fissure and extends downward and laterally to a small bony prominence on the medial surface of the ramus of the mandible called the lingula. This ligament located between the mandible and skull represents remains of the first cartilaginous bar or Meckels' cartilage, of the first branchial arch, the mandibular arch. This ligament has been suggested to act to check the angle of the mandible from sliding as far forward as the condyles do during the translatory cycle.[19]

The above ligaments receive their nerve supply from the auriculotemporal and masseteric branches of the mandibular nerve, the third and only motor branch of the trigeminal nerve.

Malleomandibular Ligament or Pinto's Ligament

Pinto's ligament arises from the neck of the malleus of the inner ear and runs in a mediosuperior direction to insert into the posterior aspect of the TMJ capsule and disc as well as connecting onto the sphenomandibular ligament.[20] Ermshar has suggested that the association of this ligament to the middle ear and TMJ may serve as rationale for associated ear symptoms associated with temporomandibular joint dysfunction.[21]

MUSCLE STRUCTURE AND FUNCTION

Skeletal muscles are composed of many bundles (fasciculi) of fibers. Each fiber is made up of myofibrils. The thicker myofibrils are composed of myosin, a protein with enzymatic properties acting as adenosine triphosphatase. The thinner myofibrils contain actin and are responsible for the contraction and relaxation of muscle tissue. Each fiber is ensheathed in a delicate envelope called the sarcolemma, which provides for the elastic recoil of muscle tissue. Each muscle fiber, or muscle cell, encloses approximately 2,000 myofibrils.

The basic unit of the neuromuscular system is the motor unit, which consists of a single motor neuron and a group of muscle fibers. Each neuron joins with the muscle fiber at the motor end plate. When the neuron is activated, the motor end plate is stimulated to release small amounts of acetylcholine, which initiates depolarization of the muscle fibers. The number of fibers contained within a motor unit relates to the complexity of the action involved: the more precise the movement required, the fewer the fibers per motor neuron.

Muscle fibers are classified as type I and type II. The type I fibers contract slowly and resist fatigue. Type II fibers contract rapidly and are of two categories: Type IIA fibers are fatigue resistant, whereas type IIB fibers fatigue quickly. The motor unit, a number of muscle fibers that are innervated by one motor neuron, differ from each other not only in size but also in biochemical and physiologic properties of their muscle fibers.

Masticatory muscles contain all three fiber types. The masseter muscle consists of 50 to 60 percent type IIB fibers.[22] It is therefore capable of a strong rapid contraction but fatigues readily. The lateral pterygoid muscle consists of about 70 percent Type I slow-twitch fibers throughout.[23] This suggests that the lateral pterygoid muscle is more resistant to fatigue.

Contractile activity may shorten a muscle under constant loading; such a contraction is termed isotonic. Contractile activity may increase tension within the muscle while maintaining a constant muscle length, thereby producing a holding action; this is termed isometric. Coordinated muscle action consists of various combinations of such contractile activity in agonist and antagonist muscle groups. Muscles are most efficient at generating force when they are at their physiologic resting length.[24]

Forms of striated muscles vary according to situation and function. They may be straplike (flat), fusiform (bellied), fanlike (triangular), or pennate (featherlike). Strap muscles have fascicles, bundles, parallel from end to end (sternohyoid). Fusiform muscles have nearly parallel bundles that converge on a tendon at one or both ends (digastrics). Fanlike muscles are relatively flat, with a wide attachment converging on an apical attachment (temporalis). Pennate muscles have bundles oriented obliquely to the line of pull. They attach to tendons, which resemble the shaft, or quill, of a feather. These muscles are termed unipennate when they run obliquely from a linear attachment to one side of a tendon, bipennate when they converge from opposite attachments to both sides of a tendon, such as the temporalis muscle, and multipennate when bundles angle in on numerous, alternate, tendinous plates, such as the masseter and medial pterygoid muscles. Muscles that contain a parallel fiber orientation have a strong potential for a greater range of motion (ROM) whereas the oblique fiber orientation has a relatively short ROM potential but appears to have a power advantage.

The intrinsic, direct mandibular prime movers include six pairs of variedly shaped muscles that directly influence mandibular movements. Although these muscles work most efficiently in groups, an understanding of the specific action(s) of the individual muscles is necessary for appreciation of their coordinated function during masticatory activity. Three of these muscles, the masseter, medial pterygoid, and temporalis exert their power in a vertical direction, acting to elevate the mandible. The lateral pterygoid muscle, oriented in a horizontal plane, pulls the mandible forward or protrudes the mandible. Of the suprahyoid group, only the digastric and geniohyoid muscles exert a direct pull on the mandible, pulling it in a posterior and inferior direction, thereby retruding and depressing the mandible.

The remaining suprahyoid muscles, the mylohyoid and stylohyoid, along with the infrahyoid group, and the cervial musculature are recognized as extrinsic muscles of mastication. The extrinsic muscles are responsible for maintenence of postural tone of the skull with respect to cervical alignment.

The individual characteristics of the paired intrinsic masticatory muscles are as follows.

Intrinsic Masticatory Muscles

The Temporalis

The large, fan-shaped temporalis muscle covers much of the side of the head. It arises from the temporal fossa and from the deep surface of the temporal fascia. Its fibers converge as they descend, and end in a tendon that passes deep to the zygomatic arch and is inserted into the medial surface, the

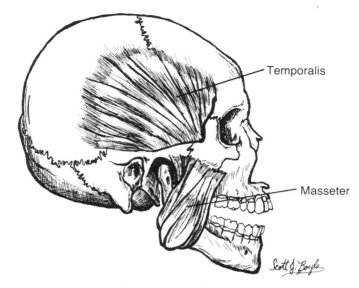

Fig. 2-6.   Temporalis and masseter muscles.

apex, and the anterior border of the coronoid process and the anterior border of the ramus of the mandible (Fig. 2-6).

The anterior fibers that form the bulk of this muscle are vertically oriented; the middle fibers are increasingly oblique, and the posterior fibers run horizontally forward to reach the coronoid process of the mandible. The flesh of the temporalis muscle is divided by deep tendinous plates which in turn are covered over by the temporalis fascia.

As the fibers converge toward their insertion a superficial tendon is observed attached to the anterior border of the coronoid process and mandibular ramus. A deep, or inner tendon inserts onto the temporal crest of the mandible and extends downward into the region of the third molor. This tendon is generally stronger than its superficial counterpart. The short, more superficial fibers of the temporalis muscles are fused with the deep fibers of the masseter muscle.[19]

The temporalis muscle is supplied by the anterior and posterior deep temporal nerves, which branch from the anterior division of the mandibular branch of the trigeminal nerve. The anterior temporal nerve is initially united with the buccal nerve, but separates from it after passing between the two heads of the lateral pterygoid muscle.

The blood supply to the temporalis muscle is furnished by the middle and deep temporal arteries. The middle temporal artery is a branch of the superficial temporal artery. The deep temporal artery is a branch of the internal maxillary artery.

All fibers of the temporalis muscle contribute to its primary function of mandibular elevation (closure). The posterior fibers are important for retrusion and lateral deviation of the mandible to the ipsilateral side. Closure to an edge-to-edge position of the anterior middle incisors involves mainly the anterior temporal fibers.

The Masseter

Both superficial and deep layers of the masseter muscle attach above to the zygomatic process of the maxilla and to the zygomatic arch. The whole muscle stretches as a rectangular plate downward and backward (Fig. 2-6). The superficial layer attaches to the external surface of the mandible at its angle and to the inferior half of its ramus. The deep layer attaches to the superior half of the ramus. The deep layer is much smaller and more muscular. It is covered over posteriorly by the parotid gland. The multipennate effect of the alternating muscle fibers and layers of tendons serves to shorten the average length of the contractile elements and to increase the total number of fibers in the muscle. This structure makes the masseter a very powerful muscle with a relatively short contractile range.

The masseteric nerve, the anterior branch of the mandibular division of the trigeminal nerve, reaches the muscle from its deep surface after passing through the semilunar notch of the mandible behind the tendon of the temporalis muscle. The nerve supplies the deep portion, perforates it, and enters the superficial portion.

The masseteric artery, a branch of the maxillary artery, and masseteric veins supply the muscle and follow the course of the masseteric nerve.

The chief action of the masseter is to elevate the mandible and close the jaws, as when clenching the molars. The superficial portion exerts pressure at a right angle to the occlusal plane of the molars, thus maximizing the crushing force between the molars. The fibers of the deep portion, oriented in a more downward and forward direction, act as retruders of the mandible when the mandible is being pulled from its most protruded position. The combined forces of both components of the masseter muscle produces a pattern of elevation and retrusion.

The Medial Pterygoid

The medial pterygoid and masseter muscles together act as a sling to suspend the angle of the mandible. The medial pterygoid muscle is a thick quadrilateral muscle situated on the medial aspect of the mandibular ramus, similar to the masseter muscle along the outer surface of the mandibular ramus (Fig. 2-7). It arises from the medial lip of the lateral pterygoid plate of the sphenoid bone, its innermost fibers arise from the pterygoid fossa and the pyramidal process of the palatine bone. Its fibers pass inferiorly, laterally, and posteriorly, and are inserted by a strong tendinous lamina into the inferior and posterior part of the medial surface of the ramus and angle of the mandible. The superior

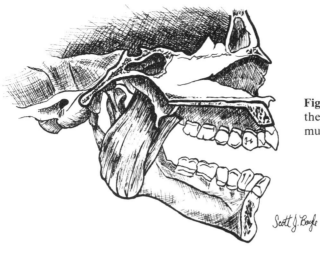

Fig. 2-7. Intraoral view of the left medial pterygoid muscles.

portion of the muscle is separated from the mandible by the sphenomandibular ligament, the maxillary vessels, the inferior alveolar vessels and nerves, and the lingual nerve. The medial surface of the muscle is adjacent to the tensor veli palatini and superior constrictor muscles of the oral pharynx.

The medial pterygoid muscle is supplied by the medial pterygoid nerve that arises from the common fused portion of the mandibular division of the trigeminal nerve. It reaches the muscle at its posterior border. Its blood supply is provided by a branch of the maxillary artery.

Bilaterally, the muscles help to elevate the mandible in concert with the masseter and temporalis muscles. The medial pterygoid activity is increased if the mandible also is protruded while it is being elevated. Acting unilaterally, the medial ptyergoid muscle deviates the mandible toward the opposite side. This muscle acts as an assist to the lateral pterygoid for protrusion of the mandible.[25]

The Lateral Pterygoid

The two divisions of the lateral pterygoid muscle lie deep to, and largely behind, the zygomatic arch. It is a short, thick muscle, somewhat conical in shape, that extends almost horizontally between the infratemporal fossa and the condyle of the mandible. It arises by two head; a larger inferior head arises from the lateral lip of the lateral pterygoid plate, and a small superior head originates from the infratemporal surface of the greater wing of the sphenoid bone. The fibers from the superior head run horizontally backward and outward, the fibers of the inferior head converge upward and outward (Fig. 2-8). The uppermost and deepest fibers of the superior head are attached to the articular capsule and to the anterior border of the articular disc. The remaining

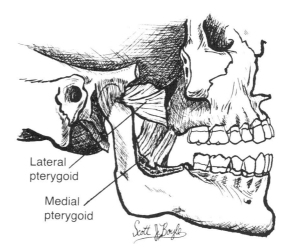

Fig. 2-8. Extraoral view of the lateral pterygoid muscle and medial pterygoid muscle.

Lateral pterygoid

Medial pterygoid

portion of the superior and the entire inferior head insert onto the roughened anterior surface of the neck of the mandibular condyle.

Both divisions of this muscle are innervated by the lateral pterygoid nerve from the anterior division of the mandibular branch of the trigeminal nerve. The muscle is supplied from branches of the maxillary artery.

The two divisions of the lateral pterygoid muscles are functionally and anatomically two separate reciprocating muscles. The inferior lateral pterygoid muscle exerts a forward, inward, and downward pull on the mandible, thereby opening the jaws, protruding the mandible, and deviating the mandible to the opposite side by the action of one muscle functioning unilaterally.

The superior belly of the lateral pterygoid muscle is inactive during the opening phase of the mandible.[26] In addition, the superior head of the lateral pterygoid inserts mostly into the condyle rather than into the disc. This suggests that the superior lateral pterygoid is an unlikely source of movement of the disc during opening. Rather, it has been demonstrated that contraction of the superior lateral pterygoid anteriorly rotates the disc on the condyle during the closing movement. The disc is rotated anteriorly only as far as the width of the articular disc space permits.[27] Further disc–condyle relationships are discussed in the section concerning functional analysis of the TMJ.

Suprahyoid Muscles

Categorically, muscles that are attached from the mandible to the hyoid bone are referred to as suprahyoid muscles and those from the hyoid bone to the scapular and sternum are called infrahyoid muscles. The supra and infrahyoid muscles play a major role in coordinating mandibular function.

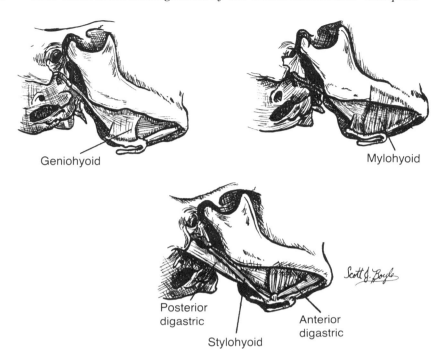

Fig. 2-9.   Right inferolateral view of geniohyoid, mylohyoid, digastric, and stylohyoid.

Geniohyoid

The geniohyoid muscle is a narrow muscle situated under the mylohyoid muscle; the latter, more superficial muscle, is more commonly referred to as the "floor of the mouth" (Fig. 2-9). The geniohyoid arises from the mental spine, a ridge of bone on the inner border of the body of the mandible and runs posteriorly and inferiorly to insert onto the hyoid bone.

The geniohyoid muscle is innervatd by fibers from the ventral rami of the lesser occipital nerve C_1. The hypoglossal nerve may be seen traveling with these fibers en route to the belly of the geniohyoid; however, the hypoglossal nerve does not innervate this muscle.

When the hyoid bone has become stablized by the infrahyoid muscles, the geniohyoid muscle exerts a downward and backward pull on the mandible, acting in concert with the digastric muscle.

The Digastric

The two bellies of the digastric muscle are united by an intervening tendon that attaches to the hyoid bone through a fibrous loop or sling. Behind and above, the posterior belly attaches to the mastoid notch deep to the attachments of the longissimus capitis, splenius capitis, and sternocleidomastoid muscles on the mastoid process (Fig. 2-9). In front and above the anterior belly attaches to the inferior border of the mandible close to its midline symphysis.

The common tendon perforates the stylohoid muscle, which lies near the front half of the posterior belly of the digastric. This common tendon of the digastric connects to the hyoid bone by sliding through a fibrous loop.

The posterior belly is innervated by a branch of the facial nerve. The anterior belly is supplied by the mylohyoid nerve from the alveolar branch of the posterior division of the mandibular nerve, the third division of the trigeminal nerve.

The digastric muscle assists in mandibular depression when the hyoid bone is fixed. With the mandible fixed, this muscle elevates the hyoid bone. Bilaterally, the digastrics assist in mandibular retrusion. This muscle is essential for forced or maximum depression. Coughing and swallowing also strongly involve the digastric muscles.

Mylohyoid

The mylohyoid muscle, flat and triangular, is located above the anterior belly of the digastric and forms, with its counterpart from the opposite side, a muscular floor for the mouth. It arises from the mylohyoid line of the mandible, extending from the symphysis mentis to the last molar tooth (Fig. 2-9). The posterior fibers pass medially and inferiorly to insert onto the body of the hyoid bone. The middle and anterior fibers with a midline fibrous raphe extend from the symphysis to the hyoid bone, where they join with fibers from the opposite side.

This muscle receives its innervation from the mylohyoid nerve from the inferior alveolar branch of the mandibular division of the trigeminal nerve. A small artery accompanies this nerve. The mylohyoid is functionally a muscle of the tongue stabilizing or elevating the tongue during swallowing.

The Stylohyoid

The stylohoid muscle is a slender muscle lying anterior and superior to the posterior belly of the digastric muscle. It arises from the posterior and lateral surface of the styloid process and, passing anteriorly and inferiorly, inserts into the body of the hyoid bone just above the omohyoid muscle (Fig. 2-9). The stylohyoid is commonly split near its insertion by the tendon of the digastric muscle.

The stylohyoid muscle is innervated by the facial nerve. This muscle draws the hyoid bone backward and upward during swallowing. The anteri_oposterior position of the hyoid bone is determined by the stylohoid, geniohyoid, and the infrahyoid muscles.

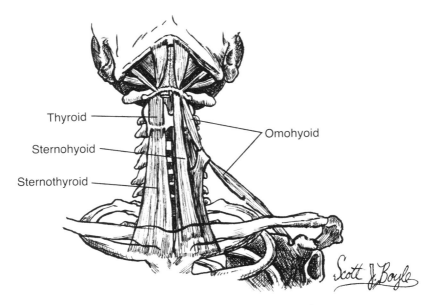

Thyroid

Sternohyoid

Sternothyroid

Omohyoid

Fig. 2-10. Infrahyoid "strap" muscles.

The Infrahyoid or "Strap" Muscles

The sternohyoid, omohyoid, sternothyroid, and thyrohyoid muscles are often referred to as "strap" muscles (Fig. 2-10). They cover the front and much of the sides of the larynx, trachea, and thyroid gland. Together with the deeper geniohyoid muscle, they represent a cervical continuation of the muscle mass that forms the "straplike" rectus abdominus muscle.[28] This straplike continuation of fiber orientation and the investment of deep fascia, therefore, provides an intermuscular continuum from the mandible to the symphysis pubis.

Superficially, and on each side of the midline, ascending from an origin on the posterior surface of the manubrium sterni and the sternal end of the clavicle, are the bilateral *sternohyoid* muscles. These thin flat muscles attach above to the body of the hyoid bone.

Lateral to the sternohyoid muscle is the superior belly of the *omohyoid* muscle, which attaches to the hyoid bone just lateral to the attachment of the sternohyoid muscle. The upper belly of this muscle parallels the sternohyoid. As it descends, it passes in front of the carotid sheath and its contents. Its fibers give way to the tendon through which it is joined to its inferior belly. The inferior belly of the omohyoid runs laterally, inferiorly, and posteriorly, across the posterior triangle of the neck, dividing this triangle into an upper occipital and a lower supraclavicular triangle, and disappears deep to the trapezius muscle. It attaches to the superior border of the scapula just medial to the scapula notch. (Omo means shoulder.) The central tendon of this muscle is held in position by deep cervical fascia. The omohyoid muscle is involved in prolonged inspiratory efforts by releasing tension on the apices of the lungs and on the internal jugular vein, which are attached to this fascial layer.[28]

Deep to the sternohyoid muscle are the *sternothyroid* and *thyrohyoid* muscles. The sternothyroid originates from the posterior surface of the manubruim and attaches above to an oblique line on the thyroid cartilage. The *thyrohyoid* runs from this line to the hyoid bone. Its lateral border usually appears posterolateral to the omohyoid muscle.

These infrahyoid muscles are innervated by fibers from upper cervical nerves. The nerves to the lower part of these muscles are given off from a loop, the ansacervicalis (cervical loop). The inferior root of the loop is a direct branch from the cervical plexus typically containing fibers from the second and third cervical nerves. The inferior root descends deep to the internal jugular vein and passes medially to form a loop (ansa) with the terminal part of the superior root; this superior root appears to take origin from the hypoglossal nerve, the twelfth cranial nerve.

The infrahyoid muscles depress the larynx and hyoid bone, a motion occurring in singing a low note and following the elevation of these structures during swallowing. Together with the suprahyoid muscles, they fix the hyoid bone, thus providing a firm base on which the tongue and mandible can be moved.

Cervical Muscles

Other major muscles, such as the sternocleidomastoid and the anterior and posterior cervical muscles, play a major role in stabilizing the skull and enabling controlled movements of the mandible. The cervical muscles can be divided

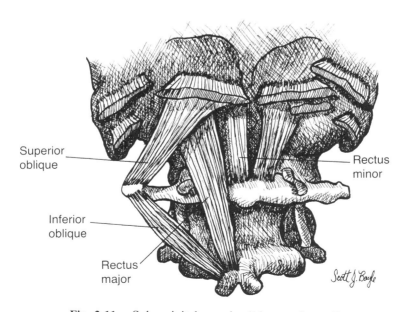

Superior oblique

Rectus minor

Inferior oblique

Rectus major

Scott J. Boyle

Fig. 2-11. Suboccipital muscles "deepest layer."

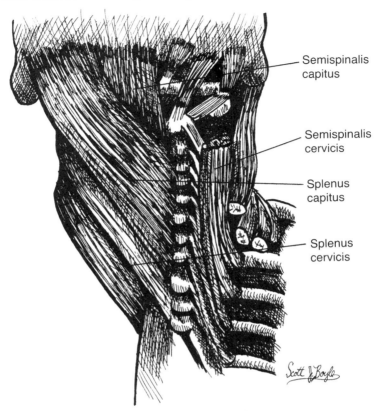

Semispinalis
capitus

Semispinalis
cervicis

Splenus
capitus

Splenus
cervicis

Fig. 2-12. Second deepest layer (semispinalis cervicis, semispinalis capitus) and third layer (splenus cervicis, splenus capitus).

into three groups by their location to the vertebral column: anterior, lateral, and posterior. The anterior group is subdivided into superficial previsceral muscles, *infrahyoid muscles,* and deep prevertebral muscles, the *longus capitus* and *longus cervicus muscles,* which lie deep to the viscera.

The lateral group consists of the deep *scalene muscles*, which descend from the transverse processes of the cervical vertebrae to the first and second ribs and the *sternocleidomastoid* muscle, which runs from the sternum and clavicle to the mastoid process.

The posterior muscles consist of four separate layers. The deepest is the shortest, containing the *rectus major* and *minor,* and the *superior* and *inferior obliques* (Fig. 2-11). These suboccipital muscles extend from the occipital bone and the atlas and axis to form a triangle known as the suboccipital triangle. Within this triangle, the vertebral artery runs its circuitous journey en route to the brain. The lower part of this layer includes the small deep muscles found all along the spine, the *multifidus, rotatores, intertransversarii,* and *interspinales.*

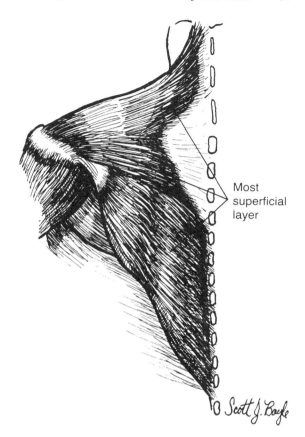

Fig. 2-13. Most superficial layer.

Most superficial layer

The second deepest layer, which is formed by the *semispinalis cervicis* and *semispinalis capitis* covers these muscles (Fig. 2-12). This layer originates from the transverse processes of vertebrae below. The semispinalis muscle fibers insert onto the spinous processes; the semispinalis capitus reaches the occipital bone in the base of the skull. Abnormal increase in tension of this muscle can entrap the greater occipital nerve, the posterior ramus of C2, which pierces it.[19] The longissimis cervicis and capitis are more lateral in this second layer.

The third layer is formed by the *splenius muscles* (Fig. 2-12). They are attached to the spines of the upper thoracic and lower cervical vertebrae and the ligamentum nuchae. They run obliquely upward and laterally to reach the transverse processes (splenis cervicis) and superiorly to reach the mastoid process and occipital bone (splenus capitis).

The last and most superficial layer in the neck is formed by the ligamentum nuchae and the cervical part of the *trapezius* muscle, which arises from the occipital bone and the spines of the inferior cervical vertebrae (Fig. 2-13).

These muscles produce the movement of flexion, extension, rotation, and lateral side bending of the cervical spine. The close proximity of these structures to the TMJ suggest a functional correlation between the cervical spine, the TMJ, and occlusion. A change in head posture produced by these cervical muscles influences mandibular position.

FUNCTIONAL ANALYSIS OF THE TMJ

Functional analysis of the TMJ depends on an understanding of the static positions that can be maintained by the TMJ as well as the dynamic motions available to the joint and its components. This section defines and describes the postures assumed by the TMJ and the motions it can perform.

Static Positions

Before functional movements and specific muscular contributions can be evaluated, the postural relationship of the mandible with the skull must first be recognized. The TMJ can assume two relative positions when the mandible is not in motion. An understanding of these positions is essential in analyzing movements of the TMJ away from these postures as well as in carrying out or communicating about an evaluation. The terminology of these positions has been confusing, controversial, and conflicting; therefore, the terminology presented is designed to describe the physiologic positions. These two mandibular postures are the rest position and the occlusal position.

Rest Position

The mandibular rest position is a natural posture that occurs because of equilibrium between forces of the gravity, or jaw-opening muscles and the antigravity or jaw-closing muscles. The residual tension of these muscles at rest is termed "resting tonus." Because of the variations in muscle tonus, this position is not constant. No occlusal contact occurs between maxillary and mandibular teeth in this position, however. Usually an interocclusal distance ranging from 2 to 5 mm can be measured between the maxillary and mandibular central incisors. This space is called the "freeway space" of interocclusal clearance. The significance of the rest position lies is that it permits the tissues of the stomatognathic system to rest and repair. This rest position is entirely dependent on the mandibular musculature, soft tissue, and gravity.

Occlusal Position

The maximum intercuspated position is the occlusal position in which all the teeth are fully interdigitated. It is a position that is dependent on the presence, shape, and position of the teeth. This is a transitional posture and one that provides a functional component for a brief period of time.

ISOLATED MANDIBULAR MOVEMENTS

Motions of the TMJ involve discrete motions of the mandible and inter-articular disc as well as relative motions between these two elements. The following details the discrete motions available to each and then outlines the complex motions of both which occur in normal opening and closing of the mouth.

Mandibular movements guided by the TMJs and muscle activity occur as a series of interrelated three-dimensional rotational and translational activities. These movements depend on four factors: (1) initiating position, (2) types of movements, (3) direction of movement, and (4) degree of movement.[29]

The first (1) *initiating position* or maximum intercuspated position is a tooth-to-tooth position. From this position (2) two *types of movement* can be executed, namely rotation and translation. Rotation is the motion of a body around its center, whereas translation is the motion of a body in which all parts move in the same direction and at the same rate. The third factor (3) is the *direction of movement* and is related to the planes of movement. There are three planes of movement with regard to the TMJ: the frontal plane, the sagittal plane, and the horizontal plane. The fourth factor (4) is the *degree of movement,* since most mandibular functions, such as chewing and talking, occur at lesser degrees of opening.

A wide range of mandibular movements require muscle activity in various synergistic and antagonistic patterns. To understand the complexities of mandibular movement better, it is necessary first to isolate the movements that occur within a single TMJ.

Two basic types of mandibular movement can be identified in the TMJ: rotation and translation.

Rotation

Rotation occurs when a body moves around a fixed point. The mandible has three axes of rotation; a mediolateral (X) axis, an anteroposterior (Y) axis, and a longitudinal (Z) axis (Fig. 2-14). Rotation around a mediolateral axis causes opening and closing and occurs between the condyle-articular disc portion of the lower joint compartment. This mediolateral axis of rotation passes through the medial and lateral condylar poles. This mediolateral axis of rotation provides a hinge movement in the sagittal plane. This hinge movement is a mandibular movement in which only rotation occurs during the first few degrees of opening.

Mandibular movement around an anteroposterior axis (*y* axis) occurs when one condyle moves inferiorly while the opposite condyle remains relatively stationary. This motion occurs in the frontal plane and produces a depression of the mandible on the moving side.

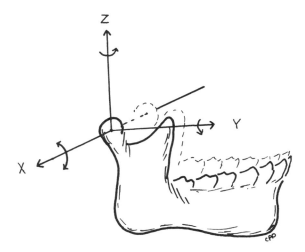

Fig. 2-14. Rotational components. Rotation around x axis is rotation in sagittal plane. Rotation around y axis is rotation in frontal plane. Rotation around z axis is rotation in transverse plane.

The longitudinal or vertical axis (z axis) of rotation occurs when one condyle moves anteriorly, rotating around an axis through the opposite condyle. This motion occurs in the horizontal plane and results in unilateral protrusive-retrusive movement. For the upper surface of the disc–condyle complex to maintain full surface contact with the temporal articular facet, the disc must rotate anteroposteriorly on the condyle. Actually, the disc rotates posteriorly on the condyle as the disc–condyle complex moves forward in relationship to the articular eminence.[30] This motion causes the forward movement of the articular disc to be considerably less than that of the condyle.

Rotary movements around each of the above mentioned axes imply separation of the jaws to a greater or lesser degree. Intercuspation influences condylar movements, thereby altering the purity of these rotational disc–condylar movements.

Translation

Translation, or gliding movements occur in the superior compartment between the inferior surface of the articular fossa and eminence of the temporal bone and the superior surface of the articular disc (Fig. 2-15). The superior shape of the disc is compatible with the fossa-eminence articular facet. The flatness and compatibility of the articular surfaces, the absence of collateral ligaments, and the loose attachment of the capsular ligament ensure freedom of gliding movement in all directions.[30] Translation occurs during the downward and forward movement of the disc–condyle complex, a protrusive movement. A return of this complex in the upward and backward position is called a retrusive movement. During translation, the teeth, condyles, and rami all move in the same direction and to the same degree. A partially lowered mandible

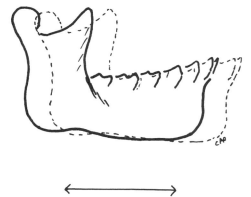

Fig. 2-15.   Translation of mandible.

can move forward or backward over the articular eminence, with all points of the jaw moving in the same direction at the same rate at any given instant.[31]

ISOLATED MOVEMENTS OF THE INTERARTICULAR DISC

The size and shape of the disc are determined by the shape of the condyle and articular eminence. The lower articular surface of the disc is contoured in both dimensions to fit the condylar facet to permit uninterrupted rotary gliding movements around a horizontal axis. The upper articular surface of the disc is shaped to fit the temporal articular facet. These compatible surfaces permit linear gliding movements in all directions.

Interarticular pressure imposed on the disc by the articulating bones narrows the articular space and exerts pressure on the disc. This pressure results in a rotational movement of the disc which introduces a thinner portion of the disc between the articulating bones. Reduction of this pressure results in a widening of the articular disc space and a resumption of a thicker portion of the disc to fill in the space (Fig. 2-16).

The contour of the disc also prevents excessive sliding between disc and condyle without inhibiting rotatory movements. The thicker posterior margin of the disc prevents linear displacement of the disc anteriorly; likewise, the thicker anterior margin prevents excessive posterior displacement. Therefore, the contour of the disc provides harmonious translation of disc and condyle without displacement.[10]

FUNCTIONAL MOVEMENTS

Combinations of the basic movements of the disc and mandible comprise the functional movements of the TMJ. The biomechanics of this joint are determined by the morphology and structural arrangement of its parts as they

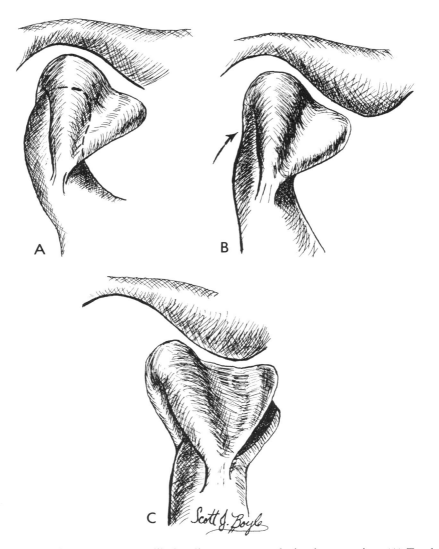

Fig. 2-16.   Right temporomandibular disc movement during jaw opening. **(A)** Teeth in maximum intercuspation. **(B)** Midopening, disc rotating posterior on condyle. **(C)** Full opening, both disc and condyle have translated forward; disc has rotated posteriorly in relation to condyle.

relate to the demands of function. The bilateral hinge joints, suspended by strong temporomandibular ligaments, are capable of linear sliding movements down and around the articular eminence.

Opening and *closing* movements of the jaw are a combination of rotary and translatory movements of the mandible and disc. During the first several

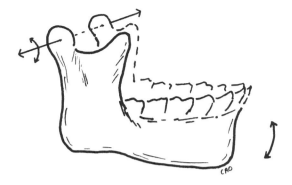

Fig. 2-17. Rotation around *x* axis occurring in first few degrees of jaw opening and closing.

degrees of the opening phase, the mandible rotates around a fixed axis that passes through the centers of the two condyles (Fig. 2-17). As the condyles continue to rotate, the condylar ridge moves forward on the intermediate zone of the disc. The intermediate zone of the disc remains interposed between the anterior slope of the condylar articular surface and the articular eminence. The relationship between the disc and condyle is that of rotation of the disc posteriorly on the condyle. As the translatory phase begins, the upper surface of the articular disc slides down against the articular eminence. Excessive translation occurs when the disc and condyle pass over the crest, and move forward along the anterior plane. During the closing phase, the upper surface of the disc retraces the sliding movement back to the resting position. During this return phase, the disc rotates anteriorly until the cycle is completed. During this closing phase, the condyles rotate onto the bicondylar axis, and the condylar ridge returns to the intermediate zone of the disc.

Protrusion occurs when the mandible is moved forward with the teeth separated. Protrusion is a forward movement of the mandible occurring in the superior joint compartment. It is a smooth symmetrial motion that reflects smooth contiguous articular surfaces. Protrusion consists of the disc and condyle moving downward and forward along the posterior slope of the articular eminence. The disc moves forward along the articular plane that forms the anterior surface of the articular eminence. As the condyle moves forward onto the intermediate zone of the disc, the bilaminar retrodiscal tissue stretches 6 to 9 mm to allow this movement.

The return phase of the translatory cycle is a retracing of the disc and condyle back to the rest position. From this position, the maximally intercuspated position can be assumed.

Retrusion is initiated from the maximally intercuspated position. Retrusive range is limited and rarely amounts to more than 3 mm. This position must be voluntarily achieved only after the teeth have been disengaged. The limitations to further retrusion are also imposed on by the taut temporomandibular ligaments. The most retruded position is not an integral part of functional masticatory movement but instead provides a dimension for joint play.

Lateral shift of the mandible results when the translatory cycle is unilateral. During lateral excursion, the disc and condyle of the nonworking joint

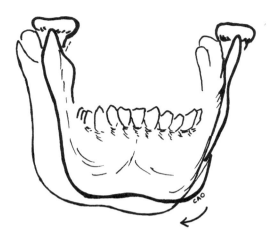

Fig. 2-18.   Lateral deviation to the right. Right condyle moves downward, backward, and laterally. Left condyle moves downward, forward, and medially.

move medially as they approach the articular eminence (Fig. 2-18). This deviation displaces the disc and condyle in an inferior direction. Simultaneously, on the opposite or working side, the disc and condyle pivot until the inner horizontal band of the temporomandibular ligament arrests further posterior movement of the lateral pole. From that point on, the disc and condyle rotate around a vertical axis that passes through the lateral pole of the working condyle. During a simple lateral movement, a motion occurs at the sagittal, horizontal, and vertical axes. Each axis is simultaneously tilting to accommodate to the movement occurring around the other axes. These movements are intricately controlled by the neuromuscular system.

FUNCTION OF THE MASTICATORY SYSTEM IN MASTICATION, DEGLUTITION, AND VOCALIZATION

The three major functions of the masticatory system are chewing, swallowing, and talking. Its role in each is described below.

Mastication (Chewing)

The bipedal human has had the face rotated downward and backward under the brain case. The skull base at the foramen magnum and occipital condyles is now below the level of the temporomandibular articulations, bringing the tympanic bone and elongated mastoid process far down and close behind the ramus of the mandible. A wide opening of the jaw in a pure hingelike rotation is no longer feasible. To compensate for this restriction in hinge movement, the lateral pterygoid muscles pull the condyle and the disc forward and downward along the articular eminence, thus providing a greater arc for bicondylar axial rotation.

The biomechanics involved in TMJ movement require synchronous activity of the masticatory muscles while these muscles actively shift their role from movers to balancers to stabilizers. Stability of the joint is maintained by constant activity of the muscles that pull across the joint. Even in a resting state, these muscles are in a mild state of contraction, or tonus. Unconscious mandibular activity is guided largely by preconditioned habit patterns that become resistant to change. Normal function depends on harmony between the forces imposed by the muscles and the occluded dentition.

As the intrinsic prime movers for mandibular elevation (the temporalis, masseter, and medial pterygoid muscles) contract to execute the power stroke, contraction of the inferior lateral pterygoid muscle exerts a strong holding action on the condyle. During chewing, the interarticular pressure on the biting side is decreased as the power stroke is applied to the food rather than to the joint. The tension on the superior retrodiscal lamina tends to retract the disc. To counter this posterior force on the disc, the superior lateral pterygoid becomes active during this power stroke, rotating the disc forward on the condyle so that the thicker posterior border of the disc maintains articular contact. As the teeth pulverize the food, the cusps approximate each other and the interarticular pressure in the joint is increased. With increased pressure, the disc is mechanically rotated posteriorly so that the thinner intermediate zone fills the space. Once the chewing cycle has ceased, the disc–condyle relationship returns to the rest position. The disc, at rest, occupies its most anterior position on the condyle permitted by the articular disc space. The muscles relax, assuming a state of muscular equilibrium represented by a resting muscle tonus. Synovial fluid penetrates the articulating surface, and the joint is lubricated and made ready for the next movement.

Chewing is a complex function that uses muscles, teeth, lips, cheeks, tongue, palate, and salivary glands. The opening and closing movements of the jaw represent chewing strokes. The closing, or elevation movements may be subdivided into *crushing* and *grinding* components. Both crushing and grinding can be divided into three phases: (1) the first, or preparatory phase is a free movement of the mandible; (2) the second phase ends as tooth contact is initiated; and (3) the third phase is the articulatory movement that occurs under tooth contact.[33]

As food becomes trapped between the teeth, the crushing phase is initiated. Once the food is firmly situated between the teeth, the grinding phase begins. The mandible is guided by the occlusal surfaces of the teeth, and the cuspal inclines pass across each other, permitting shearing and grinding of the bolus of food. Under normal conditions, contact of the lateral teeth, particularly in the first molar region, can be maintained only on one side. If the mandible is shifted to the right, the right molars and premolars maintain contact. The occlusion of the teeth during the grinding movement is not balanced due to the forward, downward, and lateral shift of the "moving condyle." When food is initially introduced into the mouth, few occlusal contacts occur; however, in the final stages of mastication prior to swallowing, contacts occur during every stroke.[34]

Deglutition (Swallowing)

Swallowing, like chewing, can be initiated voluntarily or reflexly. During swallowing, a bolus of food is moved from the oral pharynx through the esophagus to the stomach. This motion consists of voluntary, involuntary, and reflex muscular activity. Stimulation of sensory receptors around the oropharynx carry impulses to the swallowing center in the brain stem, which relays motor signals to the appropriate muscles. The act of swallowing is divided into three phases: the oral, the pharyngeal, and the esophageal phase.[34]

The first phase involves voluntary separation of the bolus of food by the tongue. This bolus is placed on the dorsum of the tongue and is pressed against the hard palate. The pressure of the bolus against the mucosa of the hard palate initiates a reflex wave of contraction in the tongue which results in a backward displacement of the bolus. The bolus is then transferred to the pharynx. During this phase, the soft palate elevates, closing the pathway to the nose while the tongue prevents reentry of food into the mouth. Respiration is inhibited briefly.

During the second stage, the bolus of food is caught in a peristaltic wave produced by the contraction of the pharyngeal constrictor muscles and carried down to the esophagus. The hyoid bone is elevated upward and posteriorly in rapid sequence, and the epiglottis is tilted over the glottis. Food is prevented from entering the trachea by inhibition of respiration, narrowing of the laryngeal vestibule, elevation of the larynx, approximation of the vocal cords, and tilting of the epiglottis. The distal portion of the pharynx is narrowed by the constrictor muscles, thereby creating a pressure that forces food into the esophagus. In the uppermost portion of the esophagus, passive elastic tension creates a closed sphincter exerting a pressure of 40 cm H_2O higher than atmospheric. This inhibits large volumes of air from entering the stomach during normal respiration. During swallowing, this sphincter is passively opened by the upward movement of the pharynx and larynx permitting food to be forced into the esophagus. Subsequent return of the sphincter pressure prevents food reflux from the esophagus.

The third stage of swallowing consists of passing the bolus through the esophagus by peristalsis; liquids are shot through the esophagus by the force of swallowing and by gravity. Peristaltic waves take 6 to 7 seconds to carry the bolus of food through the length of the esophagus. In the upper section of the esophagus, the muscles are mainly voluntary and can be used to return food to the mouth when necessary for more complete mastication. In the lower section, the muscles perform involuntarily.

Vocalization (Speech)

Speech is created when a volume of air is forced from the lungs by the diaphragm through the larynx and oral cavity. The desired pitch is obtained by controlled contraction and relaxation of the vocal cords of the larynx. Resonance and articulation of sound is determined by the posture of the lips as the air is expelled through the mouth. Prolonged expiration permits a resultant series of syllables, words, and phrases.

A variety of sounds can be accomplished by varying the relationship of lips and tongue to palate and teeth. During the sounding of the letters M, B, and P, the lips come together and touch. The S sound is created as the air passes between the incisal edges of the maxillary and mandibular teeth. The D sound is made as the tip of the tongue reaches up to touch the palate behind the teeth. For sounds like K and G, the posterior portion of the tongue rises to touch the soft palate. The lower lip touches the incisal edges of the maxillary teeth to form the F and V sounds. Once speech is learned, it becomes an unconscious activity of the neuromuscular system, a learned reflex activity.

In conclusion, the normal functions of the TMJ are essential to the normal execution of some of a human's most basic activities: chewing, swallowing, and vocalization. Motion provided by the TMJ is the sum total of an elegantly orchestrated set of movements performed by the synergistic activity of several muscles. Normal function depends on smooth symmetrical alignment of complex joint surfaces and on the congruency of an equally complex intraarticular disc. Such specialization within this complex allows such diverse activities as chewing bubblegum, sipping champagne, and hollering at a ball game. It also allows for subtle dysfunctions within any individual component. Thus, it is incumbent on the clinician treating temporomandibular dysfunction to have a sound understanding of the morphology and biomechanics of this unique functional unit.

ACKNOWLEDGEMENT

I would like to express my gratitude to two artists, Scott J. Boyle and Carol A. Oatis, for their rendering of the illustrations in this chapter.

REFERENCES

1. Dolwick MF: The temporomandibular joint. In Helms CA, Katzberg RW, Dolwick MF (eds): Internal Derangements of the Temporomandibular Joint. University of California Press, San Francisco, 1983
2. Sicker H: Oral Anatomy. CV Mosby, St. Louis, 1949
3. DuBrul EL: Sicher's Oral Anatomy, 7th Ed. CV Mosby, St Louis, 1980
4. Rees LA: The structure and function of the mandibular joint. Br Dent J 96:125, 1954
5. Glineburg RW, Laskin DM, Blaustein DI: The effects of immobilization on the primate temporomandibular joint. J Oral Maxillofac Surg 40:3, 1982
6. DeBont LGM, Boering G, Havinga P, et al: Spatial arrangement of collagen fibrils in the articular cartilage of the mandibular condyle: A light microscopic and scanning electron microscopic study. J Oral Maxillofac Surg 42:306, 1984
7. Mohl DN: Functional anatomy of the temporomandibular joint. in The President's

Conference on the Examination, Diagnosis and Management of Temporomandibular Disorders, American Dental Association, Chicago, 1983

8. Moffett B: Histologic aspects of temporomandibular joint derangements: Diagnosis of Internal Derangements of the Temporomandibular Joint. Vol. 1. University of Washington, Seattle, 1984

9. Rees LA: The structure and function of the mandibular joint. Br Dent J 6:125, 1954

10. Dolwick MF, Katzberg RW, Helms CA, Bales DJ: Arthrotomographic evaluation of the temporomandibular joint. J Oral Surg 11:793, 1979

11. Hansson T, Oberg T, Carlsson GE, et al: Thickness of the soft tissue layers and the articular disc in the temporomandibular joint. Acta Odontol Scand 35: 1977

12. DuBrul ET: The biomechanics of the oral apparatus. In DuBrul ET, Menekratis A: The Physiology of Reconstruction. Quintessence, Chicago, 1981

13. Kopp S: Topographic distribution of sulphated glycoaminoglycans in the surface layers of the human temporomandibular joint. J Oral Pathol 1978

14. Toller PA: Opague arthrography of the TMJ. Int J Oral Surg 3:17, 1974

15. Moss M: A functional cranial analysis of centric relation. Dent Clin North Am 19:431, 1975

16. Dolwick MF: Surgical Atlas of Dental Implant Techniques. WB Saunders, Philadelphia, 1980

17. Thilander B: Innervation of the temporomandibular joint capsule in man. Trans R. School Dent 7:9, 1961

18. Hollinshead WH: Textbook of Anatomy, 3rd Ed. Philadelphia: Harper & Row, 1974

19. Friedman MH, Weisberg J: Temporomandibular Joint Disorders. Quintessence, Chicago, 1985

20. Pinto OF: A new structure related to temporomandibular joint and middle ear. J Prosthet Dent 12:95, 1962

21. Ermshar CB: Anatomy and neurology. In Margan DH, House LR, Hall WP, et al (eds): Diseases of the Temporomandibular Apparatus. 2nd Ed. CV Mosby, St. Louis, 1982

22. Manns A, Miralles R, Palazzi C: EMG bite force and elongation of the masseter muscle under isometric voluntary contractions and variations of vertical dimension. J Prosthet Dent 42, 1979

23. Taylor A, Cody FW, Bosley MA: Histochemical and mechanic properties of the jaw muscles of the cat. Exp Neurol 38: 1973

24. Basmajiian JV: Muscles Alive. 4th Ed. Williams & Wilkins, Baltimore, 1978

25. Carlsoo S: Nervous coordination and mechanical function of the mandibular elevators: an electromyographic study of the activity, and an anatomic analysis of mechanics of the muscles. Acta Odontol Scand 11, 1952

26. McNamara JA, Jr: The independent function of the two heads of the lateral pterygoid muscle. Am J Anat 138: 1973

27. Mahan PE, Wilkinson TM, Gibbs CH, et al: Superior and inferior bellies of the lateral pterygoid muscle: EMB activity at basic jaw positions. J Prosthet Dent 50: 1983

28. Gray H: Anatomy of the Human Body. Lea & Febiger, Philadelphia, 1973

29. Neff PA: Occlusion and Function: A Teaching Aid. 4th Ed. Georgetown University, Washington, DC, 1980

30. Okeson JP: Fundamentals of Occlusion and Temporomandibular Disorders. CV Mosby, St. Louis, 1985

31. Bell WE: Temporomandibular Disorders: Classification, Diagnosis, Management. 2nd Ed. Year Book Medical, Chicago, 1985

32. Gibbs CH, Mahan PE, Wilkinson JM, et al: EMG activity of the superior belly of the lateral pterygoid muscle in relation to other jaw muscles. J Prosthet Dent 51:691, 1984
33. Moller E: The chewing apparatus. Acta Physiol Scand, 69 suppl. 280:00, 1966
34. Ahlgren J: Mechanism of mastication. Acta Odontol Scand, 24 suppl. 44:5, 1966

3 | TMJ Disorders

Frank Benson

The purpose of this chapter is to provide the reader with a sound understanding of various afflictions that affect the TMJ. These include growth, disease, arthritic, macrotrauma, and dysfunctional disorders. Some of these conditions can be quite painful and can even cause severe dysfunction.

To cover the variety of disorders that may involve the TMJ, each is discussed briefly covering the etiology, occurrence or pathology, evaluation, and overview of treatment. This type of presentation attempts to provide the reader with an awareness of disorders that may be present in any given patient. Emphasis of the evaluation and treatment is placed on the disorders that are most common in a typical clinical setting.

GROWTH DISORDERS

The TMJ develops during the fourteenth week of gestation.[1-3] Most synovial joints develop from a single condensation of cells. The TMJ develops from two condensations or layers of cells: One condensation is on the condyle of the mandible; the other is in the temporal region. These two groups of cells proliferate and grow toward each other during the eighth and twelfth weeks of gestation. A third condensation or layers of cells develops between these two layers and forms the disc.[1-3]

This developmental sequence of the TMJ is very complex and must occur with precision if a normal TMJ is to develop. This process can be disrupted, resulting in a growth disorder.

Condylar Hypoplasia

Etiology

Condylar hypoplasia may develop due to an alteration of one of the condensations of cells of the TMJ at an early stage of development.[4]

51

Occurrence

Condylar hypoplasia is relatively rare. It is seldom painful and causes no problem unless the ipsilateral mandible is underdeveloped as well. The ramus may be reduced in vertical height, and the mandibular neck may lean posteriorly.

Evaluation

Condylar hypoplasia is best evaluated using radiographs such as the orthopantomograph. The most severe problem with bilateral hypoplasia is a severe malocclusion characterized by a retruded mandible and on anterior open bite.[5]

Treatment

No treatment is indicated unless esthetics are a concern of the patient. If so, an orthodontic evaluation is indicated.

Condylar Hyperplasia

Etiology

The etiology for condylar hyperplasia is unknown, but is probably due to a continuation of growth in the subchondral growth center.[6] Biopsies of affected TMJs show that the cartilage has a well-developed blood supply and no subchondral bony plate.[4]

Occurrence

Condylar hyperplasia is generally noted in adolescence.[7] At this time, facial growth has ceased, but the continued growth of the condyle produces a facial asymmetry in which the mandibular midline is displaced to the opposite side. The body of the mandible is displaced downward and laterally, which may stimulate a compensatory growth of the maxilla with a tilting of the teeth and occlusal plane.[4] This condition is relatively rare. It is most notable in teenagers and has been called "the orthodontist's nightmare."[5]

Evaluation

Appropriate radiographs, such as a Panorex and anteroposterior (AP) views, should be ordered for patients who complain of their "bite shifting to one side" or for those whose midline has changed over time. Radiographs might show a normal condyle with an elongated condylar neck or a greatly enlarged condyle.[5] A bone scan will show the affected TMJ to be "hot" relative to the opposite unaffected side.

Treatment

Surgical treatment for this condition can be relatively simple to remarkably complex. If the deformity is treated before the maxilla is involved, surgical correction may be limited to the mandible. If the defect is moderate, the affected condyle may need to be excised, and an osteotomy of the contralateral side may be needed to treat the facial and occlusal discrepancies. Severe deformities may involve excision of the condyle, along with maxillary and mandibular osteotomies.[7]

Neoplasms

Etiology

Neoplasms of the TMJ can arise from various cell populations within the joint, or can metastasize from primary tumors elsewhere or invade from nearby adjacent tissues.

Occurrence

TMJ tumors are very rare.[8,9] Their signs and symptoms are quite similar, however, to those of other disorders that affect the TMJ. Clinicians should be very suspicious of TMJ pain that remains refractory to treatment and increases.

Benign tumors, such as myxoma, osteoma, hemangioma, chondroma, and osteochondrama are much more common than primary malignant neoplasms. These latter tumors include chondrosarcoma, osteosarcoma, and multiple myeloma. Metastases that have been reported include bronchogenic carcinoma[10] and adenocarcinoma.

Evaluation

Patients with tumors may have chronic pain that may be exacerbated during jaw movement or function. Limitation of jaw movement and an open bite on the affected side may be noted.

Radiographs should be ordered for suspected cases. Benign tumors may show bony protruberances on x-ray studies. Malignant tumors can manifest either osteolytic or osteoblastic radiographic changes. Swelling over the lateral aspect of the joint may be present. Hearing loss has also been noted.

Treatment

The surgical treatment of tumors of the TMJ is governed by the principles of all tumor surgery. Excisions should have wide enough margins to increase the chances for a cure. The need for a prosthesis can be determined at the time of surgery if the extent of the tumor margin is unknown prior to surgery.[7]

After surgery, muscle activity, occlusal forces, and joint stability must be addressed. Various physical therapy modalities can be used to regain jaw function and movement.

DISEASES OR ARTHRITIC DISORDERS

Infectious Arthritis

Etiology

Any pathogenic bacteria can infect the TMJ. Older children and adults are most commonly infected with gonococci, staphylococci, streptococci, and pneumococci.[11] These bacteria may infect the TMJ at any age, but are most common in the second, third, and fourth decades of life because antecedent infections due to these bacteria are most prevalent at these ages.[12]

Bacteria usually seed the joint space through a hematogenous spread of an infection located in another organ of the body. An open wound or direct extension of an infection from a neighboring region such as the ear may be responsible. Direct innoculation may also occur at the time of surgery or medication or dye injection.

Pathology

The anatomic changes in the TMJ consist of a nonspecific, acute suppurative infection. Depending on the virulence of the organism, the synovium may ulcerate and involve the articular surfaces.[13] The result may be extensive destruction of the joint surfaces. Fibrous adhesions between the disc and articulating surface or scarring of the capsule may produce significant TMJ hypomobility.

Evaluation

The signs and symptoms of a patient with TMJ infectious arthritis usually consist of a fever and complaints of pain in the joint. The joint is usually extremely painful to passive or active movements. There is usually evidence of septicemia and local symptoms of the primary focus.

Treatment

Any suspicion of septic involvement requires immediate referral to an oral surgeon or physician, who should perform a synovial fluid aspiration and subsequent Gram stain and culture for antibiotic sensitivity testing. Physical therapy may be necessary for restoration of joint function once the acute phase has been successfully treated.

Traumatic Arthritis

Etiology

The term traumatic arthritis is best reserved for joint lesions produced by acute direct trauma.[11] This may include blows to the mandible sustained during motor vehicle or sports accidents.

Pathology

The amount of trauma sustained by the TMJ depends on the magnitude, duration, and direction of the insult. Minor trauma may cause strain of the ligaments or capsule with subsequent edema. Healing is usually rapid and complete due to a rich blood supply.[13]

More severe injuries may traumatize the synovium, which may upset the dynamics of the TMJ. As a result, the injury may persist but usually heals uneventfully.

Very severe blows may traumatize the articular surfaces and/or subchondral bone to such a degree that posttraumatic degenerative joint disease develops.[13] An irregular joint surface may result.

Evaluation

The diagnosis of traumatic arthritis may be obvious from history and examination. The TMJ is usually painful, tender, and swollen. Interincisal (mandibular depression) opening may be severely impaired.

Hanlon and Estes have introduced four criteria for the diagnosis of traumatic arthritis:[14]

1. The trauma must be severe enough to produce synovitis with pain, swelling, effusion, and dysfunction.
2. The traumatized joint must be only one showing such inflammation.
3. Normal articular function must have been present before the injury.
4. Progressive articular changes may occur, which in time may be demonstrated by radiographs.

Treatment

Treatment of traumatic arthritis is best accomplished with conservative measures. Soft diet, local moist heat, and analgesics for pain should be part of the treatment. A full-coverage interocclusal appliance may help decrease pain and aid healing by relieving the affected joint of stress. R. Meyer (personal communication) stresses that traumatic arthritis is one of the few indications for the use of intraarticular steroids. Studies have shown that irresponsible use of intrajoint corticosteroid injections may produce progressive degeneration of the TMJ.[15] Physical therapy treatments such as the use of modalities to help control pain and swelling are indicated. Once the acute stage has subsided, physical therapy treatments to regain capsular extensibility can be offered if indicated.

Metabolic Joint Disease (Gout)

Etiology

Gout is a recurrent acute arthritis of a peripheral joint, such as the TMJ, due to deposition of crystals of monosodium urate from supersaturated hyperuricemic body fluids.[16]

More than 95 percent of gouty patients are hyperuricemic. Gout strikes men nine times more frequently than women and tends to strike in the third decade.[16]

Pathology

The deposition of urate crystals in and about joint components results in the activation of the complement system. White blood cells that have migrated to the scene attempt to engulf the crystals. Lysosomal enzymes are then released and tend to destroy the integrity of the articular surfaces.[12]

Evaluation

The signs and symptoms of an acute attack usually appear without warning, but may be precipitated by trauma, overindulgence in food or alcohol, fatigue, or infection.[13]

When examined, the joint appears red, swollen, tender, and warm. The metatarsophalangeal joint of the big toe is the most commonly affected joint (podagra). Very few cases of gouty TMJ involvement have been reported.

Treatment

The objectives for treatment of a gouty TMJ are similar to those of other joints. First, the patient should be referred to a physician for confirmation of the suspected diagnosis. Rest and antiinflammatory medications are the cornerstone of treatment for the acute attack. A full-coverage interocclusal appliance may be indicated to produce more favorable joint loading.

Degenerative Joint Disease (Osteoarthritis, Arthrosis)

Degenerative joint disease (DJD) is an arthritide characterized by degenerative loss of articular cartilage, subchondral bony sclerosis, and cartilage and bone proliferation at the joint margins in the latter stages.

DJD is primarily a noninflammatory disease and has been termed osteoarthrosis in this stage.[17] Clinical symptoms of joint pain and stiffness is believed to be due to secondary inflammation of the capsular tissue.[18] This results from proteoglycans that are released into synovial fluid as a result of degeneration of joint surfaces and that are capable of causing the chronic synovitis.

Four different tissue layers can be found on the condyle and temporal component. These layers include bone, cartilage, undifferentiated mesenchymal cells, and fibrous connective tissue. A thickening of the subarticular soft tissue layer results from cellular proliferation with cartilage formation from the undifferentiated mesenchyme.[19] Studies point to variations in biomechanical loading of the TMJ as stimulating the mesenchyme to a proliferative response.[20-22]

Etiology and Pathology

Several theories have been offered as an etiology for DJD. No unanimous agreement has been reached concerning the causative factors, however.

Repetitive Loading Theory. Degenerative changes can be produced in joints that have received repetitive or impact loads. This has been demonstrated in the laboratory. Clinically, degenerative changes are more common in the elbows and shoulders of pneumatic drill operators. This suggests that a breakdown of the joint occurs when the articulating surfaces are subjected to repetitive overloading in excess of the functional capacity. The joint surface may begin to break down, however, when it is subjected to normal loads and a reduced functional capacity, due to such processes as aging or prior bouts of rheumatoid arthritis.[23]

This theory of repetitive joint loading has been investigated by many researchers, such as Mongini[24] and Hansson.[25] Hansson contends that occlusal discrepancies may be significant in adversely loading the TMJ. Mandibular elevator muscle hyperactivity and/or altered activity as a result of nocturnal or diurnal bruxism, stress (emotional or physical), and or cervical spine influences might also load the TMJ, however, in lieu of occlusal dysharmony. Mechanical factors such as lack of posterior support, "overclosed" complete dentures, or class II malocclusion may also overload the TMJ due to distalization of the condyles from their functional position on the eminence. Sound research is still lacking to prove or disprove these proposed etiologies.

Perforation Theory. An intact articulating disc is generally agreed to be essential for the health of the joint. During TMJ surgery, osteophytes are frequently noted to be protruding into a perforation of the disc or retrodiscal pad. The question that remains to be answered, however, is whether the osteoarthritic changes caused the perforation or the perforation brought about the degenerative changes.

Internal Derangement Theory. In a case of TMJ internal derangement, the condyle functions off the disc on the retrodiscal pad unless the condyle can translate far enough anteriorly to reduce the displacement. If this condition persists long enough, the articulating surfaces may be adversely affected to the extent that they no longer keep pace with functional demands and begin to degenerate.

Regardless of etiology, once the first histologic changes take place at the joint surface, it begins to degenerate by developing horizontal fissures (called flaking) and vertical fissures (called fibrillation). Subsequent to degeneration of the articular surface, free bodies of the joint surface migrate to the synovial fluid and from there to the synovium. The fragments may elicit an inflammatory response, termed synovitis. The breakdown of the joint surface may then allow biomechanical forces to be transmitted to the underlying bone. The bone may become reactive, forming a dense layer immediately beneath the articular surface. Medullary compartments or Ely's cysts may form as a result of osteoclastic resorption of the subchondral bone.[26] The periosteum at the articular periphery may be stimulated to produce bony spicules or lipping. As the degenerative process progresses, exposed bone may undergo resorption.

Repair of the degenerated TMJ can occur.[20] Fibrous connective tissue, under the right conditions, can migrate across the denuded joint surface. Bony tissue may be deposited as well, resulting in a condyle with a flattened articular surface as seen on x-ray studies. Such a TMJ is usually painless but may exhibit crepitus.

Occurrence

The incidence of TMJ DJD varies greatly from study to study. Blackwood performed one of the first studies of DJD in 1963.[27] Dissection of 530 cadavers revealed that approximately 40 percent of the specimens aged more than 40 years showed evidence of remodeling or DJD. Toller reported an incidence of 8 percent in a study of 1,573 cases.[28]

Osteoarthritis may not necessarily be an age-related process. Studies, noted above, generally point to TMJ DJD peaking in the fourth and fifth decade and occurring most frequently in persons aged more than 50 years. TMJ DJD is definitely found, however, in persons in their twenties and thirties. TMJ DJD should be part of the differential diagnosis in any patient with TMJ pain and/or dysfunction.

Evaluation

A primary symptom of TMJ DJD is pain on condylar translation, not only on biting or attempted wide opening, but at any point in the range of movement. Pain symptoms may develop as the day progresses and become more obvious with advancing tiredness.[28] Maximum opening is typically impaired. Opening produces deflection to the affected side.

Clinical exam reveals tenderness on the lateral surface of the TMJ. Auscultation reveals joint sounds best described as grating, grinding, or crunching—termed crepitus. These sounds should not be confused with popping or clicking; they may be sensed by the patient and may be palpable by the examiner.

TMJ DJD generally affects a single TMJ. Both TMJs, however, may occasionally exhibit signs of the active disease state. Most diagnosed cases exhibit signs and symptoms for approximately 9 to 12 months, followed by a gradual "burning out" of the disease process with a decrease in pain and dysfunction.[28] A small percentage of patients may continue to have signs and symptoms for years, however, despite vigorous attempts at conservative management. Younger patients are typically more refractory to treatments.

Treatment

Conservative treatment comprises four general items—reassurance, medications, physical therapy to deal with muscle imbalances of the mandible and cervical spine, and splint management.

A kind and sympathetic attitude on the part of the treating clinician is a must. The problem and course of treatment should be explained in terms that the patient can understand. As explained previously, most patients experience a profound resolution of signs and symptoms in 9 to 12 months. The patient should also be made aware that an exacerbation of pain and dysfunction may be encountered before a decrease in symptoms is noted, and that a small percentage of patients have continuing pain and dysfunction for years.

Medications play a major role in pain relief of patients with TMJ DJD. Patients should be given the option of taking medications, provided that potential side effects are discussed. There is little evidence that the standard nonsteriodal antiinflammatory drugs (NSAIDs) alter the natural progression of the disease process. Aspirin is a key drug due to its analgesic and antiinflammatory properties. Other nonsteroidal analgesics also reduce pain, edema, and inflammation.

Intraarticular injections of corticosteroid should be used only as a last recourse after more conservative measures have failed. Toller reported 160 patients who had had steroid injections.[29] He concluded that patients aged more than 30 years were more likely than younger patients to respond favorably. Steroid injections are frequently associated with a prolonged, if variable, and frequently permanent reduction in symptoms. Toller concluded that steroid injection resulted in an acceleration of the degenerative process with beneficial side effects of greatly decreased pain and dysfunction. Poswillo, however, noted that repeated steroid injections may cause significant damage to the TMJ.[15]

Empirically, joint overload from parafunction, such as clenching and grinding or muscle hyperactivity, or morphologic factors, such as lack of posterior support, or lost vertical dimension contributes to the degenerative process. Muscle hyperactivity may also play a major role in the disease process. A maxillary, full-coverage interocclusal appliance is a simple, reversible, and relatively inexpensive modality that can be used to address these factors. There is no evidence, however, that occlusal therapy per se is of any value in the treatment of TMJ DJD.

Joint rest is the key to DJD treatment and can best be achieved by voluntary rest and self-awareness of any parafunctional habits. Self-massage is a very simple method to achieve short-term pain relief.

Physical therapy treatments consist of various modalities and mandibular exercises as covered in detail in chapter 6. If muscle hyperactivity involves both the mandibular and cervical spine musculature, physical therapy is indicated. Clinically, physical therapy is quite effective in the management of muscular involvement that adversely loads the TMJ, especially when physical therapy is used in conjunction with an interocclusal appliance.

Surgery should be reserved for patients who have failed to respond favorably to the above conservative modalities. Approximately 2 to 12 percent of TMJ DJD patients are subsequently treated surgically. In carefully selected cases in which surgery was performed correctly, very favorable responses have been noted. Surgery consists of reshaping the condyle and repairing or replacing the disc when indicated. After surgery, all predisposing factors such as inadequate occlusion and muscle hyperactivity related to parafunctional habits, occlusion, and cervical spine involvement should be addressed. Complicated reconstruction may not be indicated, because as Toller has demonstrated, striking clinical improvements may not result from extensive dental treatment.[28]

Rheumatoid Arthritis

Rheumatoid arthritis (RA) is a chronic syndrome characterized by nonspecific, usually symmetric inflammation of the peripheral joints, potentially resulting in progressing destruction of articular and periarticular structures.[16]

Etiology and Occurrence

The etiology of RA is unknown, but most likely involves both genetic and environmental factors. Alleles such as H1A-DR4 have been shown to exist in 70 percent of patients with RA.[30] Not all patients with this gene develop the disease, however. The environmental factor generally accepted at present is the Epstein-Barr virus (EBV).[31]

Approximately 1 to 3 percent of the general population is affected.[12] Assessments of the incidence of involvement of the TMJ, based on clinical and radiological evidence, vary. In a study of 100 unselected patients, Franks found that 86 percent had either clinical or radiographic evidence of TMJ involvement.[32] Only 53 percent gave a history of TMJ complaint. Russel and Boyles[33] reported 51 percent, whereas Hatch found that 58 percent of patients with RA had TMJ involvement in the course of their disease.[35] The TMJ is usually one of the last joints to be affected in the course of the disease process.

Pathology

The histopathologic changes observed in the TMJ are similar to those observed in other joints. Blackwood observed that the synovial tissues of the lower joint compartment are affected first.[34] The synovial membrane may become hyperplastic, with thickened villi. It may then spread over the articular surfaces of the TMJ, resulting in erosion of the fibrocartilage, subchondral bone, articular capsule, and ligaments. Small adhesions may form between the condylar surface and disc.

The joint is destroyed in varying degree. The result in some cases is fibrous ankylosis, which may be partial involving the lower joint space or complete with fibrous union of articular surfaces.[27] Bony ankylosis is not an unknown finding and may be a complication in younger patients.

Evaluation

Patients with RA of the TMJ, as well as those with other inflammatory pathologies, are often unaware that their symptoms originate in the TMJ itself. To many patients, the pain seems to arise in the ear, and they may complain to their physicians of ear trouble.

Hatch found that the initial symptoms of patients with RA with TMJ involvement were pain and limitation of jaw motion.[35] The pain typically is worse in the morning and decreases as the day progresses. The pain most typically is dull, aching, and deep-seated over the involved joint. Many patients have referred pain to the temporal region, ear, or angle of the mandible.

The clinical signs of joint noise and pain, masticatory muscle tenderness, limited mandibular movement, and pain with movements are similar in TMJ DJD and rheumatoid arthritis. Subtle differences are noted: Pain may involve both joints in rheumatoid arthritis, and symptoms may worsen as the day progresses in DJD.[17]

Treatment

Any suspected case of RA should be referred to a rheumatologist to confirm the diagnosis and to determine the extent of systemic involvement. The rheumatologist will order appropriate blood tests to confirm the presence and extent of the disease. The sedimentation rate may be elevated. Rheumatoid factors may be present. A high titer generally indicates a poor prognosis and is often associated with progressive disease. Antinuclear antibody tests can be ordered. Aspiration reveals synovial fluid to have decreased viscosity.

The principal aims of treatment are suppression of the active disease process, preservation of function, and relief of pain.

Various treatment measures are available. Conservative measures such as mandibular awareness exercises to encourage rest, physical therapy modalities, and manual procedures to control pain and maintain as much as possible capsular extensibility and jaw mobility, (covered in chapters 6 and 11), and NSAIDs should be tried first. Failure of this regimen may call for more aggressive treatment, but not without increased risk of side effects.

As the pannus migrates across the affected condyle, erosion may occur, significantly shortening condylar height. The result of this shortening is creation of an anterior open bite as the shortened condyles ascend into the glenoid fossa. Two approaches are available to the clinician for management of this sequelae. The first approach is for the patient and clinician to accept the disability and to use conservative measures to keep the patient as comfortable as possible. The second is a surgical approach. The decision for surgery must be based on the extent of condylar destruction and subsequent open bite. The severity of the patient's pain, together with the age and overall health of the patient, must be weighed and considered.

Rheumatoid arthritis in children can also result in fibrous or bony ankylosis. As a result, facial growth is disturbed, resulting in mild to severe retrognathism. Generally, physicians agree that the ankylosis should be treated. Controversy exists, however, as to the appropriate procedure.

Psoriatic Arthritis

Etiology and Occurrence

The cause of psoriasis is presently unknown. Heredity is a factor in a small percentage of patients. Psoriasis may occur in either sex and at any age.[16]

Evaluation

The onset of psoriasis is generally quite gradual. The course of this disease varies widely, with the frequency and severity of the recurrences varying from patient to patient and even within the same patient.[16] The skin lesions are sharply demonstrated erythematous papules or plaques covered with overlapping, shiny, scales. Areas infected include the elbows, knees, scalp, and nails. The nails of affected patients look as though they are infected by a fungus.

Psoriatic TMJ arthritis is similar in many respects to rheumatoid TMJ arthritis. However, serological findings for psoriatic arthritis are negative.

TMJ radiographs of these patients reveal rapid or extensive destruction of the articular surface of the mandibular condyle. Farrar and McCarty state that the condition appears to be radiographically similar to osteoarthritis.[5] The degree of destruction is more extensive. It may be continuous and cause complete necrosis of the condyle.

Treatment

Treatment for patients with joint involvement is similar to the treatments for RA. Remarkable improvements in both skin and joints occur following use of folic acid antagonists or mercaptopurine. The use of these drugs, however, is still in the experimental stage.

Osteochondritis

Etiology and Incidence

The cause of osteochondritis is unknown. It is best defined as an acute necrosis of the mandibular condyle that can result in its shortening 2 to 3 mm.[5] It occurs primarily in females aged from 14 to 17 years.

Evaluation

The disease process is characterized by a phase consisting of intercapsular edema and rapid necrosis of the articular surface of the condyle. The intracapsular edema can give rise to a posterior capsulitis. The initial phase has been termed the inflammatory necrotic phase and lasts from 6 to 8 weeks. Up to 25 percent of the cases in this phase may be RA-positive and may remain so throughout this phase. The positive RA sign typically does not recur.

The healing phase lasts 10 to 12 weeks. The condyle gradually becomes reconstructed in this phase.[5] The condyle may flatten, as evidenced by radiographs.

Treatment

A full-coverage splint is indicated in the inflammatory necrotic phase to reduce condylar encroachment on the inflamed retrodiscal tissues. In addition, NSAIDs can help with the pain and inflammation. Jaw use should be restricted and/or controlled through patient education and mandibular awareness exercises.

Osteochondritis is self-limiting. It also allows healing to take place to the extent that the joint returns to a healed condition.

MACROTRAUMA DISORDERS

The TMJ can be traumatized by both acute and chronic causes.

Condylar and Temporal Fracture (Involving the Fossa and or Articular Eminence)

Severe blows to the mandible can result in condylar and or temporal bone fracture. A careful history can be very helpful in making the diagnosis.

Patients with this condition may have greatly restricted or even inability to open the jaws. Swelling and tenderness to lateral palpation may be noted.

Radiographs are indicated in suspected cases of condylar fracture. Fracture lines may be noted in the condyle. Treatment is based on the location and extent of such a fracture. Controlling for secondary edema and muscle hyperactivity through the use of medication, interocclusal appliances and physical therapy treatments is indicated. Surgery may be indicated depending on the extent and location of the fracture.

TMJ DYSFUNCTION

A dysfunction can be defined as a disturbance, impairment, or abnormality of the functioning of an organ that is not related to growth disorders, disease, or macrotrauma.[36] This definition can easily be applied to the TMJ.

Disc–condyle derangements are covered in this section. Of the various dysfunctions that may occur, they are the most common. Dysfunctions involving subluxation and dislocations are also covered. Dysfunctions involving capsular inflammation and tightness as well as retrodiscal inflammation are covered in chapters 4 and 6 where appropriate.

Disc–Condyle Derangements

An internal derangement can best be defined as an abnormal relationship of the articular disc to the mandibular condyle, fossa, and articular eminence, without regard to condylar position.[37] In actuality, the disk is anteromedially displaced due to the direction of contraction of the superior head of the lateral pterygoid muscle.

The term displacement is used here to describe disc position relative to other joint structures. The term dislocation should be reserved for condylar position relative to eminence.

Internal derangements can be viewed as a natural progression of events that occur as a result of changes in the integrity of the disc–condyle assembly. The etiologies that must be considered include trauma, both macrotrauma and microtrauma. Macrotrauma includes external forces such as blows to the mandible sustained in sports or motor vehicle accidents. These forms of trauma can result in an elongation of the collateral ligaments. A thorough history will reveal when macrotrauma is a "cause" of an internal derangement. Microtrauma due to forced movements on the part of the patient, such as a yawn or bruxism, can play a role in internal derangement etiology.[38] Muscle hyperactivity and/or altered muscle activity is an incoordination among agonist, antagonist, and synergistic muscle groups that influence mandibular movement and positioning. Microtrauma owing to occlusal imbalances such as balancing interferences or a slide from initial contact to maximum intercuspation may play a role, but strong experimental evidence is lacking. Excessive muscle activity from parafunctional habits or even chronic gum chewing or ice biting can adversely load the TMJ. One should remember that the superior head of the lateral pterygoid muscle contracts in conjunction with the mandibular elevator muscles. This chronic loading of the collateral ligaments can lead to a forward positioning or displacement of the disc and set the stage for the elongation of these ligaments.[38]

Normally, the disc–condyle assembly stays intact due to the morphology of the disc (i.e., the posterior band, intermediate zone, and anterior band that keep it centered on the condyle). The disc is tightly bound to the lateral poles of the condyle by the collateral ligaments. This prevents translation of the disc relative to the condyle. Any translation of the disc relative to the condyle takes place only after elongation of the collateral ligaments.

Disc Displacement

The result of the various etiologies is that the morphology of the disc may become flattened and the collateral ligaments elongated, with the disc then translating over the condyle (Fig. 3-1). The degree of this translation is a function of the flatness of the disc and the amount of elongation of the collateral ligaments. Thus, prior to a complete displacement, it is possible to have various degrees of displacement. The final determinant of disc position is interarticular pressure as a function of biting pressure, which is directly related to the amount of muscle activity.

Once the collateral ligaments have become elongated, the disc can be pulled forward and anteriorly by the pull of the superior head of the lateral pterygoid muscle. The posterior band of the disc can then become further

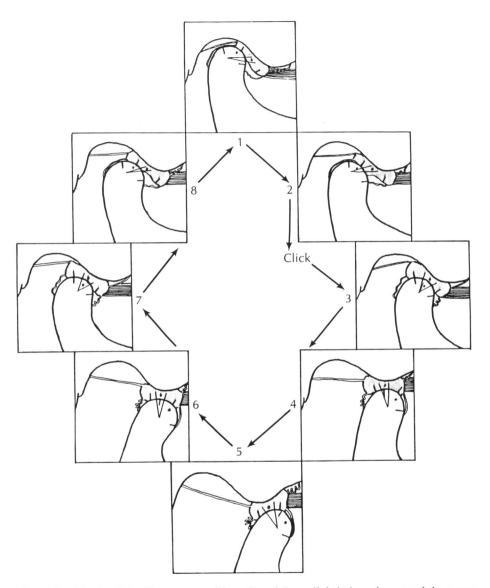

Fig. 3-1. Single click. Between positions 2 and 3, a click is heard as condyle moves across posterior border into intermediate zone of disc. Normal disc–condyle function occurs during remaining opening and closing movement. In closed joint position (1), disc is again displaced forward (and medially) by activity of superior lateral pterygoid muscle. (Reproduced by permission from Okeson JP: Fundamentals of Occlusion and Temporomandibular Disorders. CV Mosby, St. Louis, 1985.)

thinned. As the disc becomes thinned, and the collateral ligaments stretch, the superior elastic lamina may begin to be stretched to the point at which it can no longer return to its original length. The disc may then maintain its anteriorly displaced position with the teeth in maximum intercuspation. The condyle may begin to function on the posterior band as the condition becomes more chronic.

Once the condyle functions on the posterior band, the disc is said to be displaced.[38] Patients may have pain at this stage of the degenerative process. The pain may be related to functional pressures on the retrodiscal pad, as in biting, due to the pull of the superior head of the lateral pterygoid muscle contracting and elongating the already compromised collateral ligaments. The translation of the condyle as during jaw opening from its position on the posterior band can give rise to a very subtle click as the condyle becomes seated in the thin intermediate zone. This subtle click is usually the first sign of an internal disc–condyle derangement. No further sound is heard as the disc–condyle complex is carried intact to maximum opening and during turn around. If the disc maintains its position on the condyle, no subtle closing click is heard. Therefore, such patients may have intermittent joint noises. The opening click will be heard more consistently if, prior to opening, muscle activity is increased, thereby loading the joint and displacing the condyle on the posterior band of the disc. If, however, the pull of the superior head of the lateral pterygoid muscle with an additional increase in muscle activity causing additional loading of the joint is greater than the remaining elastic properties of the superior elastic lamina and collateral ligament integrity, the disc will be pulled forward on the condyle. No click is heard as the condyle assumes its position on the posterior band due to low interarticular pressure. Such patients primarily have only an opening click with either no click or a very subtle closing click.

Anteriorly Displaced Disk With Reduction

As this condition becomes more chronic, the disc may continue to thin and the collateral ligaments may continue to elongate (Fig. 3-2). The condyle may assume a position in a herniated sac in the retrodiscal tissues. Due to this latest position, the condyle may push the disc ahead of it until the condyle slides under the posterior band and seats in the intermediate zone, creating an opening click usually somewhere at the beginning or middle range of opening. The closing click occurs because the elasticity of the superior elastic lamina is less than the tonicity of the superior head of the lateral pterygoid muscle. As the condyle moves backward and upward into its herniated position, the closing click may be heard.

The click that is heard during opening can occur at any point during opening. The point at which the click occurs depends on various factors, such as the thickness of the posterior band, the degree of elongation of the collateral ligaments, the contraction of the superior head of the lateral pterygoid muscle, and the elasticity of the superior elastic lamina.

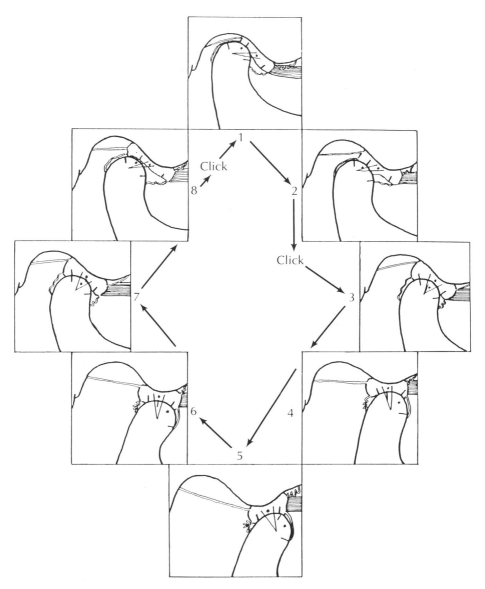

Fig. 3-2. Reciprocal click. Between positions 2 and 3, a click is heard as condyle moves across posterior border of disc. Normal disc–condyle function occurs during remaining opening and closing movement until closed joint position is approached. Then a second click is heard as condyle once again moves from intermediate zone to posterior border of disc (between positions 8 and 1). (Reprinted by permission from Okeson JP: Fundamentals of Occlusion and Temporomandibular Disorders. CV Mosby, St. Louis, 1985.)

The longer the disc is in a more anteriorly displaced position, the more likely it is that further damage will occur to the disc–condyle complex. The posterior band may slowly thin, and the collateral ligaments may continue to elongate. In addition, the superior elastic lamina remains in a stretched condition and may elongate to such a degree that it no longer has the ability to retract the disc fully.

Anteriorly Displaced Disk Without Reduction

The disc may assume an anterior position in which no clicking or popping is heard. The disc then is maintaining its displaced position during opening and closing movements of the mandible. This condition is called an anteriorly displaced disc without reduction (Fig. 3-3). Patients may be able to reduce the displacement temporarily with side-to-side movements of the mandible. If the displacement without reduction occurs occasionally, it is termed intermittent. An acute anteriorly displaced disc without reduction may be noted months or even years after a patient has noticed popping and/or clicking. This condition may be painful and depends on the status of the innervated structures within the TMJ. Compression of the retrodiscal pad or elongation of the collateral ligaments can cause pain. In addition, a reflex muscle splinting may also contribute to the pain pattern.

Patients can usually tell which TMJ is involved. Astute examiners can confirm their suspicions from the history, the patient's observations, and the clinical examination. Interincisal opening is usually restricted to condylar rotation or 25 mm during the initial stages of the acute disc displacement that does not reduce because the disc is blocking translation. In the acute anteriorly displaced disc without reduction, opening results in deflection to the affected side. In addition, mandibular movements to the opposite side are restricted due to inability of the condyle to translate. This condition may be painful only during the limits of mandibular movement.

As the condyle functions on the retrodiscal tissue, the interarticular forces may cause it to degenerate. This degeneration may manifest itself as a retrodiscitis and pain. Continual function of the condyle on the retrodiscal pad may result in its ultimate breakdown and perforation. Once the articulating surfaces of the condyle and eminence become functionally apposed, they may undergo remodeling. If the articulating surfaces fail to keep up with the biomechanical demands, they may begin to degenerate.

Some patients may progress to this final stage of degeneration, in which they have essentially pushed the disc completely forward of the condyle to the point of having near-normal mandibular dynamics. Therefore, a patient may be able to open and close to maximum opening as the discs are pushed down the eminence. These patients will then have joint noises of crepitus heard

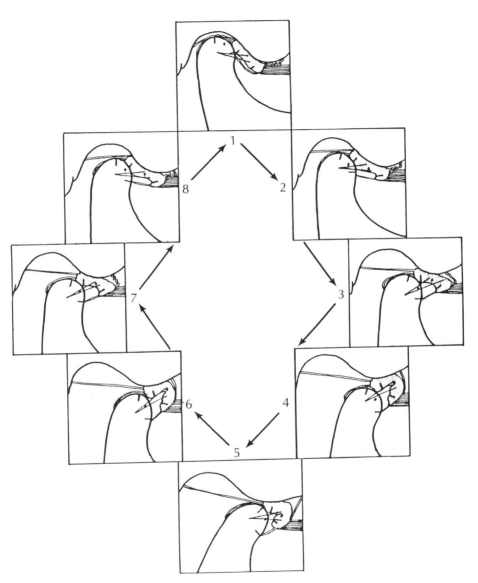

Fig. 3-3. Closed lock. Condyle never assumes a normal relationship on disc but instead forces disc forward ahead of it. This condition limits distance it can translate forward. (Reprinted by permission from Okeson JP: Fundamentals of Occlusion and Temporomandibular Disorders. CV Mosby, St. Louis, 1985.)

throughout full opening and closing movements, and x-ray studies may show DJD.

Capsular Tightness

Details of the etiology pathology, evaluation, and treatment of capsular tightness are covered in detail in chapter 6.

Condylar Subluxation

Condylar subluxation manifests itself due to the intact disc–condyle assembly translating past the crest of the eminence. Patients presenting with this condition may say, "My jaw joint jumps out."

Pain is seldom noted with subluxation unless there is an associated capsulitis. If pain exists, treatment for the capsulitis is indicated. Treatment for the subluxation consist of neuromuscular reeducational exercises, which are discussed in chapter 6, and an awareness of any prognathic mannerisms during speech or parafunction.

Condylar Dislocation

Condylar dislocation may be either an acute or chronic condition. The mechanics are similar to that of condylar subluxation, except that the condyle and disc assembly is "locked" anterior to the crest of the eminence.

Patients typically have a history of having had their mouths open for a relatively long time, as during a dental appointment. Yawning or opening widely while eating can also be inciting events. The patient typically complains of inability to close from a fully opened position.

Treatment consists of relocating the condyle manually by distracting the condyle and guiding the condyle onto the eminence and instructing the patient on restricting full jaw opening. Hand placement for relocating the condyle and exercises to help in prevention are discussed in Chapter 6.

CURRENT CONCEPTS AND SCHOOLS OF THOUGHT

Confusion and Controversy

The state of the art of craniomandibular practice is virtually in a state of disarray.[40] Controversy and confusion abounds in this field. No consensus of opinion concerning the causes and treatments has been reached among the various practitioners, researchers, and insurance carriers. Consequently, the field is in a state of flux, making communication and cooperation among these groups difficult and even frustrating at times.

Many reasons exist for this continuing controversy in the field. One of the main problems is the extremely complex anatomy and the interdependency of function of various regions in the upper quarter.

A second reason for this confusion and controversy is that signs and symptoms are classified and interpreted according to the philosophy of the researcher or clinician. Various built-in biases then begin to play a role in the interpretation of patient or research data. These biases are evident in the multitude of terms that have arisen. These include mandibular dysfunction syndrome,[41] TMJ occlusal dysfunction syndrome,[42] TMJ–pain dysfunction syndrome,[43] and myofascial pain dysfunction (MPD) syndrome.[44]

It does appear reasonable to agree on a general term to designate the constellation of signs and symptoms of patients who have problems of the TMJ and/or muscle problems of the upper quarter. Bell has proposed that the term ''temporomandibular disorders'' be adopted as a

> general clinical term for the morbid conditions, derangements and abnormalities of function that involve the temporomandibular joints, the associated articular ligaments, and the muscles that furnish power for stability and movement, the muscles being the masseters, the temporals, the medial pterygoids, and the lateral pterygoids.[15]

A key omission in this general definition is that of the muscles of the shoulder girdle and posterior cervical regions, which contribute both directly and indirectly to pain and dysfunction in the cranial region. I believe that proper recognition of these muscles groups requires that the term or the definition be changed to include them.

Bell proposes the use of the term temporomandibular disorders as a general clinical term. On the basis of similarity of clinical symptoms, temporomandibular disorders are then classified into five major groups: (1) acute muscle disorders, (2) disc-interference disorders, (3) inflammatory disorders, (4) chronic mandibular hypomobilities, and (5) growth disorders.[45] Each of these groups is then subgrouped to help the clinician arrive at a correct diagnosis.

A third factor in this controversy is the dilemma of pain. There is a lack of agreement as to measuring and assessing it. Pain is uniquely subjective. It tends to be transient,[46] and its reproducibility varies within and among individuals.[47] Studies have been performed based on a subjective complaint of pain,[48] whereas other researchers base their results on pain elicited by palpation.[49] The validity and value of much of the literature in this field is thereby limited.

Treatment, however, is not based on subjective complaints only. The examiner can achieve additional insight into the patient's pain and/or dysfunction etiology by asking specific questions regarding other closely associated adjacent areas, such as the cervical spine and shoulder girdle region.

One theory stating that facial pain and temporomandibular dysfunction is caused by emotional stress is the widely accepted MPD syndrome.[44] Laskin named one or more of the following positive symptoms: clicking or popping noises in the TMJ, pain of unilateral origin felt in the preauricular area, limitation of jaw movement, and muscle tenderness. Two negative symptoms that comprise the syndrome are an absence of clinical, radiographic, or biochemical evidence of organic changes in the TMJ, and lack of tenderness of the TMJ on palpation through the external auditory meatus.[44]

The advocates of the MPD syndrome state that treatments such as mock equilibration, biofeedback, placebo therapy, and psychological counseling can greatly diminish the subjective symptoms. The objective symptoms of clicking and popping, however, may not be altered by these treatment modalities. If the MPD syndrome is defined as consisting of four cardinal symptoms, and if the primary etiology is emotional stress, successful treatment of the emotional etiology should eliminate the objective symptoms as well as those that are more subjective.[40] The objective symptoms such as clicking and popping and limitation of jaw movement are often caused by internal derangements that have been discussed earlier in this chapter.

If the MPD syndrome is still a valid concept, it must be redefined with terms that are clinically accurate so that practitioners will know which patients have MPD syndrome as opposed to something else, such as internal derangements. Travell and Simons[50] propose use of the term myofascial pain syndrome and define it as pain and/or autonomic phenomena referred from active myofascial trigger points with associated dysfunction. This term is synonymous with myofascial syndrome and myofasciitis. The word dysfunction is dropped from the term, and the definition makes no mention of preauricular pain and mandibular dysfunction such as clicking or popping and limitation of jaw movement. This term and definition is concerned only with muscular imbalance.

Communication can thus be made easier between clinicians using this term. A descriptive and accurate diagnosis can be made to describe muscle and/or TMJ pain and/or dysfunction. For example, a diagnosis could be made of myofascial pain syndrome of the shoulder and posterior cervical muscles with an anteriorly displaced disc with reduction of the left TMJ. This diagnosis leaves no doubt as to the sources of pain and/or dysfunction for the patient. Remember that all displaced discs do not result in pain or even in significant dysfunction for the patient.

Considerable controversy currently exists between those who believe in the MPD syndrome and those who believe in an occlusal etiology. Four theories have been offered by various groups of the occlusionists to support their viewpoints.[51] These theories tend to point to the teeth, directly or indirectly, as contributing to the signs and symptoms of temporomandibular disorders.

The first theory is that of mandibular displacement. This theory was offered by Costen and is thus called Costen's syndrome.[52] The syndrome was thought to be due to compression of the chorda tympani nerve and pressure on the auriculotemporal nerve due to distalization of the condyle on these structures. Costen believed that overclosure of the mandible due to loss of teeth was the primary cause. Sicher has shown this theory to be invalid based on anatomic dissections.[53] Today, mandibular displacement still occurs but involves tissues different from those described by Costen.

A neuromuscular theory postulates that occlusal discrepancies combine with emotional tension and bruxism to create hypertonicity of the masticatory muscles, resulting in pain.[1] Impulses from joint receptors and periodontal ligament receptors are believed to produce the dysfunction.

Occlusal disharmony theory has been in existence for more than 40 years. Many practitioners believe that occlusal discrepancies are the primary cause of masticatory pain: Because of occlusal disharmonies and muscle hypertonicity, TMJ pain results.[54] This theory is based on the assumption that most patients with pain and dysfunction also manifest occlusal disharmonies.[51] Treatment of the occlusal discrepancies frequently decreases or even eliminates presenting symptoms.

The psychophysiologic theory offers masticatory muscle spasm as the primary factor giving rise to symptoms. The initiating factors are thought to be emotional rather than physical.[44] Muscle fatigue and pain results from parafunctional habits such as nocturnal and diurnal bruxism.

Although malocclusion may play an important role in muscular and TMJ dysfunctions, there is no consistent meaning for the terms.[51] Definitions of malocclusion vary considerably. Many clinicians use the Angle classification scheme, which breaks malocclusions into classes of I, II, and III. Bell has used the term acute malocclusion to describe a condition in which inflammation of the TMJ produces a slight posterior open bite on the ipsilateral side.[45] Other practitioners describe malocclusion in terms of a slide from initial tooth contact to maximum intercuspation.[55]

The purpose of this chapter is not to provide a literature review on the role of occlusion as an etiologic agent for neuromuscular disorders. The concept that malocclusion, loss of teeth, and occlusal interferences play a major role in dysfunction is not always well supported by the evidence. Muscular imbalances should be viewed as having multiple etiologies. To focus on the occlusion as the primary etiology for muscle imbalances of the upper quarter and TMJ dysfunction is to fail to recognize the abundant literature stating otherwise.

Musculosketal disorders may affect the cervical and craniomandibular regions simultaneously.[56] Symptoms of headache and TMJ pain can be caused by referred pain from cervical muscular imbalances.[57] Temporomandibular disorders frequently exhibit extensive involvement of the muscles of the upper quarter.

Physical therapy plays an important and substantial role in the treatment of upper-quarter muscle imbalances and TMJ dysfunction. Treatment of patients who have these complaints is difficult if not impossible without the services of a physical therapist who is well versed in and knowledgeable of upper-quarter musculoskeletal disorders.

REFERENCES

1. Moffet BC: The morphogenesis of the temporomandibular joint. Am J Orthod 52:401, 1966
2. Symons NBB: The development of the human mandibular joint. J Anat 86:326, 1952
3. Keith DA: Development of the human temporomandibular joint. Br J Oral Surg 20:217, 1982
4. Keith DA: Etiology and diagnosis of temporomandibular pain and dysfunction: organic pathology (other than arthritis). p. 118. In Laskin D, Greenfield W, Gale E, et al (eds): President's Conference on the Examination, Diagnosis and Management of Temporomandibular Disorders. American Dental Association, Chicago, 1983
5. Farrar WB, McCarty WL: A Clinical Outline of Temporomandibular Joint Diagnosis and Treatment. 7th Ed. Walker, Montgomery, 1983
6. Rushton MA: Unilateral hyperplasia of the mandibular condyle. Int Dent J 2:51, 1951
7. Guralnick W: Treatment of organic temporomandibular joint disease (excluding arthritis). p. 129. In Laskin O, Greenfield W, Gale E, et al (eds): President's Conference on the Examination, Diagnosis, and Management of Temporomandibular Disorders. American Dental Association, Chicago, 1983
8. Thoma KH: Tumors of the mandibular joint. J Oral Surg 22:156, 1964
9. Nwoku AL, Koch H: The temporomandibular joint: a rare localization for bone tumors. J Maxillofac Surg 2:113, 1974
10. Peacock TR, Fleet JD: Condylar metastasis from a bronchogenic carcinoma. Br J Oral Surg 20:39, 1982
11. Mayne J, Hatch G: Arthritis of the temporomandibular joint. J Am Dent Assoc 79:125, 1969
12. Robbins S: Pathologic Basis of Disease. WB Saunders, Philadelphia, 1974
13. Freyberg R: The Joints. In Sodeman W, Sodeman W (eds): Pathologic Physiology: Mechanisms of Disease. WB Saunders, Philadelphia, 1967
14. Hanlon C, Estes W: Osteo-arthritis aggravated by trauma. Am J Surg 78:555, 1949
15. Poswillo DE: Experimental investigation of the effects of intraarticular hydrocortisone and high condylectomy on the mandibular condyle. J Oral Surg 30:161, 1970
16. Berkow R: The Merck Manual of Diagnosis and Therapy. Merck, Sharp and Dohme Laboratories, Rahway, 1977
17. Zarb GA: Non surgical treatment of rheumatoid and degenerative arthritis of the TMJ. p. 133. In: Keith DA: Etiology and Diagnosis of Temporomandibular Pain and Dysfunction: Organic Pathology (Other Than Arthritis). p. 118. In Laskin D, Greenfield W, Gale E, et al (eds): President's Conference on the Examination, Diagnosis and Management of Temporomandibular Disorders. American Dental Association, Chicago, 1983
18. Hart FD: Pain in osteoarthritis. Practitioner 212:244, 1974
19. Hansson TL: Current concepts about the temporomandibular joint. J Prosthet Dent 55:370, 1986
20. Blackwood HJ: Cellular remodeling in articular tissue. J Dent Res, (Suppl.), 3:480, 1966
21. Hansson T, Oberg T, Carlsson GE, et al: Thickness of the soft tissue layers and articular disk in temporomandibular joints. Acta Odontol Scand 35:77, 1977
22. Hansson T, Nordstrom B: Thickness of the soft tissue layers and articular disk in temporomandibular joints with deviations in form. Acta Odontol Scand 35:281, 1977

23. Toller P: The transpharyngeal radiography for arthritis of the mandibular condyle. Br J Oral Surg 7:47, 1969
24. Mongini F: Remodeling of the mandibular condyle in the adult and its relationship to the condition of the dental arches. Acta Anat 82:437, 1972
25. Hansson T: Temporomandibular joint changes related to dental occlusion. In Solberg W, Clark G (eds): Temporomandibular joint problems. Quintessence, Chicago, 1980
26. Kreutziger K, Mahan P: Temporomandibular degenerative joint disease. Part I. Anatomy, pathophysiology and clinical description. J Oral Surg 40:165, 1975
27. Blackwood H: Arthritis of the mandibular joint. Br Dent J 115:317, 1963
28. Toller P: Osteoarthrosis of the mandibular condyle. Br Dent J 134:223, 1973
29. Toller P: Use and misuse of intra-articular corticosteroids in the treatment of temporomandibular joint pain. Proc T Soc Med 70:461, 1977
30. Winchester RJ: B-lymphocyte allo-antigens, cellular expression and disease significance with special reference to rheumatoid arthritis. Arthritis Rheum 20:1595, 1977
31. Ford OK, Smiley JP: Continuous culture of a B-immunocyte from rheumatoid synovium. Arthritis Rheum 16:341, 1973
32. Franks A: The temporomandibular joint in adult rheumatoid arthritis. J Dent Res 46:108, 1966
33. Russel L, Boyles T: The temporomandibular joint in rheumatoid arthritis. J Am Dent Assoc 28:533, 1941
34. Blackwood H: Pathology of the temporomandibular joint. J Am Dent Assoc 79:118, 1969
35. Hatch G: Clinical and radiographic findings of the temporomandibular joint in patients with rheumatoid arthritis. Thesis, Mayo Graduate School of Medicine (University of Minnesota), Rochester, 1967
36. Dorland's Illustrated Medical Dictionary, WB Saunders, Philadelphia, 1974
37. Dolwick MF: Diagnosis and etiology of internal derangements of the temporomandibular joint. p. 112. In Laskin D, Greenfield W, Gale E, et al (eds): President's Conference on the Examination, Diagnosis and Management of Temporomandibular Disorders. American Dental Association, Chicago, 1983
38. Okeson JP: Fundamentals of Occlusion and Temporomandibular Disorders. CV Mosby, St. Louis, 1985
39. Katzberg RW, Dolwick MF, Helms CA, et al: Arthrotomagraphy of the temporomandibular joint. AJR 134:944, 1980
40. Farrar WB: Craniomandibular practice: the state of the art: definition and diagnosis. J Craniomandib Pract 1:1, 1982
41. Molin C: Studies in mandibular dysfunction syndrome. Svensk Tandlak Tidskr 66:7, 1973
42. McCarty W: Diagnosis and treatment of internal derangements of the articular disc and mandibular condyle. p. 145. In Solberg WK, Clark GT (eds): Temporomandibular Joint Problems: Biologic Diagnosis and Treatment. 1st Ed. Quintessence, Chicago, 1983
43. Ramfjord SP, Ash MM: Occlusion. 2nd Ed. WB Saunders, Philadelphia, 1971
44. Laskin, DM: Etiology of the pain-dysfunction syndrome. J Am Dent Assoc 79:147, 1969
45. Bell WE: Classification of TM disorders. p. 24. In Laskin D, Greenfield W, Gale E, et al (eds): President's Conference on the Examination, Diagnosis and Management of Temporomandibular Disorders. American Dental Association, Chicago, 1983

46. Kopp S: Clinical findings in temporomandibular joint osteoarthritis. Scand J Dent Res 85:434, 1977
47. Gale EN, Corah NC: Changes in pain upon muscle palpation after treatment for TMJ syndrome. J Dent Res 60A: (abstr. 351) 1981
48. Norheim PW, Dahl BC: Some self-reported symptoms of temporomandibular joint dysfunction in a population in northern Norway. J Oral Rehabil 5:63, 1978
49. Carraro J, Caffesse RG: Effect of occlusal splints on TMJ symptomatology. J Prosthet Dent 40:563, 1978
50. Travell JG, Simons DG: Myofascial Pain and Dysfunction: The Trigger Point Manual. Williams & Wilkins, Baltimore, 1983
51. Bush FM: Occlusal etiology of myofascial pain dysfunction syndrome. p. 95. In Laskin D, Greenfield W, Gale E, et al (eds): President's conference on the examination, diagnosis and management of temporomandibular disorders. American Dental Association, Chicago, 1983
52. Costen JB: Syndrome of ear and sinus symptoms dependent upon disturbed function of temporomandibular joint. Ann Otol Rhinol Laryngol 1:15, 1934
53. Sicher H: Temporomandibular articulation in mandibular overclosure. J Am Dent Assoc 36:131, 1948
54. Krough-Poulsen WG, Olsson A: Occlusal disharmonies and dysfunction of the stomatognathic system. Dent Clin North Am 10:627, 1966
55. Sadowsky C, Begole EA: Long-term status of temporomandibular joint function and functional occlusion after orthodontic treatment. Am J Orthod 78:201, 1980
56. Kreisberg M: Headache as a symptom of craniomandibular disorders II: management. JJ Craniomandib Pract 4:220, 1986
57. Travell J: Temporomandibular joint pain referred from muscles of the head and neck. J Prosthet Dent 10:745, 1960

4 | Evaluation of Temporomandibular Disorders

Charles G. Widmer

The history and clinical examination of patients with temporomandibular disorders provides the basis for differential diagnosis and subsequent rational treatment of these patients. Refinement and enhancement of techniques for obtaining an accurate history and clinical examination of patients with temporomandibular disorders must always be the goal of any health care practitioner, particularly since these patients may have a background of various signs and symptoms. Differential diagnosis of temporomandibular disorders from neurologic, otolaryngologic, psychological, cervical, or dental sources of pain must be determined from the initial patient contact to direct proper referrals or undertake treatment procedures that will provide the most positive response and also gain the patient's confidence. Establishing an accurate differential diagnosis, however, requires a knowledge of such areas as gross anatomy, neuroanatomy, and neurophysiology so that signs and symptoms may be correlated with their sources. These correlations, based on signs and symptoms, cannot be memorized without knowing their implications. Therefore, the purpose of this chapter is (1) to delineate the frequently observed signs and symptoms and explain their rationale and (2) to define the limitations of history and clinical examination for differential diagnosis of temporomandibular disorders.

HISTORY

The history is one of the most important sources of information and cannot be overemphasized. The method of obtaining an accurate and thorough history can be a way of establishing good rapport with patients, who are often appre-

Table 4-1. Approach for Obtaining History of Illness

I.   Question the patient regarding common signs and symptoms associated with temporomandibular disorders, such as: (a) Difficulty in opening the mouth (b) Noises from the TMJ with mandibular movement (c) Inability to open the mouth ("locked") (d) Spontaneous pain around the ears, cheeks, eyes, head, or neck (e) Functional pain associated with chewing, yawning, or opening wide (f) Ear noises, tinnitus, or vertigo (g) Headaches (h) Clenching or grinding the teeth during the day or night
II. Question the patient regarding the pain, such as: (a) Where does it occur? (b) Does it start in one location and spread to other locations? (c) When does it occur (morning, afternoon, evening)? (d) How frequently does the pain occur? (e) When is the pain worse (morning, afternoon, evening)? (f) How long does the pain last? (g) What type of pain is it (lancing, dull ache, throbbing, burning)? (h) How severe is the pain (scale of 1 to 10)? (i) What aggravates the pain (chewing, jaw movement, yawning)? (j) What helps relieve the pain (heat, rest, soft diet)?
III. Question the patient regarding the sequence of events that led up to the manifestation of the chief complaint, such as: (a) When did the problem start and was it associated with trauma to the head or an emotional event? (b) Whom did you see regarding the problem, what treatment was performed, and was the treatment successful? (c) What medications have you been taking or are you currently taking for the problem?

(Data from President's Conference on the Examination, Diagnosis, and Management of Temporomandibular Disorders. J Am Dent Assoc 106:75, 1983)

hensive and uncertain. The history itself consists of obtaining the patient's chief complaint, medical history, and history of present illness.

The chief complaint is a description of the patient's reason for seeking the services of a health care professional and is normally only a sentence in the patient's own words. This information will often refer the clinician to the area that is most bothersome to the patient and should be the central theme of discussion at the end of the evaluation. This discussion will acknowledge to the patient that the clinician has listened and has understood the problem and can address the patient's concerns in the diagnosis and treatment plan. Often, the physical therapist or dentist may encounter a chief complaint that is not in their area of expertise. It is important for the health practitioner to recognize general signs and symptoms related to other specialties such as neurology, otolaryngology, or orthopedics and to refer the patient to the appropriate health specialist.

The medical history is extremely important for identifying systemic disorders that may be related to the patient's chief complaint. The medical history may alert the clinician to the necessity for prophylactic antibiotic coverage for certain cardiac disorders and also identifies a patient who may be medically compromised and who requires special care. Certain systemic disorders deserve special attention since their presence may also involve the TMJ or refer pain to the facial areas. Cardiac pain associated with angina or myocardial infarction can be experienced as the common substernal pain and can involve the jaw, throat, back, shoulder or arm.[1] Systemic autoimmune disorders such as lupus erythematosus,[2] psoriasis,[3] Reiter's syndrome,[4] or rheumatoid arthritis (RA)[5] may also involve the TMJ. Hyperthyroidism, diabetes, and other endocrine disorders can cause headaches that may sometimes be misdiagnosed as a temporomandibular disorder.[1] These few examples stress the importance of an accurate medical history; additional information on this topic can be found in any physical evaluation text.[6]

The most detailed portion of the history involves the history of present illness. This information establishes the groundwork for evaluating the patient's chief complaint. A standardized, methodical approach for obtaining this information may include items as shown in Table 4-1.[7]

Using a standardized format for obtaining the history of present illness will prevent the clinician from missing important information that may not be obvious initially but may be necessary for diagnosis and treatment of the patient. After the chief complaint, medical history, and history of present illness are obtained, the clinical evaluation can proceed, with patient rapport established.

SUBJECTIVE AND OBJECTIVE TESTS FOR EXAMINATION OF TEMPOROMANDIBULAR DISORDERS

The structures that should be examined in patients with temporomandibular disorders include: the TMJ; the muscles of mastication; the suprahyoid, infrahyoid, and cervical muscles; and the teeth. Ideally, the evaluation of these structures should be conducted with objective testing procedures independent of the patient's verbal response. With regard to pain, however, no objective measure currently exists. Thus, the pain report from the patient is an interpretation that may not accurately reflect the patient's condition and that must be carefully analyzed for consistency with objective signs. One method for evaluation of the patient's response involves testing control sites. Control sites are sites that should not elicit a positive response by the patient since there are no underlying structures that should be tender or painful. Areas that have been suggested as control sites are (1) posterior to the mastoid process avoiding the attachment of the sternocleidomastoid muscle or posterior cervical muscles (Fig. 4-1A) and (2) the infraorbital rim[8,9] (Fig. 4-1B).

A second method for evaluation of the patient's response involves rating the patient's reaction to the palpation. One rating system ranges from 0 to 3 with lack of reaction rated as 0, mild pain reported by the patient rated as 1, facial expression in response to the palpation rated as 2, and retreat of the head prior to the palpation rated as 3.[9] This method allows future reevaluation of the patient to document changes of symptoms associated with treatment. Although the ideal rating system would not involve the patient's response, the

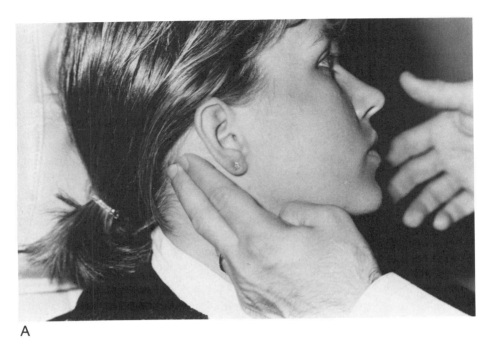

A

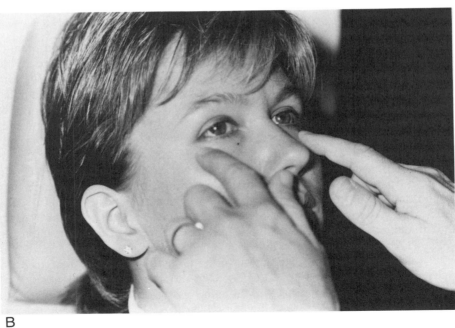

B

Fig. 4-1. **(A)** Control site: posterior to mastoid process. **(B)** Control site: infraorbital rim.

evaluation of pain currently cannot be achieved independent of the patient's verbal report. Some patients will respond to all palpation sites, which suggests that the palpation scores must be critically evaluated.

Muscle Examination

Masticatory and cervical muscle tenderness is a common symptom in patients with temporomandibular disorders. One example of masticatory muscle symptomology associated with TMJ pain can be observed in patients with muscle hyperactivity of jaw-closing muscles, such as chronic bruxism patients. Chronic bruxism may cause excessive loading in the TMJs and can result in pain in the TMJ as a clinical symptom. Conversely, pain from the TMJ may cause secondary muscle splinting in an attempt to minimize rotational or translational movement in the TMJ.[10] The differentiation of primary from secondary muscular involvement is important for appropriate treatment techniques and requires a detailed examination.

Palpation of muscles requires a standardized approach for site of palpation, delivery of palpation, and palpation pressure. These three variables must be kept constant if changes in signs and symptoms are to be monitored from one appointment to the next. Gross and Gale[9] recommend using bimanual palpation using three fingers with a pressure of approximately 3 pounds. For structures that cannot be accessed by both hands (e.g., intraoral sites), it is important for the patient to compare side-to-side responses. A control site for intraoral palpation, similar to a control site for extraoral palpation, should be used for the patient to experience the palpation pressure only (e.g., the buccal mucosa overlying the roots of the maxillary anterior teeth is an appropriate intraoral control site since this structure is not commonly symptomatic in patients with temporomandibular disorders).

Muscle palpation may elicit pain in localized areas known as active trigger points. Travell defines a trigger point as a "hyperirritable locus within a taut band of skeletal muscle, located in the muscular tissue and/or its associated fascia."[11] The trigger point may cause referral of pain to other structures and should be closely evaluated as a primary source of the patient's pain.

The next sections describe the muscles commonly associated with temporomandibular disorders that are innervated by the motor division of the trigeminal nerve. Particular emphasis is placed on muscle fiber orientation and muscle function since clinical examination evaluates the static muscle form as well as the dynamic muscle function.

Masseter

The masseter muscle is composed of two portions: superficial and deep fibers. Functionally, the masseter acts to apply a crushing force and is more active on the side of chewing.[12-15] Examination of the superficial fibers is performed by bilateral manual palpation starting slightly inferior to the zygomatic arch and working inferiorly and posteriorly to the angle of the mandible (Fig. 4-2A). The deep fibers can be palpated intraorally by placing a finger in the buccal vestibule lateral to the maxillary second and third molars and pressing superiorly towards the origin of the muscle on the zygoma (Fig. 4-2B). This location can be verified by having the patient clench the teeth and palpating the rigidity of the muscle. Tenderness to palpation of superficial fibers and particularly deep fibers of the masseter muscle have been highly associated with bruxism, which is defined by Ramfjord and Ash as clenching or grinding of the teeth.[16] Bruxism has been implicated by many investigators and clinicians as one of the primary etiologies of temporomandibular disorders.[17,18]

Temporalis

The temporalis muscle is a fan-shaped muscle composed of three portions: anterior, middle, and posterior fibers. The anterior fibers are oriented vertically; the posterior fibers have a more horizontal direction. The middle fibers occupy an oblique orientation. The action of the anterior fibers is to elevate and position the mandible rather than provide a crushing force. The posterior fibers on the side of chewing cause a lateral and vertical movement of the jaw, whereas the contralateral posterior fibers are activated during the final stages of closing by retruding the jaw towards the midline.[12-15] Palpation of these fibers should include all three portions of the muscle, starting with the origin and working downward towards the zygomatic arch (Fig. 4-3A through C). Palpation of the insertion on the coronoid process is best achieved intraorally by having the patient open the mouth and move the jaw laterally toward the side of palpation. The coronoid can be located by placing the finger lateral to the first mandibular molar and following the ramus of the mandible in a posterior direction until the tip of the coronoid can be felt (Fig. 4-3D). Tenderness of the coronoid process, like the deep fibers of the masseter, is commonly associated with bruxism. Pain in the anterior temporalis may be associated with the primary complaint of headache pain. Pain in the posterior fibers has been observed in persons with a deep overbite or lingually inclined maxillary incisors in whom the mandible must be retruded prior to completion of closure to intercuspation of the teeth.[14,15]

Medial Pterygoid

The medial pterygoid muscle is composed of two portions: a superficial and deep head. The fibers are oriented in a posterior and lateral direction. The action of the medial pterygoid muscle is to elevate the mandible and move the jaw contralaterally.[14] Palpation of the insertion of the muscle can be performed extraorally at the medial side of the angle of the mandible or intraorally, posterior to the mandibular retromolar pad (Fig. 4-4A and B). This jaw-closing

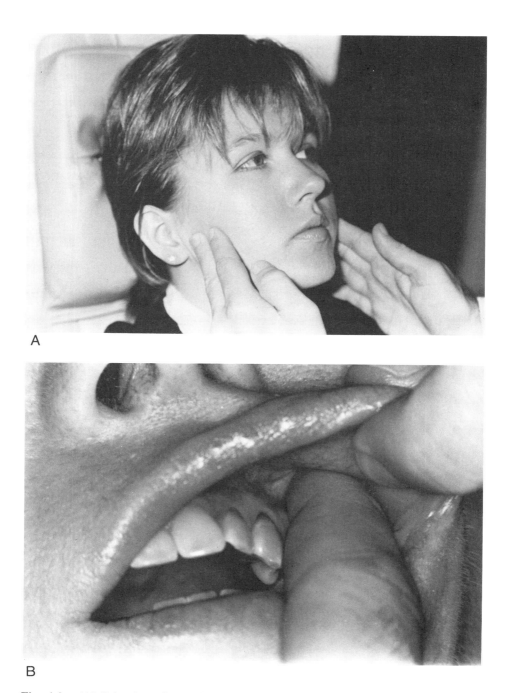

Fig. 4-2. (A) Palpation of superficial fibers of masseter muscle. (B) Palpation of the deep fibers of masseter muscle.

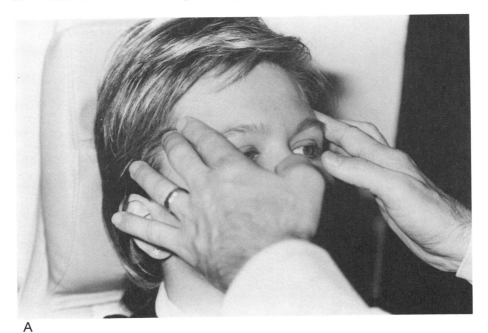

A

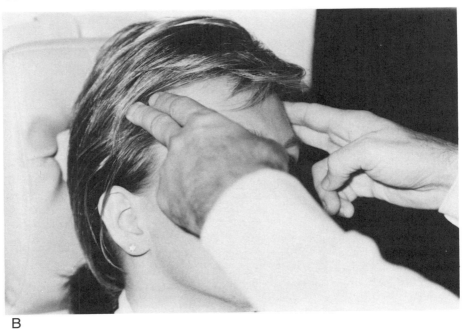

B

Fig. 4-3. **(A)** Palpation of anterior/vertical fibers of the temporalis muscle. **(B)** Palpation of middle/oblique fibers of temporalis muscle. (*Figure continues.*)

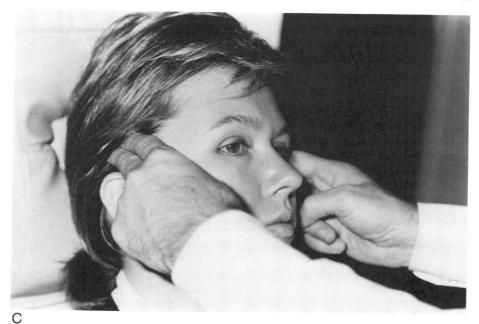

C

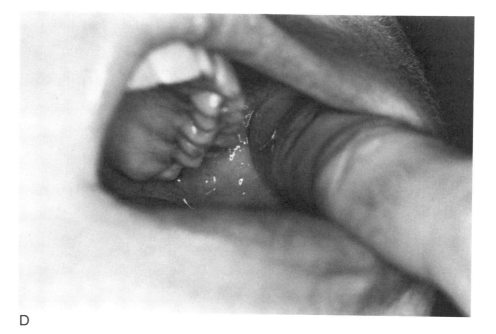

D

Fig. 4-3. (*Continued*). (**C**) Palpation of posterior/horizontal fibers of temporalis muscle. (**D**) Palpation of coronoid process.

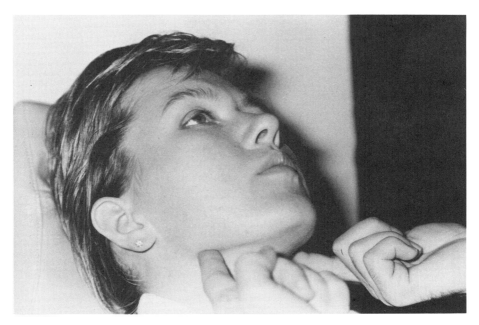

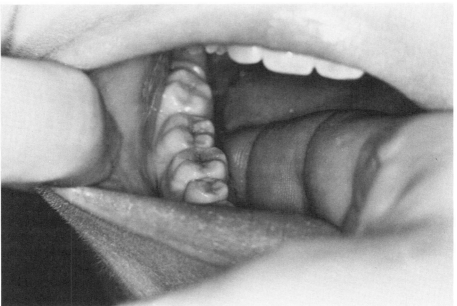

Fig. 4-4.   Palpation of medial pterygoid muscle insertion.

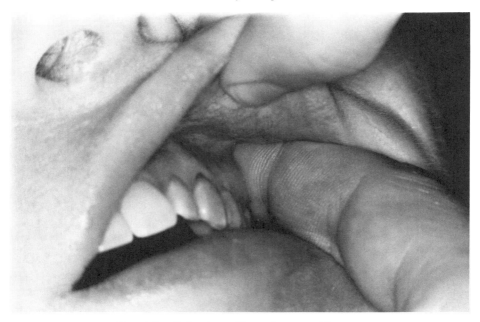

Fig. 4-5. Palpation of lateral pterygoid area.

muscle, like the masseter muscle, largely contributes to the crushing force applied near maximum intercuspation of the teeth.

Lateral Pterygoid

This fourth muscle of mastication is a major jaw-opening muscle that is composed of two portions: a superior and inferior head. The superior head originates from the infratemporal surface of the greater wing of the sphenoid bone and inserts into the articular disc and neck of the mandibular condyle.[19] The inferior head arises from the lateral surface of the lateral pterygoid plate and inserts into the neck of the mandibular condyle in a posterior, superior, and lateral direction. The function of the inferior head is to pull the condyle in an anterior, inferior, and medial direction, causing the jaw to open, protrude, or move laterally.[20] The superior head functions during the time of jaw-closing[19,21] and is hypothesized to stabilize the articular disc and mandibular condyle against the articular eminence. Traditionally, the lateral pterygoid has been palpated by placing the finger in the maxillary buccal vestibule at the third molar area and pushing in a superior, posterior, and medial direction behind the maxillary tuberosity (Fig. 4-5). This approach, however, does not directly palpate the body of the muscle because this muscle is located at least 2 to 3 cm deep to the palpation site.[22] Indeed, palpation of this area will also put pressure on fibers of the medial pterygoid muscle. Many investigators and

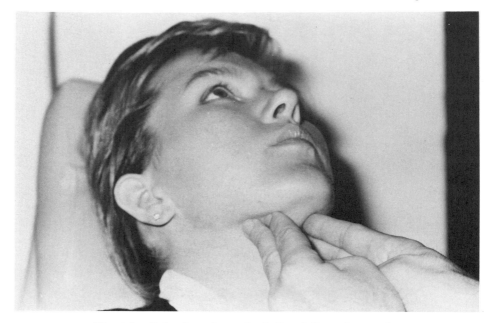

Fig. 4-6. Palpation of anterior belly of digastric muscle.

clinicians have reported tenderness to palpation of this area and have correlated this symptom with other signs and symptoms of temporomandibular disorders. This palpation site is also tender to palpation in patients who do not have clinical signs and symptoms of temporomandibular disorders.[9] Therefore, the significance of tenderness to palpation of this area is not completely understood.

Digastric

The digastric muscle is composed of two portions: an anterior and posterior belly. These two bellies join around the hyoid bone, forming a thick tendon. The muscle fibers of the anterior belly are directed inferiorly, laterally, and posteriorly; the posterior belly has an inferior, medial, and anterior direction. The anterior belly of the digastric muscle is innervated by the trigeminal nerve (V); the posterior belly has its innervation from the facial nerve (VII). The function of the anterior belly is to assist with jaw opening after stabilization of the hyoid bone by the infrahyoid muscles. Both bellies assist with swallowing by elevating the hyoid bone.[12-15,23] Palpation of the anterior digastric is accomplished by having the patient open the jaw against resistance and finding the body of muscle medial and almost parallel to the inferior border of the mandible (Fig. 4-6).

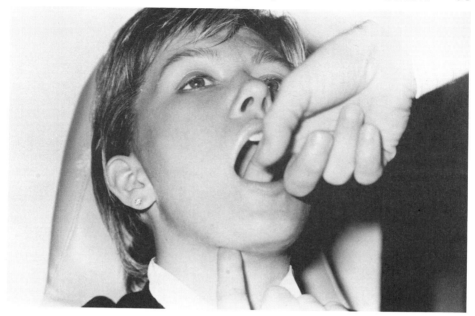

Fig. 4-7.   Palpation of mylohyoid muscle.

Mylohyoid

The mylohyoid muscle originates from the medial surface of the mandible at the mylohyoid line and joins at a median fibrous raphe for the anterior and middle fibers. The fibrous raphe blends into the posterior fibers attaching to the hyoid bone. This muscle, which forms the floor of the mouth, can be easily palpated by trapping the muscle between the forefingers, using both an intraoral and extraoral approach (Fig. 4-7). This muscle functions as a minor jaw-opening muscle as well as assisting with swallowing.[13,14] One example of mylohyoid muscle soreness can be observed after excessive tongue protrusion against the anterior teeth or against an intraoral appliance. These symptoms can be minimized by having the patient control the tongue and suprahyoid hyperactivity. Swallowing difficulties may also be reported by the patient and may be a sequella of mylohyoid or digastric hyperactivity.

TMJ Examination

Differentiation of intracapsular and extracapsular signs and symptoms that contribute to the patients' chief complaint is important for an accurate differential diagnosis and appropriate treatment. Many times, however, distinction of these two areas is hindered by the diffuse presentation of symptoms. Therefore, periodic reevaluation of the patient is necessary to determine if the signs

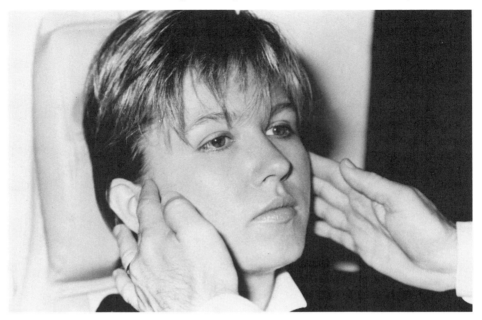

Fig. 4-8.   Palpation over lateral pole of condyle bilaterally.

and symptoms are still consistent with the primary diagnosis or are related to an underlying problem that only becomes obvious after reduction of acute symptoms.

Techniques useful in evaluation of signs and symptoms attributable to intracapsular and capsular involvement include: (1) palpation of the TMJ, (2) loading the TMJ, (3) mandibular dynamics and position, (4) joint sounds, and (5) radiographic examination and imaging of the TMJ. These evaluations must be combined with the history to provide supporting evidence for the differential diagnosis.

TMJ Palpation

Examination of the TMJ involves palpating lateral and posterior to the joint. Palpation of these areas applies pressure to the dense population of TMJ receptors located in the posterior and posterolateral portions of the joint and allows the clinician to determine the sensitivity of the joint. Bimanual palpation is performed over the lateral pole of the condyle in a closed mandibular position, using firm pressure for a few seconds (Fig. 4-8). The patient's response should be scored on a rating scale of 0 to 3. Next, the clinician has the patient open the jaw and palpates the same area, which is now a concavity since the condyle has translated anteriorly in the glenoid fossa (Fig. 4-9). This technique applies

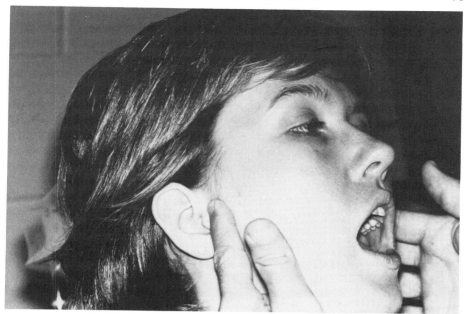

Fig. 4-9. Palpation posterior to lateral pole of condyle with mouth opened.

pressure over the capsule and posterolateral aspects of the condyle and retrodiscal tissue.

Palpation of the posterolateral portion of the retrodiscal tissue can be applied by the examiner through the external auditory meatus. This is performed by asking the patient to open the jaw and place the little fingers in the ear canal with pressure toward the back of the TMJ; the patient is then instructed to close slowly (Fig. 4-10A and B). Prior instructions should be given to the patient so that they will cease the closing activity when pain is experienced. This technique gives the patient control of the discomfort that is experienced. Continuation of the examination should be performed for the non-painful TMJ after removal of the examiner's finger from the external auditory meatus on the pain side. External auditory meatus palpation will reveal a retrodiscitis and can simulate ear pain that may be reported by the patient. A retrodiscitis is usually present with the sudden occurrence of an anterior displaced disc or trauma to the mandible. Clicking in the TMJ may be noted by the clinician when palpating the posterior aspect of the TMJ through the ear canal and is due to the close proximity of the disc-condyle complex and ear canal.

TMJ Loading

Selective loading of the TMJ can aid in determining intracapsular pathology. Dynamic loading of one TMJ can be obtained by having the patient chew or bite forcefully on a cotton roll on the side contralateral to the TMJ examined

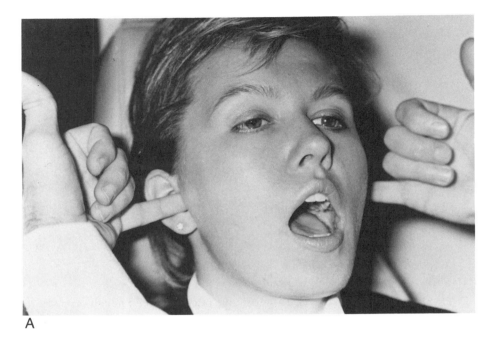

A

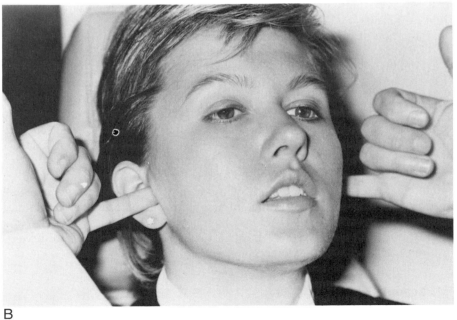

B

Fig. 4-10. **(A)** Palpation through external auditory meatus. **(B)** Palpation through external auditory meatus with teeth together.

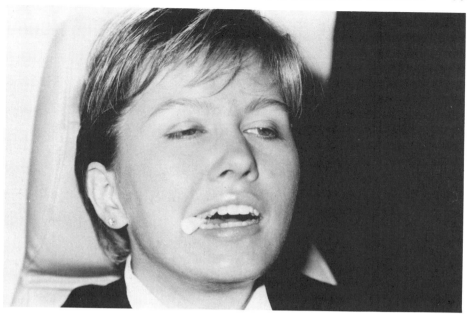

Fig. 4-11.   Dynamic loading of left TMJ.

(e.g., to load the left TMJ selectively, the patient is asked to bite forcefully on a cotton roll between the molars on the right side) (Fig. 4-11). This procedure loads the contralateral TMJ and may elicit pain in that TMJ if the condyle is functioning on the retrodiscal tissues due to an anteriorly dislocated disc. Many patients will chew on the same side as the TMJ pain because the ipsilateral joint is not loaded like the contralateral TMJ. Posterior loading of the TMJ can be accomplished by grasping the patient's chin between the thumb and forefinger of one hand and steadily pushing the mandible posteriorly while moving the mandible in an opening and closing motion (Fig. 4-12). Superior loading of the TMJ is accomplished by using Dawson's technique.[24] This technique requires standing or sitting behind the patient and supporting the patient's head, placing the fingers along the inferior border of the mandible on both sides and placing the thumbs on the patient's chin. A torquing action is used by pushing downward by the thumbs and lifting superiorly with the fingers, thus placing a superior loading force in both TMJs (Fig. 4-13). This force can be maintained while moving the mandible in an opening and closing motion. Both superior and posterior loading forces will elicit pain if a retrodiscitis is present. Unloading the TMJ is a technique that allows differentiation of a capsulitis from a retrodiscitis because the capsulitis pain will be intensified by unloading or distracting the condyle and a retrodiscitis pain will be enhanced with posterior or superior loading of the condyle in the TMJs. Unloading the TMJ is easily accomplished by placing the thumb over the mandibular molars on the side of the TMJ to be unloaded and pulling inferiorly while supporting the inferior

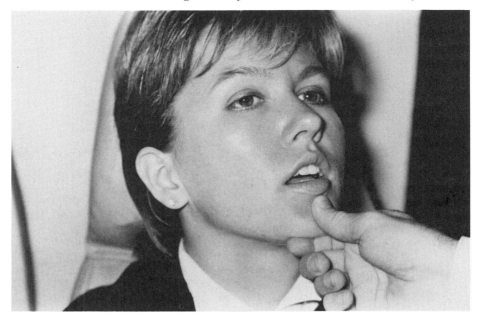

Fig. 4-12. Posterior loading of TMJ.

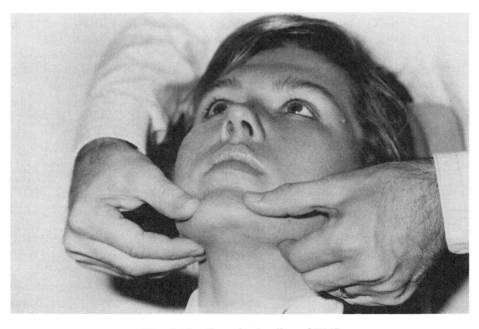

Fig. 4-13. Superior loading of TMJ.

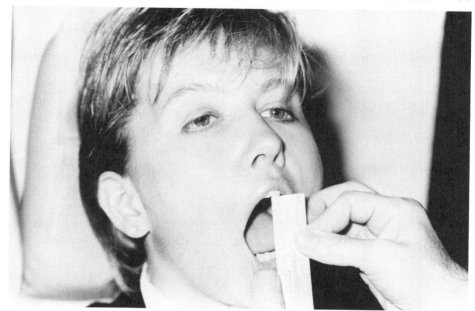

Fig. 4-14. Mandibular vertical opening measured between maxillary and mandibular incisal edges.

border of the mandible on the opposite side with the other hand (see Fig. 6-1 in Ch. 6).

Mandibular Dynamics

Mandibular dynamics or kinematics can be helpful in determining the limitation of rotation or translation for each temporomandibular joint as well as incoordination of mandibular movement. Mandibular movement should be recorded in both the vertical and horizontal planes for accurate representation of rotation and translation. Measurement of the maximum voluntary mandibular vertical opening can be obtained by measuring between the maxillary and mandibular incisal edges with ruler scaled in millimeters (Fig. 4-14). Normal mandibular opening has been reported to be between 40 and 50 mm,[9,25] and limitation of mandibular depression has been advocated as a classic sign of temporomandibular disorders.[17,26,27] A second static mandibular position to be recorded is the vertical opening where the pain begins. This information can be valuable when comparing the timing of a click associated with an anteriorly displaced disc and the occurrence of pain. The vertical path of the mandible during opening and closing should be recorded for deviations or deflections. A deviation is defined as a lateral movement of the mandible that returns to the midline prior to maximum opening, whereas a deflection is a lateral movement without return to the midline. The observation of deviations or deflections in vertical opening must also be compared with the movement of the jaw during horizontal movements such as lateral excursions or protrusion. For example, movement of the mandible in a left lateral motion will require translation of the condyle in the right TMJ. Lateral movement is normally 8 to 10 mm when the midlines of the maxillary and mandibular incisors are viewed. Movement of 50 percent (5 mm) or less is usually indicative of an intracapsular restriction such as an anteriorly dislocated disc without reduction in the TMJ contralateral to the side of lateral movement. Protrusion is usually 8 to 10 mm, and a lateral deflection of protrusive movement can often be observed when no deflections are evident during a vertical movement of the jaw. This is because a protrusive (horizontal) movement forces translation in the TMJs, whereas vertical movement can occur as a pure rotation movement in the TMJ with minimal translation and may allow a patient to have the appearance of a normal vertical opening. In patients with restricted translation in one TMJ, a protrusive movement will deflect toward the side with reduced translation.

TMJ Noises

TMJ noises are commonly of two types: clicking or popping and crepitus. Clicking or popping is the single sound associated with mandibular opening; crepitus is a multiple, grinding sound much like that of automobile tires rolling over gravel. Reciprocal clicking, or a click that occurs during reciprocal movements such as opening and closing the mandible, has been associated with the diagnosis of an anteriorly dislocated disc. The click is heard with a stethoscope as an opening click that occurs at a greater vertical mandibular opening than the closing click. The difference of the timing of the opening and closing clicks associated with an anteriorly dislocated disc can be attributed to the resistance of the movement of the condyle over the posterior band of the disc during the opening movement. After the condyle has reduced beneath the posterior band of the disc, the disc is positioned in a relatively "normal" disc–condyle relationship. During the closing phase, the disc remains stable over the condyle until the condyle retrudes to a point at which the stability can no longer be maintained, and the disc becomes anteriorly dislocated again. The stability of the disc in the closing phase accounts for the difference in the timing of the reciprocal clicking pattern. Often, a closing click cannot easily be detected; an easy method to enhance the sound of clicking or crepitus is to load the TMJs superiorly while the patient opens and closes the mandible. This technique does not require much force and can be performed by placing the fingers on the inferior border of the mandible and maintaining a constant upward pressure in the TMJs while the patient voluntarily opens and closes the mandible (Fig. 4-15). A click occurring at the same vertical opening in the opening and closing movement may be indicative of an irregularity in the path of the disc–condyle complex, in contrast to an anteriorly dislocated disc, and this sound is also detected in the same horizontal position in a protrusive-retrusive motion of the

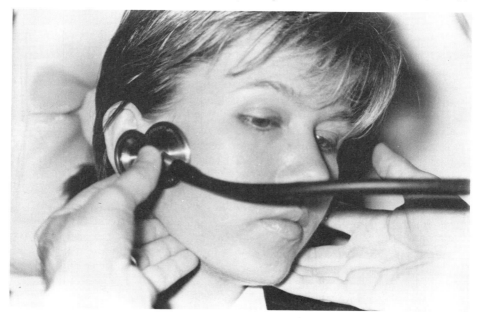

Fig. 4-15. Superior loading of TMJ during voluntary opening and closing movements of mandible.

mandible.[30] Crepitus can be heard as a soft sandy sound or as a loud grinding sound. The loud grinding sound is usually associated with degenerative joint disease (DJD) or osterarthritis owing to bone-to-bone contact. The soft sandy sound may be heard as the condyle moves over the retrodiscal attachments of the disc and may not be indicative of bone-to-bone contact. The vertical mandibular opening for the opening and closing click should be recorded as well as the horizontal position of the protrusive-retrusive clicking. One easy test to determine if the clicking is due to an anteriorly dislocated disc is first to have the patient open the mandible and click onto the disc and then to have the patient close so that the maxillary and mandibular incisors are edge to edge. Next the patient is asked open and close the mandible at the edge-to-edge position and verify that the clicking is no longer detectable and would be consistent with a normal disc–condyle relationship. Finally, the patient is asked to start from the edge-to-edge position and slowly retrude the mandible until a reciprocal or second click is detected. Accentuation of the retrusive click can be obtained by manually loading the TMJs using a mild upward force on the inferior border of the mandible as previously described.

Clicking can be graded as an early, middle, or late opening click; this grading roughly corresponds to the amount of translation needed before the condyle reduces beneath the anteriorly dislocated disc.[30] The occurrence of the closing click in the retrusive direction (approaching the maximum intercuspation of the teeth) can be an indication of the stability of the disc over the condyle and can have certain prognostic indications. The disc that has stability over the condyle over a range of protrusive-retrusive movements of the mandible has a better prognosis for conservative therapy than a disc that cannot be easily stabilized. This is not the only indicator regarding the prognosis for successfully recapturing an anteriorly dislocated disc, however, since TMJ pain, masticatory and cervical muscle dysfunction, and occlusal disorders can also have an impact on the prognosis. A clicking TMJ in itself is not an indicator for treatment unless pain or limitation of mandibular movement also exists. This treatment approach is based on epidemiological studies that have established that approximately one-third of the asymptomatic population has TMJ sounds; it is uncertain what percentage of these patients will progress to a condition involving pain and dysfunction.[9,31-33] Educating the patient regarding the cause of the click and informing the patient of possible indicators for treatment such as pain in the TMJ, muscular pain and limitation of mandibular movement will allow the clinician and patient to monitor signs and symptoms to determine if conservative treatment is indicated for the patient.

Another TMJ sound that can be confused with a late anteriorly dislocated disc is the sound from subluxation of the condyle beneath the crest of the eminence. This sound is duller and occurs at the same point in the opening and closing movements near the extreme of the jaw-opening movement. The patient may have a large vertical opening associated with this sound and may also report having occasionally been "stuck open" after opening wide.

Differentiation of pain associated with the TMJ from pain associated with surrounding structures can be difficult to ascertain from the clinical examination. One very useful technique for making this determination is the use of a local anesthetic injection of the auriculotemporal nerve which supplies the posterior and postereolateral portions of the TMJ. This diagnostic injection blocks the pain fibers from the capsule and retrodiscal tissue and, combined with palpation, can selectively determine the source of the pain. A full evaluation of palpation, mandibular kinematics, and joint sounds are necessary for comparison to the results of the preanesthetic evaluation so that the patient's interpretation of relief of the pain can be corroborated with objective signs, thereby minimizing the possibility of a false-positive report.

Radiography and Imaging of the TMJ

Radiographic examination of the TMJ can be performed by a variety of techniques, all of which have advantages and disadvantages. Indications for radiographic evaluation include differential diagnosis of bony deformaties, traumatic injuries, degenerative changes, or tumors. Evaluation of reduced or enlarged joint spaces for diagnosis of temporomandibular disorders has not been supported by multiple studies and therefore should not be used as criteria for differential diagnosis.[34,35] Common types of TMJ imaging include panoramic, transcranial, tomographic, computerized tomography (CT scan), arthrography and, more recently, magnetic resonance imaging (MRI). The panoramic and transcranial techniques are the most common modalities available to dentists and are good screening techniques for the TMJ. Neither technique aligns the x-ray tube down the long axis of the condyle; therefore, they show a distorted view of the TMJ (e.g., the transcranial radiograph shows an image of the superior and lateral aspect of the condyle, which is a common site for bony pathology). If a thorough bony evaluation of multiple planes down the long axis of the condyle is required, tomography or CT scans are indicated. Some clinical conditions such as osteoarthritis and RA of the TMJ can be localized on the condyle or glenoid fossa using multiple plane imaging and can be beneficial for locating bony spurs or localized areas of resorption. These techniques can provide a three-dimensional view of the TMJ but require additional radiation exposure and are more costly to the patient. Because only bony tissue can be observed in the radiograph, injection of a radiopaque contrast media is required to visualize soft tissue components of the TMJ such as the disc; this procedure is called arthrography. A recent technique, MRI, uses a magnetic field rather than x-radiation for soft tissue visualization. This technique has the advantage of being noninvasive, and recent studies are encouraging for its use as a soft tissue imaging for the TMJ.[36-38] The only contraindications known for MRI studies are with patients with ferrous-containing implants, pacemakers, or patients who are unable to remain stationary for 10 to 15 minutes.

Jaw-Tracking Instrumentation

Jaw-tracking instrumentation is currently used clinically to determine the velocity, acceleration, and limits of mandibular movement. These devices have been advocated as a means for obtaining pertinent diagnostic information regarding mandibular kinematics. Investigators have questioned the reliability and validity of the measures from these devices within the range of mandibular movement however.[39] There is also a question of the impact that these measures will have on the decision-making process for differential diagnosis and treatment of patients.[40] Finally, no measure of the reactivity of the instrumentation or of how the instrumentation affects the behavior of the patient is available to establish the validity of the data.[41] Further investigations are required to address these questions of instrumentation prior to their use as a diagnostic tool.

Electromyography

Electromyography (EMG), or the recording of electrical potentials generated by muscle fibers, has been used for many years to document the coordination of muscle function with various tasks and to investigate reflex activity. EMG recordings have not, however, been able to differentiate muscles that are painful or in spasm based exclusively on the EMG activity.[42] Long silent-period durations, observed in the isometric EMG recordings of jaw-closing muscles after a tap to the chin, is another EMG parameter that has been suggested as a diagnostic indicator for temporomandibular disorder patients. The silent-period duration, however, appears to be more closely related to the bite force than to the dysfunction of the patient[26] and can be observed in patients with dentures,[27] and orthodontic patients[43] and in non-pain subjects.[44] Therefore, EMG, like jaw tracking, requires rigorous testing from multiple, independent laboratories to establish the clinical usefulness of the methodology.

Correlation of History and Clinical Examination

The importance of using both the history and clinical examination for establishing a differential diagnosis cannot be understated for patients with temporomandibular disorders. After the history and clinical examination are completed, formulation of the diagnosis follows. Specific diagnoses are discussed in the following paragraphs, which relate history and clinical presentation for various disorders. Any one or a combination of problems may be encountered, but for the sake of clarity, specific disorders will be detailed.

Anteriorly Dislocated Disc With Reduction

The history of a patient with an anteriorly dislocated disc with reduction may show either that clicking has existed for many years in one or both TMJs or that the clicking may have started recently. In either case, a history of clicking is usually reported by the patient. An anteriorly dislocated disc with reduction may cause pain in the patient who experiences sudden onset, whereas a patient who has been clicking for many years may not have pain directly related to the dislocated disc. One example is a TMJ capsulitis caused by excessive loading, which may be attributed to muscle hyperactivity such as bruxism and may not require treatment specifically for the dislocated disc. Differentiation of a capsulitis from a retrodiscitis is important in these cases. The opening path of the mandible will deviate toward the side of the dislocated disc until it reduces, as noted by the opening click, and the mandible will return to the midline on full opening. These patients usually will not have a restricted maximum opening unless a muscular component is associated with the dislocated disc. The vertical opening measured at the time of the opening click will be greater than the opening measured at the closing click, thus differentiating an anteriorly dislocated disc with reduction from an irregularity in the path of the condyle–disc complex. In addition, a soft crepitus may be heard with a stethoscope prior to the click and is due to the condyle moving over the posterior attachments of the disc. Verification of this condition can usually be obtained with arthrography, but this radiographic technique is not indicated for routine confirmation of an anteriorly dislocated disc with reduction. Indications for arthrography of the TMJ include evaluation of disc position, disc morphology, tears or perforations of the disc, or adhesions of the disc.[45]

Anteriorly Dislocated Disc Without Reduction

The patient with an anteriorly dislocated disc without reduction usually has a history of clicking in the involved TMJ prior to the incidence of "locking" or not having the ability to open wide. Acute trauma patients may also have this condition. These patients will usually have a retrodiscitis and a deflection toward the involved TMJ with vertical mandibular opening and protrusion. A muscular spasm causing a restriction of mandibular movement can be differentiated from an intracapsular component if a horizontal deflection is apparent when the patient protrudes the mandible. An intracapsular restriction or capsular tightness will not allow much translation in the involved TMJ, whereas a patient with muscular symptoms will have unrestricted horizontal movement (i.e., translation within the TMJ) as long as there is no change in the muscle length. Vertical opening will stretch the muscles and, in patients with muscular symptoms, a deflection of the mandible toward the side of the shortened muscle will be observed. Some patients with anteriorly dislocated discs without reduction may gradually regain their normal maximum opening over a period of months, but feel a restriction, pulling, or blockage in the TMJ at the extreme of opening. The history of a "locked" incident that slowly resolved but continues to be painful is an important indicator for diagnosis of an anteriorly dislocated disc without reduction. Sometimes, with this condition, a soft crepitus that is associated with the movement of the condyle over the retrodiscal attachments may be detected during opening. Overt, loud crepitis is usually indicative of a bone-to-bone contact associated with an osteoarthritic condition. Because an anteriorly dislocated disc without reduction is a soft tissue condition, radiographic findings of the hard tissue will usually be within normal limits.

Retrodiscal Inflammation

Many patients with retrodiscal inflammation will report a history of intermittent clicking in the TMJ which is not detected on the day of the clinical examination. Intermittent clicking may be due to an intermittent masticatory muscle hyperactivity or may only occur during yawning or chewing. These patients may have pain simulating an earache or localized to the area around the TMJ. Clinical examination usually reveals tenderness with palpation of the external auditory meatus and no significant limitation of maximum opening, lateral excursions, or protrusion of the jaw. Muscular symptoms may be commonly found with retrodiscitis and may complicate differentiation of the primary source of pain. No positive radiographic findings are observed with this clinical presentation.

Capsulitis

A capsulitis without any other presenting intracapsular pathology may be associated with muscular hyperactivity such as bruxism or other contributing factors that can cause prolonged or excessive loading in the TMJ. Pain is experienced with palpation lateral to the TMJ and with distraction of the condyle in the TMJ. Muscular tenderness often exists, particularly in the jaw-closing muscles. No restriction of mandibular depression is observed unless there is muscular involvement. Radiographic examination will show normal bony anatomy.

Capsular Tightness

Capsular tightness can usually be observed after surgical intervention in the TMJ. This occurs due to the close reapproximation of the capsule flaps and scar tissue formation. These patients have a limited amount of translation in the TMJ even though no intracapsular structures are causing the restriction. Postsurgical physical therapy can have a significant impact on decreasing the restriction caused by capsular tightness and is discussed in Chapter 6.

Subluxation

Patients with hypermobility of the mandible may subluxate the condyle beneath the crest of the eminence. This subluxation occurs at the end of the maximum opening and some patients report a history of locking open or not having the ability to close after maximum opening. Subluxation can be heard as a dull sound as compared with the traditional sharp sound associated with an anteriorly dislocated disc with reduction. Patients with bilateral subluxation will present with a sigmoid or S-shaped mandibular opening path because the subluxation will occur first in one TMJ, causing the mandible to shift toward the opposite side, and then in the second TMJ, causing the mandible to change direction and shift toward the side oposite that TMJ. The sound of subluxation will occur at the same vertical dimension in the opening and closing path, suggesting that the obstruction is fixed and is not an anteriorly dislocated disc. Radiographically, the condyle will appear anterior to the crest of the eminence when the mandible is maximally open. These patients can have pain owing to chronic stretching of the capsule and retrodiscal tissue, although many patients will experience no pain and may not require treatment if they have not experienced pain or locking.

Other Conditions

Arthritic conditions affecting the TMJ are explained in detail in Chapter 3. Although rare, tumors may occur in the TMJ and can be primary tumors or secondary metastasis. These tumors can usually be observed radiographically as radiopaque or radiolucent areas in the condyle or fossa area.

Occlusion and Muscle Factors

The relationship of occlusion of the teeth and its affect on muscular function has been a major topic of investigation for many years in the dental field. Three theories postulate the interactions of the occlusion, the TMJ, and the muscles and their role as an etiology for temporomandibular disorders. The first theory regards the occlusion as being the major etiology. The interdependency of the occlusion and muscular function has traditionally been considered so closely associated that minor discrepancies of tooth-to-tooth contacts were reported to have major implications as an etiology for muscular dysfunction.[16,24] Unfortunately, these opinions were based on clinical observations and have not stood the test of well-standardized experimental studies that included control groups and placebo treatments.[27,46] Neither has epidemiological evidence supported the occlusal theory as being a major etiology for temporomandibular disorders. Indeed, the occlusal contacts associated as the *cause* of the dysfunction may in reality be a *result* of the dysfunction and should be evaluated only in the absence of symptoms.[47]

A second theory postulates that the maxillomandibular positioning is abnormal and causes a strain on the muscles of mastication and the TMJ and that this strain creates a neuromuscular imbalance. The improper positioning, according to this theory, can be due to the position of the teeth, deficiency or excess of the maxilla or mandible, or improper position of the condyle in the TMJ. Various radiographic procedures have evaluated condylar position in nonsymptomatic and symptomatic patients and have not supported an ''ideal'' position that should be used for diagnosis of temporomandibular disorders. Neither has definitive evidence regarding skeletal malocclusions (deficiency or excess of the maxilla or mandible) and their role as an etiological factor been supported by various epidemiological studies.[48] Therefore, treatment for temporomandibular disorders should not be directed primarily at correcting the abnormal jaw positioning unless a true cause and effect can be demonstrated for that patient.

The third theory involves abnormal neuromuscular patterns that develop due to central nervous system (CNS) influences such as with chronic bruxism. A recent investigation has found that chronic nocturnal bruxism that produces pain may be closely associated with rapid eye movement (REM) sleep. A much lower correlation was found with non-pain bruxers and REM sleep suggesting multiple categories for nocturnal bruxers.[49] Bruxism has also been highly correlated with stress, either as anticipatory stress or as a response to stress.[50] This demonstration of limbic system influences over masticatory muscle activity emphasize the role of the CNS in facial pain. Additional investigations will be necessary to determine the significance of the CNS influences over muscular hyperactivity.

Conditions Mimicking Temporomandibular Disorders

Various pathological and dysfunctional conditions that are not associated with an intracapsular involvement of the TMJ and do not involve the muscles of mastication can produce facial pain or limitation of mandibular movement.

Although many of these conditions are not commonly encountered, a working knowledge of the basic signs, symptoms, and pathophysiology are required to formulate an accurate differential diagnosis. Complete descriptions of each condition can be found in various texts that detail the pathophysiology[1] and will not be covered here.

Trigeminal Neuralgia

Trigeminal neuralgia consists of an intense shocking or burning pain that lasts a few seconds to minutes and is associated with light sensory contact of the skin (trigger zone). This condition is usually unilateral, usually involves a single division of the trigeminal nerve, and is more commonly observed in older women. Anesthetic blocking of the appropriate sensory nerve that triggers the pain is a good diagnostic test to differentiate the pain from muscular sources.

Atypical Facial Neuralgia

Pain that is continuous and intolerable and may be unilateral or bilateral without the characteristics of trigeminal neuralgia has been termed atypical facial neuralgia. This condition also predominantly affects women and is usually not accompanied by a trigger zone. This diagnosis is made after exclusion of other patterns of facial pain.

Central Nervous System Lesions

Some brain-stem lesions or lesions involving motor cortex may cause masticatory or cervical muscle rigidity or trismus. Tumors may also present as pain, usually on the same side as the location of the tumor. The patients may have pain that is vague and, if a tumor is suspected, the patient should be immediately referred to a neurologist for further evaluation. Anesthesia of a whole division of the trigeminal nerve is another indicator for immediate neurological evaluation.

Odontogenic Pain

Pain from the teeth will usually be felt as localized and will frequently be enhanced by the drinking of hot or cold fluids or by percussion of the involved teeth. Local anesthesia of the suspected tooth followed by a significant relief of pain will help confirm a diagnosis. Radiographic changes at the apex of the tooth will also aid in the differential diagnosis of odontogenic pain.

Sinus Pain

Pain from the sinuses may be felt on the same side in the maxillary teeth or may begin as a frontal headache. Radiographic findings of a cloudy sinus or excessive drainage from the sinus will help differentiate this pain from odontogenic pain. Changes in head position will often enhance the pain felt in the maxillary teeth underlying the maxillary sinus, such as the bicuspids or molars.

Otological Pain

Ear pain as the primary complaint may be mistaken for middle ear infection (otitis media) or other ear sources of pain and may in fact originate from the TMJ or from the masticatory or cervical muscles. *Primary* ear pain should first be addressed by a physician to exclude ear pathology; only after exclusion of this source should the patient be examined for TMJ or muscular sources.

Developmental Abnormalities

Mandibular hyperplasia involves a slow, progressive enlargement of the condyle that introduces facial asymmetry and a shift of the mandibular midline *away from* the affected side. This condition can be observed radiographically as well as clinically when it has progressed further.

Mandibular hypoplasia is a underdevelopment of one or both condyles and is usually evident in early life. This condition may be either congenital or acquired and can be visualized radiographically and clinically as a shift of the mandible *toward* the affected side.

Chondromatosis is a rare condition that involves metaplasia of cartilage within the synovial membrane. Diagnosis of this condition may require radiographs and a 99m technetium bone scan.[51] A clinical presentation may show preauricular swelling, pain, and deviation and limitation of mandibular movement.

Neoplasias

Primary neoplasias of the TMJ are rarely encountered and when found are more commonly benign than malignant. Benign tumors include chondroma, chondroblastoma,[52] osteoma, and osteoblastoma. Malignant tumors include osteosarcoma, chondrosarcoma, and mesenchymal chondrosarcoma. Another malignant tumor located in the nasopharynx and involving the pterygoid muscles causes Trotter's syndrome. This syndrome consists of unilateral deafness, defective mobility of the soft palate on the affected side, ipsilateral pain in the lower jaw, tongue, and side of face, and trismus of the medial pterygoid muscle, causing inability to open the mandible.[53] Although the bony tumors can be observed radiographically, the differential diagnosis of non-bony tumors requires a careful history, thorough clinical examination, and specialized radiographic studies such as CT scans.

Parotid Diseases

Most salivary gland pain is due to inflammation or blockage of the salivary duct, and the source of the pain can be easily localized to the particular salivary gland. The pain usually is intensified during eating and must be differentiated from masticatory muscle pain.

Vascular Diseases

Pain of vascular origin includes common and classic migraine headache, cluster headache, and temporal arteritis. The migraine and cluster headaches may respond to vasoconstricting agents such as ergotamine tartrate or caffeine, thus reducing the pulsating character. Temporal arteritis involves inflammation and tenderness of the superficial temporal artery with giant cell infiltration and a conclusive diagnosis can only be obtained by biopsy. This condition, if not discovered, can further progress to blindness.

Myofascial Pain

Examination for myofascial pain has been previously described and is currently attributed to prolonged muscle activity causing an associated inflammatory response within the muscle. Bell[54] characterized the muscular pain as muscle splinting pain, trigger point pain, or muscle spasm pain. Muscular impingement on nerves can also elicit neurological symptoms such those that occur with greater occipital nerve entrapment.

Cervical Muscle Dysfunction

Cervical muscle symptoms have commonly been identified when patients have masticatory muscle and TMJ pain. Many persons have implicated the cervical muscle symptoms as causing the masticatory muscle or TMJ dysfunction, but no controlled scientific studies have established a true cause-and-effect relationship. The central excitation theory is one possible explanation of cervical muscle structures *referring* pain to cephalad structures; however, this theory does not directly explain the symptomatic involvement of cephalad structures unless by a secondary effect such as generalized muscle tension as a reaction to the experienced pain.[55] The influence of cervical muscle and cervical spine dysfunction as an etiological factor for temporomandibular disorders needs to be critically evaluated by well-designed scientific investigations rather than clinical interpretation if the true influence of these structures is to be ascertained.

Others

Eagle's syndrome is the calcification of the stylohyoid ligament, with pain associated with swallowing or turning the head.[56] If the calcification is oriented in a medial or lateral direction, then possible impingement of the internal or external carotid arteries may occur causing carotidynia. Radiographic evidence of an elongated styloid process by itself is not diagnostic for Eagle's syndrome. Clinical examination must confirm the source of pain as originating from the styloid process.

SUMMARY

In conclusion, the importance of an accurate history and thorough clinical examination for differential diagnosis of temporomandibular disorders cannot be overstated. After establishment of an accurate diagnosis, appropriate treatment must be provided that will address the primary sources of pain and dysfunction.

REFERENCES

1. Isselbacher KJ, Adams RD, Braunwald E, et al (eds): Harrison's Principles of Internal Medicine. 9th Ed. McGraw-Hill, New York, 1980
2. Jonsson R, Lindvall A-M, Nyberg G: Temporomandibular joint involvement in systemic lupus erythematosus. Arthritis Rheum 26:1506, 1983
3. Stinson CW, Leban SG: Recurrent ankylosis of the temporomandibular joint in a patient with chronic psoriasis. J Oral Maxillofac Surg 40:678, 1982
4. Bomalaski JS, Jimenez SA: Erosive arthritis of the temporomandibular joint in Reiter's syndrome. J Rheumatol 11:400, 1984
5. Larheim TA, Dale K, Tveito L: Radiographic abnormalities of the temporomandibular joint in children with juvenile rheumatoid arthritis. Acta Radiol [Diag] 22:277, 1981
6. Bates B: A Guide to Physical Examination. 3rd Ed. JB Lippencott, Philadelphia, 1983
7. President's Conference on the Examination, Diagnosis, and Management of Temporomandibular Disorders, J Am Dent Assoc 106:75, 1983
8. Libman E: Observations on individual sensitiveness to pain. J Am Med Assoc 102:335, 1934
9. Gross A, Gale EN: A prevalence study of the clinical signs associated with mandibular dysfunction. J Am Dent Assoc 107:932, 1983

10. Broton JG, Sessle BJ: Effects of temporomandibular joint (TMJ) afferent stimulation on masticatory muscle activity. J Dent Res 65:334, 1986
11. Travell J, Simons D: Myofascial Pain and Dysfunction: The Trigger Point Manual. Williams & Wilkins, Baltimore, 1983
12. Alghren J: Mechanisms of mastication. Acta Odontol Scand, 24:suppl. 44, 1–109, 1966
13. Moller, E: The chewing apparatus: an electromyographic study of the action of the muscles of mastication and its correlation to facial morphology. Acta Physiol Scand, 69:suppl. 280, 1–229, 1966
14. Moller E: Action of the muscles of mastication. Front Oral Physiol 1:121, 1974
15. Moller E: Human muscle patterns. p. 128. In Sessle BJ, Hannam AG (eds): Mastication and Swallowing: Biological and Clinical Correlates. University of Toronto Press, Toronto, 1976
16. Ramfjord SP, Ash MM: Occlusion. WB Saunders, Philadelphia, 1971
17. Laskin DM: Etiology of the pain-dysfunction syndrome. J Am Dent Assoc 79:147, 1969
18. Clark GT, Beemsterboer PL, Rugh JD: Nocturnal masseter muscle activity and the symptoms of masticatory dysfunction. J Oral Rehabil 8:279, 1981
19. McNamara JA: The independent functions of the two heads of the lateral pterygoid muscle. Am J Anat 138:197, 1973
20. Mahan PE, Wilkinson TM, Gibbs GH, et al: Superior and inferior bellies of the lateral pterygoid muscle EMG activity at basic jaw positions. J Prosthet Dent 50:710, 1983
21. Gibbs CH, Mahan PE, Wilkinson TM, Mauderli A: EMG activity of the superior belly of the lateral pterygoid muscle in relation to other jaw muscles. J Prosthet Dent 51:691, 1984
22. Johnstone DR, Templeton M: The feasibility of palpating the lateral pterygoid muscle. J Prosthet Dent 44:318, 1980
23. Munro RR: Activity of the digastric muscle in swallowing and chewing. J Dent Res 53:530, 1974
24. Dawson PE: Evaluation, diagnosis and treatment of occlusal problems. CV Mosby, St. Louis, 1974
25. Agerberg G: Maximal mandibular movements in young men and women. Swed Dent J 67:81, 1974
26. Donnarumma GC, Burdette BH, McCall WD: Bite force and silent period durations: comparisons in normal subjects and TMD patients. J Dent Res 65:180, 1986
27. McCall WD, Tallgren A, Ash MM: EMG silent periods in immediate complete denture patients: a longitudinal study. J Dent Res 58:2353, 1979
28. Farrar WB: Differentiation of temporomandibular joint dysfunction to simplify treatment. J Prosthet Dent 28:629, 1972
29. Zarb GA, Thompson GW: The treatment of patients with temporomandibular joint pain dysfunction syndrome. J Can Dent Assoc 41:410, 1975
30. Farrar WB: Characteristics of the condylar path in internal derangements of the TMJ. J Prosthet Dent 39:319, 1978
31. Gale EN, Gross A: An evaluation of temporomandibular joint sounds. J Am Dent Assoc 111:62, 1985
32. Rieder CE: The prevalence of mandibular dysfunction. Part I. Sex and age distribution of signs and symptoms related to mandibular dysfunction. J Prosthet Dent 50:81, 1983
33. Agerberg G, Carlsson GE: Functional disorders of the masticatory system. Acta Odontol Scand 30:597, 1972

34. Blaschke DD, Blaschke TJ: Normal TMJ bony relationships in centric occlusion. J Dent Res 60:98, 1981
35. Katzberg RW, Keith DA, Ten Eick WR, Guralnick WC: Internal derangements of the temporomandibular joint: an assessment of condylar position in centric occlusion. J Prosthet Dent 49:250, 1983
36. Helms CA, Gillespy T, Sims RE, Richardson ML: Magnetic resonance imaging of internal derangement of the temporomandibular joint. Radiol Clin North Am 24:189, 1986
37. Katzberg RW, Bessette RW, Tallents RH, et al: Normal and abnormal temporomandibular joint: MR imaging with surface coil. Radiology 158:183, 1986
38. Harms SE, Wilk RM, Wolford LM, et al: The temporomandibular joint: magnetic resonance imaging using surface coils. Radiology 157:133, 1985
39. Clark GT, Moody D: A comparison of the accuracy of two jaw tracking methods. J Dent Res 64:340, 1985
40. Clark GT: Clinical, diagnostic and research applications of jaw tracking and electromyography. J Dent Res 65:716, 1986
41. Rugh JD: Future directions for clinical and research applications of EMG and jaw tracking. J Dent Res 65:716, 1986
42. Majewski RF, Gale EN: Electromyographic activity of anterior temporal area pain patients and non-pain subjects. J Dent Res 63:1228, 1984
43. Felli AJ, McCall WD: Jaw muscle silent periods before and after rapid palatal expansion. Am J Orthod 76:676, 1979
44. McCall WD, Hoffer M: Jaw muscle silent periods by tooth tap and chin tap. J Oral Rehabil 8:91, 1981
45. Dolwick MF, Sanders B: TMJ Internal Derangement and Arthrosis. CV Mosby, St. Louis, 1985
46. Helkimo M: Studies on function and dysfunction of the masticatory system. Swed Dent J 67:1, 1974
47. Edmiston GF, Laskin DM: Changes in consistency of occlusal contact in myofascial pain-dysfunction (MPD) syndrome. J Dent Res 57:27, 1978
48. Egermark-Eriksson I: Malocclusion and some function recordings of the masticatory system in Swedish schoolchildren. Swed Dent J 6:9, 1982
49. Rugh JD, Ware JC: Polysomnographic comparison of nocturnal bruxists with and without facial pain. J Dent Res 65:180, 1986
50. Funch DP, Gale EN: Factors associated with nocturnal bruxism and its treatment. J Behav Med 3:385, 1980
51. Blankestijn J, Pandus AK, Vermey A, et al: Synovial chondromatosis of the temporomandibular joint. Cancer 55:479, 1985
52. Spahr J, Elzay RP, Kay S, et al: Chondroblastoma of the temporomandibular joint arising from articular cartilage: a previously unreported presentation of an uncommon neoplasm. Oral Surg 54:430, 1982
53. Shafer WG, Hine MK, Levy BM: A Textbook of Oral Pathology. 3rd Ed. WB Saunders, Philadelphia, 1974
54. Bell WE: Orofacial pains: Classification, Diagnosis and Management. 3rd Ed. Year Book Medical, Chicago, 1985
55. Dalessio DJ: Wolff's Headache and Other Head Pain. 3rd Ed. Oxford University Press, New York, 1972
56. Russell TE: Eagle's syndrome: diagnostic considerations and report of a case. J Am Dent Assoc 94:548, 1977

5 | Nonsurgical Management of TMJ and Masticatory Muscle Problems

Samuel J. Razook

The criteria for initiating treatment for disturbances that involve the TMJ and mandible vary according to the practitioners' ability to diagnose and their ability to predict if the value of treatment will outweigh the time, expense, and personal demands placed on the patient now and in the future. Diagnosis entails an understanding of the physiology and pathophysiology of the dysfunctional structures and their degenerative processes. It also entails a recognition of the many facets of pain and pain behavior that may accompany the dysfunction as a primary, secondary, or independent entity. Realistic treatment goals regarding the elimination of pain and the restoration of normal function are developed with this in mind.

The differential diagnosis of pain in and around the jaws and neck includes not only those of musculoskeletal origin but also pains of vascular, neurogenic, visceral, and psychogenic origin that can overlap musculoskeletal pain in their distribution and mimic it in quality and frequency. A clinical knowledge of these other entities and access to other specialists in these areas for consultation is an absolute requisite for proper patient care.

Musculoskeletal disorders in the head and neck are multicausal and can be classified according to organic or nonorganic etiology. Although this classification is convenient to use, it is unusual to find these entities isolated in the clinical setting. Aberrant mandibular function of organic origin may be caused by occlusal disharmonies, disturbances within the TMJ, skeletal imbalances involving head posturing or maxillomandibular size discrepancies, or any combination of these factors. It is the action of muscle and reactive forces of muscle that define the interaction between these units, which otherwise would be functioning independently. Pain and stress of nonorganic origin can also affect mandibular function by altering muscle function. In this way, nonorganic problems can lead to physical use and abuse of structures that appear to be either degenerating or dysfunctional when the patient is first seen in the clinical setting. Thus, disorders of nonorganic origin can cause organic problems in much the same way that organic imbalances that cause pain and stress may initiate intolerable conditions for the patient to manage psychologically.

FACTORS INFLUENCING REST POSITION OF MANDIBLE

Key to the treatment of mandibular problems is an understanding of the factors that can influence and are influenced by the rest position of the mandible. Ligaments are structures that limit joint movement. As such, they determine the borders in three dimensions, beyond which the joint cannot move. The temporomandibular ligaments, the capsule of the TMJs, and, to some degree, the stylomandibular and sphenomandibular ligaments determine the borders of movement of the mandible. Movement of the mandible along its upper border is influenced significantly by the dental occlusion. These borders describe an envelope of motion within which the mandible functions and rests. At any particular time, the mandible at rest is in a relatively static position determined by muscle tone of the jaw-opening and jaw-closing muscles and the associated soft tissue factors as they react to gravitational pull (Fig. 5-1).

Dental Occlusion

Several factors influence the position of rest of the mandible and therefore influence masticatory muscle tone. One of these factors is dental occlusion. Ligaments attached to the roots of the teeth and to the alveolar bone not only aid in distribution of stress from the teeth to the bone during mastication but also provide an abundance of sensory input to the central nervous system (CNS) regarding the position and quality of the load. This sensory input makes possible the alteration of masticatory muscle activity to adjust the position of the mandible in function to avoid overloading of the teeth and joints at any particular time. Contact of the occluding surfaces of the teeth through these periodontal ligaments influences masticatory muscle function.

In addition, the position of the mandible at rest is also influenced by sensory input from the periodontal ligaments. When the masticatory muscles are at rest, the mandible is within the envelope of motion and the teeth are apart

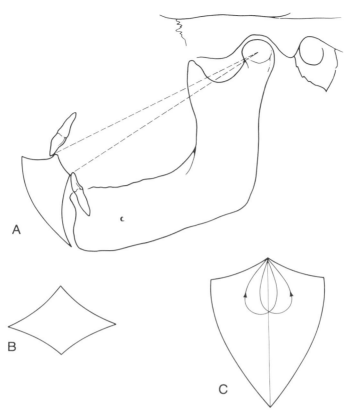

Fig. 5-1. Border movements of mandible scribed by incisal edge of the mandibular central incisor as viewed in (**A**) sagittal, (**B**) horizontal, and (**C**) frontal planes.

approximately 2 to 4 mm. During swallowing, the mandibular elevator muscles contract, moving the mandible so that the teeth come into or approach maximum intercuspation. Closure from the rest position during swallowing or during voluntary movement is in a smooth arc toward maximum intercuspation, avoiding occlusal areas that would prevent simultaneous contact of the teeth. If the position of rest does not allow smooth closure into intercuspation, the muscles will try to move the mandible to another position. This avoidance phenomenon is believed to be a protective mechanism to prevent or minimize overloading of the joints or particular teeth. This is done through the alteration of muscle activity. Muscles do not know innately where to position the mandible at rest. Instead, the mandible assumes its rest position by default as a result of avoiding other positions that are less compatible with tooth position. Consequently, altering the occluding surfaces of the teeth can alter masticatory muscle activity by causing a change in the rest position through this mechanism of avoidance.

Sensory Input from Capsule and TMJ

A second factor that can alter the rest position of the mandible is sensory input from the mechanoreceptors in the capsule of and within the TMJ. This input allows joint position sense. The etiology and sequela of capsular involvement is discussed in Chapter 6. It also has the ability to alter masticatory muscle function in such a way that it avoids allowing the TMJ and thus the mandible to achieve a border position except transiently during function. In the diseased joint, other stimuli resulting from degeneration or inflammation will act in a similar manner to reprogram muscle function and attempt to place the mandible in a position that causes the least amount of stimulation of pain receptors. This alteration of muscle function occurs during function and during rest. The resultant position of rest is one that has been found by the avoidance of all other positions that would have resulted in a greater amount of noxious stimuli being sent to the CNS.

Tongue Position and Nasal Airway

A third factor that influences the rest position of the mandible is tongue position and nasal airway. If obstruction of the nasal airway does not allow adequate flow through the nasal cavity, the tongue position will change, allowing more room for air to flow between it and the palate. The tongue will often come forward, and the mandible will be slightly more depressed. This contributes to alterations in growth of the middle and lower face. In addition, posturing the head in an extended position on the neck will also occur, allowing easier air flow by altering the position of the mandible and tongue if nasal obstruction exists. Just as an elevation in the partial pressure of carbon dioxide in the blood stream increases the respiratory rate through autonomic mechanisms, changes in tongue position to allow adequate air flow to the lungs is an adaptive response at a subconscious level. An alteration in masticatory muscle function must occur, which influences the rest position of the mandible to allow an acceptable tongue posture for adequate air flow.

Cervical Spine Positioning and Mobility

A fourth factor that alters the rest position of the mandible is cervical spine positioning and mobility. A change in head positioning will alter the rest position of the mandible. The rest position of the mandible will change slightly from day to day and from hour to hour with no apparent change in the other factors previously mentioned. Because the mandible is suspended in a sling of muscles from the cranium and because gravitational forces remain constant and in a direction perpendicular to the ground, a change in head posture alone can alter the position the mandible assumes relative to the cranium. More detail of head-neck positioning influencing the rest position (upright postural position) of the mandible is covered in Chapter 12.

Although the dentist alters tooth structure and uses prosthetic materials of an apparently unyielding nature, the teeth and dental occlusion are not part of a rigid, hard tissue system. Instead, they are truly part a soft tissue system and dynamic in all respects.

Because alterations in the occlusal contacts of the teeth affect muscular performance, the dentist is offered a mechanism to change joint position, joint loading, and muscle activity in an indirect and reasonably predictable fashion. For the masticatory system to remain functional and comfortable, however, the importance of the other factors mentioned must be appreciated in the diagnosis and treatment of the patient.

Key variables to consider that influence the patient's response to treatment for TMJ and muscle dysfunction are not only the occlusal relationships of the teeth but also cervical spine positioning and mobility. Key variables to be considered by the physical therapist in the treatment of cervical spine dysfunction must include dental relationships and temporomandibular function. The relationship is direct and predictable because both act and react to mandibular positioning through the interplay of the synergistic and antagonistic activity of the cervical and masticatory musculature.

NONSURGICAL TREATMENT OF SPECIFIC DISORDERS

Treatment of TMJ and head and neck muscle disorders should be reversible and noninvasive whenever possible. Treatment has as its goals: (1) relief of pain by resolution of muscle spasm and intra-articular inflammation, and (2) restoration of normal mandibular motion and function in the setting of a stable dental occlusion, acceptable craniocervical relationship, and normal disc–condyle relationship. If these goals are met, even with radiographic evidence of arthritic degeneration of the joint, no further treatment is required.

The basic principles of treatment of disorders of both organic and nonorganic origin are not unlike those used in the treatment of musculoskeletal pain in other joint–muscle systems in the body. Initial symptomatic treatment may include all or some of the following reversible modalities:

1. Establish rapport with the patients, letting them know you understand the problem and are willing to work through this problem with them.

2. Educate the patient as to the etiology, affected anatomy, and the need for treatment over a period of time, emphasizing that there are no "overnight cures."

3. In addition to a gross evaluation of the patient's mental status, the use of a screening evaluation (i.e., stress inventory) or more in-depth testing or psychologic consultation may be indicated.

4. Nonsteroid antiinflammatory drugs (NSAIDs) provide significant an-

algesia and antiinflammatory activity directed toward the muscles and joints. Narcotic analgesics in patients with chronic pain are indicated only rarely.

5. The application of heat to painful muscles increases blood flow and reduces spasm.

6. Application of vapocoolant sprays or the injection of local anesthetics without vasoconstrictors into muscle trigger points is effective in reversing the pain–muscle spasm cycle.

7. Muscle relaxants in small doses provide relief in some patients throughout the day. Sedative doses should be avoided.

8. Resting the jaw and adhering to the use of soft, non-chew diet is recommended.

9. Transcutaneous electrical nerve stimulation (TENS), ultrasound, and diathermy are often effective therapeutic modalities.

10. The patient should be made aware of parafunctional habits of clenching and bruxism, if suspect, and should refrain from them. Evidence or absence of evidence of wear on the occlusal surfaces of the teeth, in and of itself, is not diagnostic of bruxism or clenching.

11. It is important to encourage patients to continue with their normal work and to exercise. This helps to keep their mind off their pain. Certain postural positions and exercises can aggravate pain, however. Patients are to follow guidelines offered by their dentist or physical therapist as covered in Chapter 11.

This may be all that is necessary to reduce symptoms significantly in many patients while the underlying cause is being determined or other treatment is being planned.

Occlusal adjustment by the dentist is an irreversible modality and is rarely indicated as an initial treatment except when gross interferences prevent the effective use of occlusal splints to stabilize the desired maxillomandibular relationship. Further adjustment at a time when muscle spasm and/or intracapsular edema prevents the disc–condyle assembly from assuming its normal concentric position within the glenoid fossa or at a time when a disc is dislocated may worsen the occlusal problems after muscle spasm, edema, or disc dislocation is resolved.

Further treatment should use reversible modalities when possible until symptoms have been relieved and a stable maxillomandibular relationship is maintained. This treatment may include, separately or in combination, any of the following:

1. Occlusal splint therapy to help alter the masticatory and cervical muscle response to the existing occlusal scheme or to change the mandibular condyle position.

2. Physical therapy to modify mandibular and/or cervical posture by normalizing vertebral joint, soft tissue, and muscular relationships in the cervical and thoracic spine.

3. Behavior modification to control muscle tone and tension and stop

parafunctional habits through the use of biofeedback, hypnosis, and psychotherapy.

The following is a discussion of the application of nonsurgical therapy to specific mandibular disorders.

Nonarticular Disturbances

Neuromuscular Conditions

Increased muscle tonus progressing to acute or chronic myospasm can occur secondary to imbalances in the occlusion, cervical spine and TMJ dysfunction, and changes in the psychological state. Because of the synergistic and antagonistic relationships that exist between the masticatory and cervical musculature, it is not uncommon that both groups become involved. Depending on the degree and the amount of time the hyperactivity remains, the following muscle conditions can result.

Muscle splinting (muscle cramp, acute myospasm) is a protective reflex or guarding mechanism. This generally occurs as a result of acute trauma, causing the skeletal muscles to contract and remain in a hypertonic state, preventing further movement of the part. The trauma can be as gross as a blow to the jaw or head or as innocent as maintaining the head or jaw in one position for prolonged periods of time. Because this is of an acute nature, metabolic changes that can occur as a result of the vasoconstriction have not had time to develop. Stretching and spraying the muscle with a vapocoolant spray is often effective in breaking the spasm, restoring normal function and relieving pain almost immediately. If left untreated, the acute state can progress into a chronic state in which the metabolism of the muscle is altered.

Chronic hyperactivity, contraction, or prolonged muscle splinting can result in metabolic changes leading to chronic myospasm. Often, chronic myospasm does not develop as a result of prolonged acute spasm. Instead, it begins insidiously, developing over long periods of time, and is usually secondary to stress or the microtrauma of overuse and abuse of the neck and jaws, dental malocclusion, or maxillomandibular size discrepancies. Chronic hypercontraction of the muscle from whatever source leads to vasoconstriction, resulting in a decrease in the supply of oxygen and nutrients to the muscle. Muscle fatigue occurs as a result of ATP depletion which is critical for both muscle contraction and relaxation. Without sufficient ATP and oxygen, hypertonicity and further vasoconstriction persist. The muscle lacks the ability to eliminate metabolic waste products such as lactic acid because of the decreased blood flow. This can result in focal areas of inflammation. Pain produced by inflammation causes further muscle contraction and can initiate a self-perpetuating pain–spasm–pain cycle. Predisposing, precipitating, and/or perpetuating factors involving the TMJ, dental occlusion, head posture, or the psychological state of the patient must be identified. In addition to treatment of these factors directly, biofeedback, TENS, ultrasound, vapocoolant sprays, exercises, and NSAIDs may be necessary.

As the chronic muscle spasm persists, trigger points can develop within the muscle. These are focal areas of ischemia that exhibit altered neuronal activity that can keep the entire muscle in a hypertonic state. Trigger points are point-tender, palpable, nodular masses often felt deep within the muscle. They can develop in any skeletal muscle and are known to exist in both active and latent conditions, often lasting for years. Injection of trigger points with local anesthetics devoid of vasoconstrictors in addition to physical therapy manual techniques and modalities have proven effective in relieving pain in most patients.

Dental Malocclusion

Neurologically, the act of chewing involves an extremely complex system of motor stimulation and inhibition of various muscle groups. During mastication, the bolus of food on the occlusal surfaces of the teeth acts as a fulcrum so that the mandible acts as a class II or class III lever. Periodontal ligament receptors supply the CNS with information about the changing position of the fulcrum and the pressures being generated. This information is used to control the necessary changes in muscle contraction very rapidly during the chewing stroke to protect the teeth and joints from damage, and is accomplished through a system of reflex inhibition of muscles and muscle groups. The presence, absence, and position of teeth are a major influencing factor in the resultant load to the joints and to the muscle patterns that develop.

At times other than during the power strokes of chewing, dental occlusion still exerts a great influence on the stomatognathic system. Temporally, when one considers that actual chewing may last no longer than 1 hour a day, the effect of the dental occlusion on the resting position of the mandible during nonchewing time acquires greater significance as a factor in head and neck musculoskeletal harmony.

The mandible is said to be in centric relation (CR) to the maxilla when the TMJs are in the most anterosuperior position in the glenoid fossa with the discs in place. Centric occlusion (CO) is the tooth contact that exists when the mandible is placed in CR and closed until tooth contact occurs. Maximum intercuspation dictates the final position of the TMJs at the endpoint of chewing and at the endpoint of empty mouth closure (Fig. 5-2). When the teeth are in maximum intercuspation, the position of the mandible relative to the maxilla may be the CR position. Methods of positioning the mandible in a CR position may differ from dentist to dentist, and various techniques are described in the literature. Difficulty in passively attaining this position may be related to the force applied, the velocity and rhythm in which the mandible is manipulated, and the distance through which it is moved.

If maximum intercuspation does not exist in the CR position, and a slide

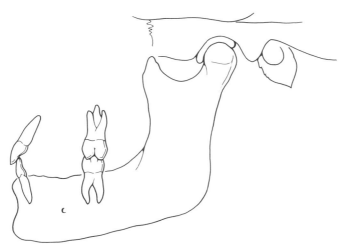

Fig. 5-2. Normal relationship of disc–condyle assembly in the centric relation position with maximum intercuspation coincidental with centric occlusion.

is detectible as the mandible moves from its initial point of contact into maximum intercuspation, a malocclusion is considered to exist. Other types of malocclusion are based on missing teeth, vertical dimension of the occlusion, and on the contact of the teeth when the mandible moves laterally or protrusively while maintaining tooth contact. A detailed discussion of these many facets is beyond the scope of this text.

When the occlusion of the teeth is not in harmony with masticatory muscle function and TMJ function, either the teeth, joints, or muscles separately or in combination will change in form, function, or position to a new point of equilibrium. If a malocclusion exists and the patient is asymptomatic with no physical findings of pathology in the dentition, muscles, and joints, adaptation has occurred and the malocclusion must be considered normal for that person. If the changes necessary are beyond the range of physiologic adaptability, degeneration or pathology will occur. This may appear as tooth mobility or wear, muscle hyperactivity associated with fatigue and pain, or degeneration of the hard or soft tissues in the TMJ.

If a malocclusion exists in the symptomatic patient, its elimination is often helpful in treatment. Occlusal disharmony is often the sustaining factor in masticatory muscle and TMJ dysfunction once the patient's adaptability has decreased. Clinical observation has shown certain occlusal conditions to be either the initiating and/or perpetuating factor responsible for disharmony in the masticatory system. The available scientific evidence confirms in general the clinical concepts that the following dental conditions are often etiologic factors in TMJ and masticatory muscle dysfunction.

Lack of Posterior Support. A lack of posterior support resulting from either missing teeth, underoccluded teeth, or restorations will increase mandibular elevator muscle activity and TMJ loading. A statistical relationship exists between the lack of posterior support and the remodeling and degenerative changes within the TMJs. Wear, mobility, and splaying of the upper anterior teeth often occur as the occlusal load is shifted to them. The spaces or diastemas resulting from tooth splaying that in some patients occur over a long time can indicate a collapse in the vertical dimension of occlusion. Patients with TMJ disc dislocations, cervical muscle symptoms, and clinically abnormal head and neck posturing often lack posterior support and/or have collapse in the vertical dimension of occlusion (VDO) (Figs. 5-3 and 5-4).

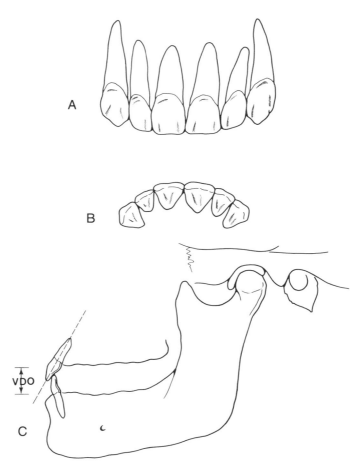

Fig. 5-3.   Maxillary anterior teeth seen in (**A**) facial and (**B**) occlusal views. (**C**) Lateral view of mandible with a lack of posterior tooth support. No collapse of vertical dimension of occlusion is apparent.

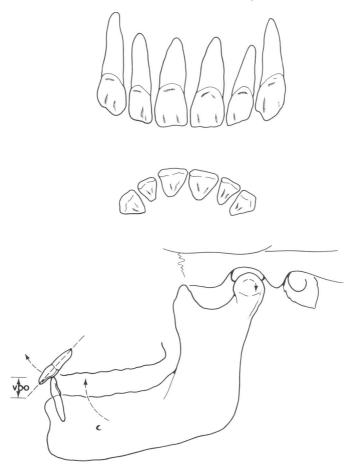

Fig. 5-4. Resultant development of diastemas and a collapse in vertical dimension of occlusion due to lack of posterior support.

Balancing Interferences. Balancing interferences (tooth contact on the side opposite to which the mandible is moving in a lateral direction with the teeth together) have also been associated with excessive wear and mobility of the posterior teeth, muscle spasm, and TMJ dysfunction. As the mandible is being guided by and/or avoiding the interference, the condyle is being distracted from the posterior slope of the articular eminence. To maintain joint stability, the disc must remain in intimate contact with the condyle and the eminence. Because the intraarticular space between the condyle and eminence has increased, the superior head of the lateral pterygoid muscle must bring the disc forward to fill the space with its thicker posterior portion. This can lead to

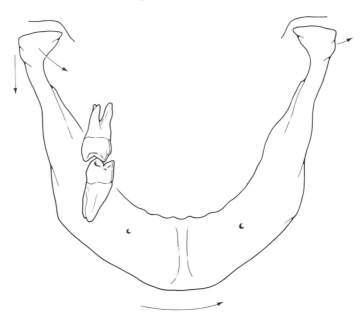

Fig. 5-5. Balancing interference of molar teeth as mandible moves into a left lateral movement. Right condyle is orbiting around left condyle, which is rotating with some lateral movement.

muscle fatigue and/or spasm and is believed to be a factor that can lead to TMJ disc dysfunction. Excessive wear of the teeth and bruxism are often believed to be caused by balancing interferences. Clinical and scientific observations do not exclusively support this view, however.

Articulation paper placed between the teeth on one side of the mouth while the patient moves the mandible in the opposite lateral direction will assess the presence of balancing interferences by marking tooth contacts. If they exist, referral to a dentist for evaluation of the occlusion is recommended (Fig. 5-5).

Maximum Intercuspation. Maximum intercuspation of the teeth can cause the TMJ to be distracted from the glenoid fossa. It can place the joint posteriorly or grossly anteriorly in the fossa or it can in some way prevent the disc–condyle complex from maintaining a position of concentricity within the glenoid fossa. This often results in muscle conditions of pain and spasm and can result in joint dysfunction (Fig. 5-6).

Detailed evaluation of the occlusion is significant with the disc in its proper position within the TMJ. The occlusal relationships of the teeth will change with change of the intracapsular relationship of the disc to the condyle. The patient who appears to have acceptable occlusal relationships with the disc out of place may have significant discrepancies when the disc is relocated. Therefore, occlusal evaluation is always made in light of the existing status of the TMJs.

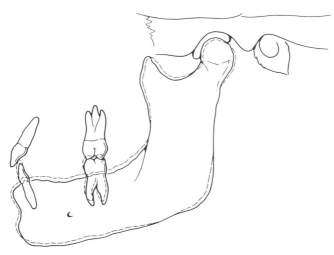

Fig. 5-6. Initial tooth contact centric occlusion (CO) as mandible maintains a centric relation position (solid line). Movement from CO into maximum intercuspation and the resultant condylar position (dotted line).

Initial treatment involves use of an intraoral orthotic appliance or "splint" to alter the existing occlusal scheme to favor more normal joint stability and muscle function. A variety of splints have been used, ranging from hard acrylic to metal to soft acrylic to fluid-filled appliances that cover all or a portion of the upper or lower teeth. One should select a particular design to fit the individual patient with full knowledge of the effects it may have on the TMJs, muscles, and teeth. The appliance can thus serve as a diagnostic tool as well as a therapeutic device. Appliances that do not cover or are not in contact with all teeth have the potential for allowing tooth movement and are not considered reversible. These splints are altered periodically until a stable maxillomandibular relationship is established, with muscle relaxation, pain relief, and a normal disc–condyle–fossa relationship. Permanent alterations to the dentition using orthodontics, prosthodontics, occlusal equilibration, or surgery can then be made to maintain the position achieved by the appliance. Sometimes either physical or emotional factors preclude the immediate transition from the splint to premanent changes in the dentition just described. In such cases, the splint can be worn until a more appropriate time.

Because of the relationship of the cervical and masticatory musculature mentioned previously, by altering masticatory muscle and joint relationships, orthotic appliances may have an effect on the pain and physical relationships in the cervical area. Favorable responses to the placement of an intraoral orthotic appliance may or may not indicate that the problem is strictly of occlusal origin. Permanent treatment of the dentition in such patients without observing head and neck posturing may be fraught with continued complaints of discomfort.

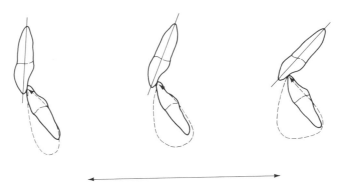

Fig. 5-7. Effect of inclination of anterior teeth on anterioposterior position of rest (posture) of mandible and its movement into intercuspation of the teeth.

An example of an appliance that fits the criteria of reversibility and that can be used diagnostically as well as therapeutically is the maxillary splint which covers all the upper teeth and makes contact with all the lower teeth. In patients who do not exhibit a loss of VDO as one of the factors in the malocclusion, the splint is made as thin as possible. This dimension can be made to be within the freeway space (1 to 2 mm) in most patients. If the VDO associated with the malocclusion shows collapse, the appliance is designed to restore the occlusion to a level approximating a normal VDO for the individual. The occlusal surface of the appliance allows for even contact of all teeth simultaneously when the TMJ is in a CR position in the glenoid fossa with the disc in place. Disclusion of the posterior teeth during protrusive and lateral movements of the mandible is off the anterior portion of the splint with the inclination of the anterior section made as minimal as possible. The inclination of the anterior portion of the splint (and anterior teeth) can restrict the range in which the mandible can rest at any particular time as head posture changes. If the inclination is too vertical or steep, the influence of the occlusion on the rest position of the mandible may not be compatible with the rest position of the mandible during changes in head posture. More freedom in this area will allow more freedom for the mandible to move from a wider variety of rest positions into maximum tooth contact and may decrease masticatory muscle activity (Figs. 5-7 and 5-8).

The importance of other modalities, physical therapy, and behavior modification in combination with the above in certain patients cannot be overstressed. Only when a continuous relief of symptoms is achieved and TMJ function is evidently optimal, should permanent changes to the dentition be considered. In achieving this, the approach should be the least invasive one that provides long-term stability in the occlusal relationship established by splint therapy. This may range from occlusal adjustment to orthodontic and prosthodontic treatment to orthognathic surgery, or any combination of treatments.

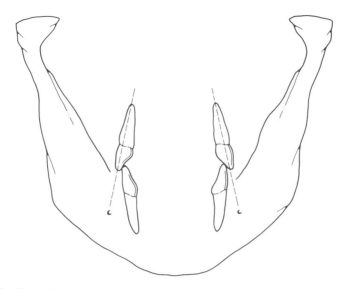

Fig. 5-8. Inclines of posterior teeth affect rest (posture) position of mandible in lateral directions and effect its path of closure into intercuspation of teeth.

Articular Disturbances

Disc Derangements

Dislocation of the disc within the TMJ has been recognized since the late 1800s. In a case report of two patients, Annandale described the surgical repositioning of the disc in 1884. Numerous reports and articles have appeared in the literature since then. Not until the mid-1970s was the concept of TMJ disc dislocation and its incidence accepted in large degree by the dental community. This was largely due to the efforts of Dr. William Farrar of Montgomery, Alabama.

Two general classifications of this disorder are the anteriorly dislocated disc that reduces during joint translation and the anteriorly dislocated disc without reduction. These two clinically evident conditions are believed to be only stages in the continuum of a disease process. Evidence implies that a disc that occasionally dislocates can develop into one that chronically dislocates but does reduce and eventually into one that does not reduce. These are believed to be clinical stages of joint degeneration that ultimately result in osteoarthritis of the TMJ.

The TMJs are naturally stressbearing. Degenerative changes are largely influenced by loads applied to the joint in excess of its ability to tolerate or its ability to adapt. Therefore, treatment is directed toward altering forces placed on the joint.

Loading is the result of muscle force. Muscle function that affects the

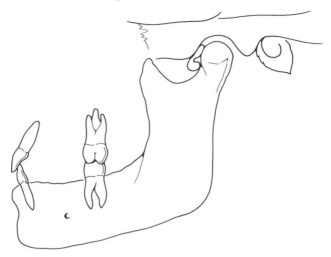

Fig. 5-9. Lateral diagram of anteriorly dislocated disc.

mandible not only involves the masticatory muscles but also muscles controlling cervical spine positioning and tongue function. Clinically, the dental occlusion appears to be the factor that most directly influences masticatory muscle function, and although it is through the occlusion that most treatment of TMJ disorders is focused, the importance of cervical involvement in the pain or dysfunction cannot be ignored.

A detailed discussion of the etiology and pathophysiology of disc dislocations and their clinical manifestations is given in Chapter 3.

Treatment of the anteriorly dislocated disc with reduction involves the use of an intraoral appliance to reposition the mandible in a more forward position to restore a normal disc–condyle relationship. The initial forward position is usually an overcorrected position. This is often effective in reducing or eliminating the muscle pain that can accompany disc dislocations. Some patients, however, cannot immediately tolerate muscularly the forward position, and it may be necessary to treat the muscle condition by using a nonrepositioning splint or physical therapy, or both.

When the disc is reduced by restoring it to its normal relationship to the condyle, the disc–condyle complex is often positioned anteriorly on the posterior slope of the articular eminence (Figs. 5-9 through 5-12). In some persons, particularly the patient with the retrognathic mandible, the condyle initially may be positioned slightly posteriorly and inferiorly within the glenoid fossa prior to treatment so that repositioning by the splint causes a concentric rather than eccentric positioning of the disc–condyle complex. The splint is worn continuously except when taken out for cleaning. During this time, efforts are made to eliminate any residual pain the patient may have. Splint therapy may last from several weeks to months as long as the patient shows signs of improvement or increasing joint stability. The ultimate goal is to adjust the ap-

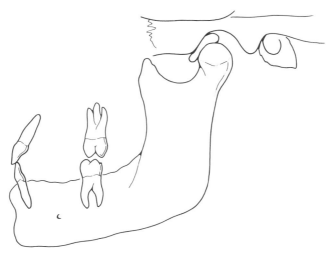

Fig. 5-10.   Reduction of disc has occurred by forward and downward advancement of the condyle around posterior band of disc; resultant occlusal relationship from this repositioning.

pliance so that the disc–condyle complex assumes a concentric position in the glenoid fossa. If this is achieved, the dental relationships are then evaluated to determine how best to restore the teeth so that they occlude evenly in the mandibular position determined by the appliance at an acceptable vertical dimension of occlusion. Dental and maxillomandibular imbalances deemed to be significant can be restored either prosthetically, orthodontically, surgically, or by occlusal adjustment, or by any combination of these. Application of the basic principles of occlusion are the basis for treatment planning. If the disc–condyle complex cannot be made to return to a concentric position, one should proceed with great caution when considering major changes to the occlusion. No scientific evidence exists to justify occlusal modification to keep the joint in an eccentric position within the glenoid fossa.

Numerous appliances have been developed to keep the mandible functioning in an anterior position for reduction of disc dislocations. These are either of a reversible or irreversible nature and must be used with caution.

Not all dislocated discs that reduce are amenable to this type of treatment. The degree of dislocation or the point at which reduction occurs is a major factor in determining how far the mandible will need to be advanced in splint therapy. If clinical judgment dictates that it will be impossible to return the disc–condyle complex to a concentric position at the end of splint therapy, treatment of this nature should not be initiated. Treatment should then be directed toward pain elimination. It is quite possible to eliminate associated muscle symptoms in many patients while leaving the disc dislocated.

If a dislocated disc is successfully treated, it should not be assumed that the joint has been made normal and that the damaged or elongated ligaments

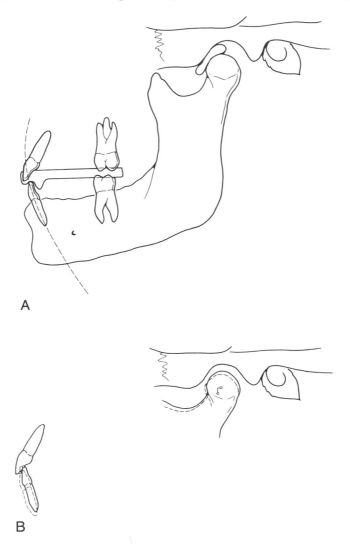

Fig. 5-11. **(A)** Orthotic appliance (splint) in place providing occlusal support at this new position. **(B)** Vertical and horizontal components of forward positioning as seen at level of condyle and anterior teeth. Vertical component represents opening that is created between the posterior teeth.

have shortened or "tightened up." This is not yet possible either in other adult joints or in the TMJ. It is more likely that success is due to alteration or redistribution of forces to the joint in such a way that they do not violate already damaged structures. Soft and hard tissue remodeling and resolution of hyperactivity of muscles may also be contributing factors.

Treatment of the anteriorly dislocated disc without reduction differs in the

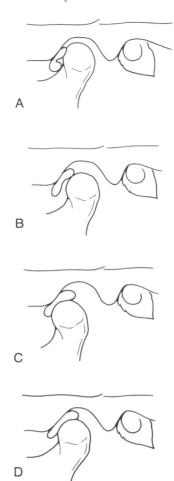

Fig. 5-12. Movement of condyle during disc reduction. **(A)** Dislocated disc and resultant function on retrodiscal tissue (not shown). **(B)** Condyle as it passes around posterior band of disc. **(C)** Disc–condyle complex at the initial time of reduction. **(D)** Slight posterior positioning of disc–condyle complex, which often can be achieved immediately; however, disc–condyle complex is not yet in a position of concentricity within glenoid fossa.

acute and chronic state (Fig. 5-13). In the acute condition, the patient usually has a history of clicking and possible locking and exhibits marked restriction of mandibular opening usually associated with deviation to the affected side. If dislocation is not a long-standing condition, one can distract the condyle, as is discussed in Chapter 6, which will allow the disc to reposition itself. Muscle injections, vapocoolant sprays, and other modalities may be necessary to block the muscle splinting often associated with this state. To manipulate the mandible, sedation or general anesthesia may also be necessary. If the dislocation is successfully reduced, an intraoral appliance must be inserted immediately to keep the mandible from shifting and allowing the disc to dislocate again.

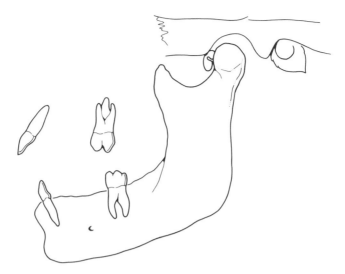

Fig. 5-13. Anteriorly dislocated disc without reduction creating an obstruction to anterior joint translation.

Treatment often follows the course of the anteriorly dislocated disc with reduction (described previously).

In the chronic condition, the dislocation is long-standing and gives a history of previous clicking and locking. The patient may have either marked restriction and deviation of mandibular opening or none. Crepitus within the joint may exist and degenerative changes may be evident on radiographs. Because the disc cannot be repositioned nonsurgically, treatment is directed toward relief of pain. Splint therapy to eliminate abnormal joint loading and establish normal occlusal relationships is the preferable dental treatment. If the pain is intolerable and cannot be managed through dental treatment, physical therapy, or any of the pain management modalities, surgery may be indicated. In patients who cannot open their mouths to an acceptable degree owing to a disc dislocation that does not reduce and when surgery is not an option, favorable results for increasing the range of motion (ROM) and minimizing masticatory muscle discomfort have been achieved in some patients by applying intraoral stretching techniques that force the disc further out of position to allow joint translation. This must be attempted with great caution and with knowledge that it may make the patient more uncomfortable. This is discussed in Chapter 6.

Inflammatory Conditions

The disc and the articulating surfaces of the mandibular condyle and glenoid fossa are nonvascularized and noninnervated and therefore cannot be the primary source of pain. Structures in and around the joint that account for pain from inflammation are the synovial membrane (synovitis), the retrodiscal tissues (retrodiscitis), and the capsule of the TMJ (capsulitis).

Inflammation of the synovial membrane may be due to infection, local trauma, or abuse, or may be secondary to a systemic connective tissue disorder such as rheumatoid arthritis. Intracapsular edema and an alteration of joint fluid occurs. Pain increases with joint movements. Undiagnosed systemic disease or locally infectious processes may require laboratory workup or referral. Treatment is based on the etiology of the problem and may involve use of antibiotics, antiinflammatory medications, or a non-chew diet to lessen loading of inflamed tissues.

Retrodiscitis may be due to external trauma or encroachment of a posteriorly positioned condyle secondary to dental malocclusion, or may occur if a disc is anteriorly dislocated. Pain will increase with joint loading. Clinically, distracting the joint manually or having the patient bite on a separator placed between the teeth on the ipsilateral side should relieve the pain and can be used as a diagnostic test. Antiinflammatory medications, restriction to a non-chew diet, and elimination of occlusal or disc discrepancies should be considered.

Inflammation of the capsule of the TMJ may be due to external trauma or may result from spread of inflammation secondary to the above two conditions. Because the capsule, including the temporomandibular ligament, functions to limit mandibular movements, thereby defining border positions, the ligament is passive unless these borders are approached. Therefore, pain will occur during wide opening, chewing of hard foods which can cause joint distraction, or anything that causes posterior displacement of the condyle.

All these conditions may cause temporary repositioning of the mandible either due to intracapsular edema or as an avoidance phenomena from nocepetive input into the CNS that alters muscular function. Permanent changes to the occlusion in the acute phase is therefore contraindicated because the mandibular position is artifactual and will change when inflammation resolves. Any of these conditions may evoke a secondary muscle response which may result in muscle pain and spasm. If the problem is long-standing, diagnosing the underlying etiologic factor may be difficult.

Arthritides

Arthritic conditions of the temporomandibular articulation are essentially the same as those of other joints, with some modifications due to specialized anatomical and functional characteristics. Arthritis of any type is a true intraarticular disease and, unlike disc derangements, may exhibit generalized involvement of many joints throughout the body. It is mentioned here for the sake of completeness. Chapter 3 contains an in-depth discussion of the classifications and treatment protocol.

Steroids given systemically have produced temporary and, often, only minor relief of intracapsular pain secondary to an inflammatory condition. The

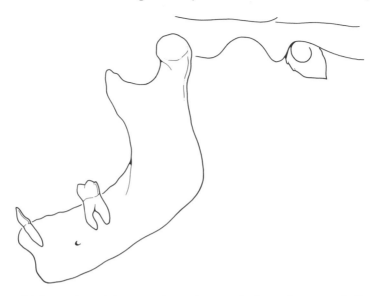

Fig. 5-14. Dislocated condyle trapped anterior to articular eminence and often elevated into infratemporal fossa.

many undesirable side effects associated with chronic use of steroids preclude their use in managing TMJ pain.

Condylar Dislocation

The capsule of the TMJ is the structure that determines the limit to which anterior joint translation can occur. Elongation of or damage to the capsular ligament may allow joint translation to occur well anterior to the articular eminence, resulting in joint dislocation.

Acute dislocation of the mandibular condyle out of the glenoid fossa demands immediate attention to relieve severe pain and minimize damage to the supporting capsule and internal ligaments of the joint. The condyle is trapped anterior to the articular eminence, and the patient is unable to close the mouth. The clinician manipulates the mandible back into the glenoid fossa by placing the thumbs over the molar teeth or retromolar pad area and applying slow, firm traction in an inferior direction to bring the condyle below the level of the eminence. The force is then directed posteriorly to seat the condyle in the glenoid fossa. Manipulating one side slightly before the other usually facilitates the reduction. It may be necessary to inject local anesthetic into and around the joint under sterile conditions or to sedate the patient with intravenous (IV) diazepam and/or narcotic to relieve pain and spasm (Fig. 5-14).

The patient should be advised to avoid wide opening of the mandible (yawning, dental treatment, large boluses of food) for at least 2 weeks. Intermaxillary fixation or elastic ligatures may be necessary after reduction if the dislocation was particularly difficult to reduce. Mild analgesic or NSAIDs may be helpful. Neuromuscular reeducation exercises are often helpful to train the patient to avoid another dislocation. Nonsurgical management will control most patients with condylar dislocations. These approaches are reviewed in Chapter 6.

Patients with recurrent dislocations should be considered for surgical treatment if the pain or condition is intolerable.

Sequence of Treatment

Once a working diagnosis is made, the modalities deemed necessary to treat will depend largely on the nature of the pain the patient is experiencing. Other than the history and physical findings, few objective tests are available to aid in diagnosing mandibular-related problems. Therapeutic tools should be used in a manner that will offer diagnostic information. The physiologic effects of all modalities described previously must be understood if they are to serve the dual role of having diagnostic and therapeutic value. If a specific treatment is successful, it is not only therapeutic to the patient but also confirms the diagnosis. If the modality is ineffective in alleviating pain or restoring function, it still offers valuable diagnostic information and will help guide further treatment. The efficacy of certain modalities often lies in the clinician's skill and judgment. The shotgun approach of offering numerous types of therapy at the same time may be temporarily successful but the tendency to overtreat and the lack of confirmation of the original diagnosis often outweigh short-term gains.

The treatment of TMJ, masticatory, and cervical dysfunction problems is not technique oriented. Treatment must be tailored to the individual patient. Patients should understand that treatment is aimed at helping them manage their problem to a level of tolerance and that "cures" rarely exist. Ideally, the level reached is one of normal function and total comfort. This should be interpreted as a level of management and not cure, however, since relapses can and do occur.

The need for a comprehensive diagnosis and coordinated treatment plan for the patient with involvement of more than one aspect of head and neck musculoskeletal dysfunction cannot be overstressed. Muscle is the common denominator to the dentist and physical therapist, and an understanding of each other's treatment principles is imperative.

The sequence of treatment for the patient with significant muscle involvement of both the neck and jaw muscles often varies depending on the location of the pain and the degree of muscle involvement. For example, a patient with an anteriorly dislocated disc with reduction may not tolerate forward repositioning of the mandible if there is concomitant severe muscle spasm in the neck or face. It may then be necessary to delay treatment of the intracapsular problem and treat the muscle condition by physical therapy or splint therapy aimed at temporary stabilization of the occlusion. Once this is accomplished, treatment of the dislocated disc may then be tolerated. Another example may be the patient who is initially under the care of the physical therapist for significant cervical muscle pain but who also has a marked malocclusion. Physical therapy may offer limited relief until maxillomandibular relationships are addressed, at which time further physical therapy becomes significantly more effective.

A general rule of thumb for sequencing treatment of patients with multiple areas of involvement is to treat the area of the greatest pain involvement first. This may require temporary disregard to physical imbalances such as malocclusions or aberrant head positioning until a later more appropriate time. The sequence of treatment modalities and the manner in which they are applied to such patients requires considerable skill and communication between the clinicians involved. If the diagnosis is correct, failure to gain relief of symptoms is not necessarily the result of an inappropriate choice of the modlitites. Instead, it can be the result of an error in the sequence or manner in which they are applied.

Numerous facets of pain, pain behavior, and musculoskeletal disturbances remain unknown. Population norms for many of the clinical guidelines to treatment now in vogue have not been established. Much information can be gleaned from treatment of other muscle–joint systems in the body and from open dialogue among the several disciplines involved in the treatment of pain. A multidisciplinary approach to such complex issues appears mandatory.

SUGGESTED READINGS

Academy of Denture Prosthetics (ADP): Glossary of Prosthodontic Terms. 3rd Ed. J Prosthet Dent 20;443, 1968

Atwood DA: A critique of research of the rest position of the mandible. J Prosthet Dent 16:848, 1966

Annandale T: On displacement of the interarticular cartilage of the lower jaw and its treatment by operation. Lancet 1:411, 1887

Beard CC, Clayton Joseph A: Effects of occlusal therapy on TMJ dysfunction. J Prosthet Dent 44:324, 1980

Bell W: Orofacial Pains: Differential Diagnosis. Year Book Medical, Chicago, 1979

Carlsson GE: Mandibular dysfunction and temporomandibular joint pathosis. J Prosthet Dent 43:658, 1980

Farrar WB: Diagnosis and treatment of anterior dislocation of the articular disc. NY J Dent 41:348, 1972

Farrar WB: Differentiation of temporomandibular joint dysfunction to simplify treatment. J Prosthet Dent 28:629, 1979

Isberg-Holm A: Temporomandibular Joint Clicking. Department of Oral Radiation, Karolinska Institute, Stockholm, Sweden, 1980

Goldstein DF, Kraus SL, Williams WB: Influence of cervical posture on mandibular movement. J Prosthet Dent 52(3):421, 1984

Kreutziger KL, Mahan PE: Temporomandibular degenerative joint disease. Part I. Anatomy, pathophysiology and clinical description. Oral Surg 40:165, 1975

Laskin DM: Etiology of the pain-dysfunction syndrome. J Am Dent Assoc 79:147, 1969

Meyer RA, Merrill RG, Razook SJ, et al: Temporomandibular Joint Disorders: Update, 1982. Continuing education course material, Emory University School of Dentistry.

McNeil C, Danzig WM, Farrar WB, et al: Craniomandibular (TMJ) disorders. The state of the art. J Prosthet Dent 44:434, 1980

Mohl ND: Head posture and its role in occlusion. NY State Dent J 42:17, 1976

Mohl ND: The role of head posture in mandibular function. In Abnormal Jaw Mechanics. Quintessence, Chicago, 1984

Posselt U: Studies on the mobility of the human mandible. Acta Ondont Scand 10:1, 1952

Ramjford SP, Ash MM: Occlusion. 3rd Ed. WB Saunders, Philadelphia, 1983

Root GR, Kraus SL, Razook SJ, Samson GS: Effect of an intraoral splint on head and neck posture. J Prosthet Dent 58(1):90, 1987

Sicher H: Structural and functional basis for disorders of the temporomandibular articulation. J Oral Surg 13:275, 1955

Travell J: Temporomandibular joint pain referred from the muscles of the head and neck. J Prosthet Dent 10:745, 1960

Travell J, Simons D: Myofascial Pain and Dysfunction: The Trigger Point Manual. Williams & Wilkins, Baltimore, 1983

6 Physical Therapy Management of TMJ Dysfunction

Steven L. Kraus

Physical therapists see many patients with head, neck, facial, and jaw symptoms. Most patients are referred by health professionals such as orthopedists, neurologists, or rheumatologists. Because health professionals may not have thoroughly evaluated the TMJ, the functional evaluation of the neuromusculoskeletal system performed by the physical therapist will need to include examination of the TMJs.

The physical therapist's *first role* in the management of TMJ disorders is evaluation of the TMJ following the guidelines established in this book. When the physical therapist is confronted with a patient with a TMJ disorder, the therapist will initiate appropriate therapy depending on what tissue(s) are involved. If the involved tissues are outside the physical therapist's expertise, or if the evaluative findings are questionable or vague, the *second role* of the physical therapist is to refer the patient to the appropriate dentist.

The *third role* of the physical therapist in the management of TMJ disorders is evaluation of the cervical spine, which has many distinguishing features pertinent to the TMJ. The cervical spine is a major source of referred symptoms in the areas of the TMJ, head, oral, and masticatory regions. The physical therapist performs a functional evaluation of the cervical spine structures (facet joints, discs, muscles, soft tissues, etc.). During the evaluation, the therapist may reproduce and/or increase the patient's symptoms. Referred symptoms that are consistently reproduced are an indication to investigate further for cervical spine dysfunction. Patients have unfortunately been diagnosed as having TMJ problems based on symptoms rather than objective signs of dysfunction. Failure to acknowledge that objective signs of cervical spine dysfunction can be a major source of referred symptoms cephalad can lead to incorrect diagnoses.

The *fourth role* the physical therapist has in the management of TMJ disorders is providing actual treatment to the cervical spine. Treatments offered for cervical spine dysfunction should attend not only to the local symptoms but to symptoms referred cephalad. Concepts in the evaluation and treatment of cervical spine dysfunction are discussed in Chapter 11. Correction of cervical spine dysfunction will diminish the adverse influences that cervical spine dysfunction has on positioning and movement of the mandible. Working directly with the cervical spine will enhance the management of TMJ disorders and myofascial involvement of the mandibular and cervical musculature. Cervical spine influences on the craniomandibular region is discussed in Chapter 12.

The *fifth role* of the physical therapist in the management of TMJ disorders is the primary emphasis of this chapter. Specific treatments offered by the physical therapist to assist in managing the position and movement of the TMJ and mandible are described.

Factors Influencing TMJ Movement and Positioning

The variety and complexity of mandibular movements is due to the bony structures of the TMJs and the associated musculature. Articulation, mastication, swallowing, yawning, coughing, and licking of the lips are all physiological activities involving movements of the condyles. A mandibular position common to all the previously mentioned movements is the so-called "rest position" (the upright postural position of the mandible). The rest position may be defined as representing the mandibular posture from which all physiological activities are initiated and automatically (reflexly) returned to when such activities are terminated.[1] Parafunctional activities such as bruxism also involve movements of the mandible from its rest position. The muscle hyperactivity associated with the parafunctional activities, however, does not allow the mandible to reflexly return to its rest position.

Factors influencing and limiting the condyles during movement, at rest, and in occlusion, are clinically important to understand, recognize, and treat. Such factors as the dentition, osseous structures, muscles and intraarticular causes such disc–condyle derangements and edema are addressed in other chapters. This chapter is divided into two sections. The first section discusses the importance of the periarticular tissues and their influence on condylar movement and positioning of the TMJ. The second section discusses the steps the physical therapist may take to assist the patient in achieving neuromuscular control over mandibular movement and positioning.

PERIARTICULAR TISSUE

Periarticular tissue refers to the capsular-ligamentous tissue of joints. The entire lateral aspect of the capsule is thickened, forming the temporomandibular ligament, and should be regarded as a part of and inseparable from the capsule.[2]

A capsule is simply a "sac-like envelope which encloses the cavity of a synovial joint by attaching to the circumference of the articular end of each involved bone. . . ."[3] The capsule of the TMJ, although somewhat deficient anteriorly, is circumferentially attached to the rim of the glenoid fossa and articular eminence of the temporal bone above and to the neck of the condyle below. The capsule is dense, irregular connective tissue with two layers. The outer fibrous layer consists mostly of collagen, and the inner layer is the synovial lining. The capsule must have an adequate blood supply in order to bring nutrients from the cells that make up the synovial membrane which, in turn, produce synovial fluid.[4]

The physiological and neurophysiological necessity of having extensibility of a joint capsule has been well documented in the literature.[5-9] Clinically, the physical therapist applying mobilization techniques to a "tight" capsule (hip, knee, spine, etc.) appreciates the therapeutic results of an increase in range of motion (ROM); a decrease in pain and a normalization of muscle tone. Scientific research regarding the etiology, sequelae, treatment, and prognosis of loss of TMJ capsule extensibility is insufficient. Therefore, further discussion on the extensibility and loss of extensibility of the TMJ capsule is based on research done on other synovial joints. The following sections on capsular change are not comprehensive but highlight those articles supporting the clinical need to evaluate and treat capsular tightness of the TMJ.

Capsular Tightness Affecting the Kinematics of the TMJ

The nature of movement at any joint is largely determined by the joint structure, including the shape of the joint surfaces. The traditional structural classification of the TMJ is ginglymoarthrodial. Ginglymus means a simple hinge joint. Arthrodia means a form of joint in which the articular surfaces are flat and glide over or against each other during movements.[10] The traditional classification of joint movement includes the following types of movement[11]:

1. Angular—indicating an increase or decrease in the angle formed between two bones (e.g., flexion-extension at the elbow).
2. Circumduction—the movement of a bone circumscribes a cone (e.g., circumduction at the hip or shoulder).
3. Rotation—movement occurring around the longitudinal axis of a bone (e.g., internal-external rotation at the shoulder).
4. Sliding—one bone slides over another with little or no appreciable rotation or angular movement (e.g., movement occurring between carpals).

This type of movement classification describes movement occurring between bones but ignores the type of movement that occurs between joint surfaces. The study of movement occurring between bones and movement occurring between joint surfaces, is divided into osteokinematics and arthrokinematics, respectively.[12,13]

Osteokinematics deals primarily with the overall movement of bones (mandible) with little reference to their related joints. Arthrokinematics is concerned more with the intimate mechanics of the movements occurring between joint surfaces (condyle and the articular eminence). An essential element to having normal kinematics of the mandible and articular surfaces is to have proper extensibility of the TMJ capsule.

Osteokinematics

Three basic movements exist in the mandible. The motions can be described as (1) opening and closing, (2) protrusive-retrusive, and (3) lateral shifts in the horizontal plane.[14] These three basic movements can be combined to produce an infinite variety of mandibular movements. When osteokinematics of the mandible are examined, the relative clinical information is derived mainly from the opening, protrusive and lateral shift movements of the mandible. The range of mandibular movement, how the mandible moves through the available range, and the end position of the mandible are all observations the examiner should consider in the evaluation.

Osteokinematic testing is done with the patient's teeth apart. Before the clinician observes each movement (opening, protrusive, and lateral shifts), the patient is instructed: "Bite, bring the back teeth together, and now relax your jaw." Establishing a consistent jaw position prior to each mandibular movement tested assures the same mandibular position for repeated tests. Different jaw positions prior to movement may influence the overall movement being tested.

When osteokinematics are examined, and a series of restrictions/deflections is observed, one can suspect capsular tightness. Such a series of altered mandibular dynamics suggest a "capsular pattern." The capsular pattern of the TMJ as observed during active mandibular movements is:

1. Depression—A "C" curve deflection to the side of capsular involvement, with opening measured less than 40 mm. (Functional opening will be considered 40 mm, measured between the anterior central incisors.)

2. Protrusion—A deflection of the mandible to the side of involvement. The patient may be unable to achieve an edge-to-edge position with the anterior central incisors. (Functional protrusive range is achievement of at least an edge-to-edge position of the anterior central incisors.)

3. Lateral excursion—Lateral movement will be normal to the side of involvement. Lateral movement to the opposite side of involvement will be decreased. (Functional lateral movement is present when the bottom frenulum of the mandible moves at least the width of one full upper central incisor, approximately 8 mm wide.)

When a capsular pattern exists, the restricted osteokinematic movements may be misdiagnosed as an acute anterior disc dislocation that does not reduce. Differential diagnosis of these two conditions is essential. Guidelines to the etiology and evaluation pertaining to a capsular tightness and an anterior disc dislocation that does not reduce will assist the clinician in making the appropriate diagnosis.

Arthrokinematics

In orthopedic physical therapy, a particular jargon has evolved, as it has in many clinical specialties. Unfortunately, the use of certain terms is often inconsistent. Presented next are the most common and useful definitions.

Arthrokinematics of any joint involves a study of accessory joint movements. Accessory movements are simply those arthrokinematic movements that must occur to achieve a full, pain-free osteokinematic movement to be present. Accessory movements are occurring in response to muscle contractions, guided by the shape of the articulating surfaces and the periarticular tissues. "Active" accessory movements include: spin, roll, slide, (translation), distraction, and compression.[15–17]

Accessory movements of a joint that cannot be produced by the action of muscle contractions but instead are produced passively in response to an outside force are called joint play movements.[18] Joint play movements include any one or a combination of the spin, roll, slide, distraction, and compression active accessory movements. These joint play movements can occur in any particular joint position. Joint play movements are the inherent quality of the joint to "give." The "built-in" factor of joint play is critical to promote efficient functional movements.[19] A hinge on a door that has play between its components to allow the door to open and close smoothly and easily is analogous. A loss or decrease in the joint play movement(s) of the TMJ may be a primary restricting factor to osteokinematic movements of the mandible.

The absence of active or passive accessory movements secondary to capsular tightness can be a primary cause of dysfunction and localized pain of the TMJ. Mandibular muscle imbalance resulting from the diminished accessory movements will probably occur.

Capsular Tightness Affecting the Articular Cartilage

Joints lacking full ROM due to capsular tightness or other mechanisms of immobilization will have a distinct reduction in the supply of blood to the joint capsule.[20] The resulting reduction in supply of oxygen and nutrients to the articular cartilage can reach critical levels. Without full range of joint movement, synovial fluid will mix inadequately. Waste products of metabolism will accumulate on the surfaces of the cartilage, causing cartilage cell dystrophy. Joint immobilization can therefore initiate an arthritic process.[20]

Another area of concern occurring secondary to capsular tightness is improper loading of articular cartilage. Biomechanically, a tight capsule may not allow normal arthrokinematic movements to occur between joint surfaces and result in improper loading of the articular cartilage. The main function of articular cartilage is to distribute compressive forces to the underlying subchondral bone.[6,21] A "tight" capsule will cause certain areas of the articular cartilage to receive higher impact loads, possibly leading to fatigue failure and arthritic changes in the articular cartilage. The effects on articular cartilage of a change in impact loading secondary to capsular tightness is dependent on the amplitudes, frequency, duration, and rate of application of such loading.[22]

An article entitled, "The Effects of Immobilization on the Primate Temporomandibular Joint"[23] concluded that prolonged immobilization of the TMJ by intermaxillary wire fixation results in degenerative changes in the articular cartilage. The degenerative changes of such immobilization may be reversed once remobilization is established. A direct correlation between immobilization by intermaxillary wire fixation and varying degrees of immobilization by capsular tightness cannot yet be drawn.

Capsular Tightness Affecting Mechanoreceptor Activity

More than 20 years ago, Thilander published an excellent article on the innervation of the TMJ in humans.[24] As clinicians, we must acknowledge the importance of the mechanoreceptors of the TMJ and how mechanoreceptor activity can be altered by a loss of capsular extensibility. The sequela of altered mechanoreceptor activity must then be investigated.

The TMJ contains as do all mammalian synovial joints, four types of receptor nerve endings, which can be differentiated by their morphologic and functional characteristics.[25] TMJ synovial receptors are located in the fibrous joint capsule, the lateral ligament, and the retrodiscal pad, but not in the intraarticular disc (central portion) and synovial tissues. Terminating on the receptors are the deep temporal, masseter, and auriculotemporal nerves, which originate from the mandibular division of cranial nerve V.[26,27]

Type I receptors discharge continuously because they are low-threshhold, slow-adapting receptors. Continuous discharging occurs, even when the mandible is at rest. The type I receptors provide continuous kinesthetic and postural perception of the mandible. Type I receptors also exert powerful reciprocally coordinated facilitatory and inhibitory reflex effects on motor unit activity of the mandibular muscles.[25]

Type II receptors are low-threshhold and rapid-adapting receptors that fire briefly as mandibular movements are initiated and exert transient coordinated reflex effects on the related musculature.

Type III receptors are high-threshhold and slow-adapting receptors that do not fire under normal circumstances. Type III receptors become active only when excessive tension is developed in the lateral TMJ ligament. Type III activation has been demonstrated to result reflexly in pterygoid and mylohyoid muscle spasms and temporalis and masseter muscle inhibition.[25]

Type IV receptors constitute the pain-receptor system of the articular tissues and are entirely inactive in normal circumstances. They become active when the TMJ articular tissues (joint capsule, retrodiscal pad, and TMJ ligament) are subjected either to marked mechanical deformation and tension or direct chemical irritation.[28]

Afferent discharges from types I, II, and III, as well as other receptors in the skin, subcutaneous tissue, and muscles around the synovial joints all converge on inhibitory interneurons, segmentally and intersegmentally. This convergence modulates the centripetal flow of nociceptive afferent activity derived from the joint tissues having type IV receptors. One may assume that the degree of TMJ pain experienced by a patient depends not only on the intensity of type IV irritation but also on the frequency of ongoing afferent discharges from the various types of mechanoreceptors embedded in the same TMJ capsule and related soft tissues and muscles.[29] Deliberate stimulation of the type I, II, and III mechanoreceptors in the TMJ capsule and adjacent tissues by the use of transcutaneous electrical stimulation (TENS) or intraoral manual oscillatory techniques may help enhance the modulating effect of the primary afferent activity on the type IV receptors of the TMJ. If capsular tightness is the primary cause of type IV activation, complete alleviation of pain may occur when proper intraoral arthrokinematic techniques are applied, restoring capsular extensibility.

Deliberate stimulation of the type I, II, and III mechanoreceptors in the cervical spine or the correction of any joint, capsule, or muscle problems in the cervical spine may modulate segmentally, intersegmentally, and cortically the type IV receptor activity stemming from the TMJ. Clinical results observed by stimulating the cervical spine mechanoreceptors to modulate type IV receptor activity of the TMJ is based on the neurophysiological relationship between the cervical and trigeminal sensory neurons.[30]

Loss of capsular extensibility needs to be investigated when patients perceived that their "bite is off." Patient perception of "malocclusion" may be related to various factors. A factor often overlooked is capsular tightness. Capsular tightness affecting mechanoreceptor activity contributes to improper joint proprioceptive feedback and jaw muscle activity, thereby influencing initial tooth/teeth contact.

Various dental procedures may need to be reexamined if such procedures place the condyle in a "strained" position. An example is the condyle position for recapturing an anterior dislocation of the disc that reduces with an anterior repositioning appliance. The corrected disc–condyle relationship is often an overcorrected position anteriorly and can be considered a strained position for the joint capsule. Such an overcorrected position may not be conducive to the articular receptor system of the TMJ capsule, especially when it appears that the mechanoreceptors located in the anterior region of the joint capsule make a facilitory contribution to supramandibular muscle activity.[31] Capsular tightness influencing the patient's tolerance to such an appliance varies depending on the preexisting extensibility of the joint capsule and the amount of over-corrected position of the condyle caused by the anterior repositioning appliance.

Techniques used by dentists to establish centric relation (CR) may be a strained position for the capsule, especially if it is already tight. Centric relation depends on every dentist's conception of what CR should be, how important CR is, and what technique(s) is used to achieve such a position.

Mechanoreceptor activity will be altered not only by capsular tightness, but also by capsular distension occurring with joint effusion. The correct application of modalities (ice and ultrasound), interocclusal appliances, or medication to control the swelling will help resolve the joint effusion and thus normalize mechanoreceptor activity. Muscle imbalances can occur from a distended joint capsule. Strengthening exercises to mandibuler muscles should be used with caution when joint effusion exists if the result of such joint effusion may be reflex muscle inhibition.[32] Exercises attempting to strengthen muscles are futile if one does not recognize that muscle weakness may be pseudoweakness.[33]

In summary, proper extensibility of the TMJ capsule will help decrease the mechanical stress that can stimulate the type IV nociceptor system. Extensibility of the TMJ capsule allows proper mechanoreceptor activity to occur. In turn, this extensibility provides kinesthetic and perceptional awareness of the mandible. Normal activity of the muscles innervated by cranial nerve V that regulate mandibular movement and position is enhanced by proper mechanoreceptor activity of the TMJ.

Etiology of Capsular Tightness

Biochemical and biomechanical changes occur in the capsule when normal ROM of the joint is decreased. Biochemically, a reduction in water and glycosaminoglycans (GAG) results. GAG and water form a semifluid viscous gel that acts as a lubricant between collagen fibers making up the outer layer of the capsule. Free gliding of collagen fibers over one another is essential for the extensibility of a joint capsule. Biomechanically, when water and GAG are reduced, the capsule becomes tight because of the loss of the free gliding of the collagen fibers. This classically occurs in response to immobilization.[34-37]

Immobilization may be complete (fixated) or partial. Partial immobilization can occur if joint pain makes the patient unwilling to move the joint completely. Partial immobilization also occurs with muscle tightness, anterior disc dislocation that does not reduce, and orthodontic elastics used between the maxillary and mandibular teeth, as well as after TMJ surgery. The result is a capsule unable to experience its full extensibility, leading to biomechanical and biochemical changes in the joint capsule.

Joint capsules may also lose their extensibility with a resolution of an acute articular inflammatory process or a chronic low-grade inflammatory process.[38] Such inflammatory processes may involve the joint capsule directly. The result of either inflammatory process is an increase in collagen fiber content, contributing to the loss of capsular extensibility. The more destructive the process, the more vigorous the repair response and collagen production during resolution. More collagen production occurs with an acute inflammatory process as compared with relatively low-grade, noninfectious joint inflammation.[38] In acute inflammatory conditions, the period of immobilization is greater because of pain and because the patient is encouraged to use the jaw less. The biochemical and biomechanical changes previously described with immobilization enter into the inflammatory process cycle, compounding the loss in capsular extensibility.

When an increase in collagen production occurs secondary to the inflammatory process involving capsular tissue, resolution of the situation is more difficult. Remodeling of the excess collagen and realignment of the collagen fibers and abnormally placed cross-links among the collagen fibers are all factors possibly hampering normalization of capsular extensibility.[36,38]

Clinically, capsular tightness resulting from immobilization only will resolve rapidly. Conditions involving an increase in collagen production within the joint capsule resulting from an inflammatory process respond much more slowly to treatment. The following list briefly discusses the conditions that may cause TMJ capsular tightness (all or part of the capsule involved). Conditions are listed in decreasing order of rapidity of return of capsular extensibility in response to joint mobilization techniques.

I. Simple Immobilization
   A. *Orthognathic surgery*: The patient's maxillomandibular relationship is fixated, usually for a period of 6 to 8 weeks.
   B. *TMJ surgery*: The presence of postoperative pain, joint effusion, and reflex muscle guarding restrict joint movement.
   C. *Orthodontic banding*: Partial immobilization occurs when the maxillary arch is banded to the mandibular arch by restrictive elastics.
II. Capsular Trauma
   A. *Macrotrauma*: Macrotrauma results from a direct blow to the mandible (spraining the capsule) or from TMJ surgery. The immobilization that follows is caused by pain, joint effusion, and reflex muscle guarding. The capsule may also heal in a shortened state, or may adhere to adjacent tissues during the healing process. Adhesions may develop between the joint surfaces and the interarticular disc. The intraoral techniques used in examining and treating capsular tightness will also help resolve the intraarticular adhesions occurring between the joint surfaces and the interarticular disc.
   B. *Microtrauma*: Microtrauma may occur with a "malocclusion of the teeth resulting in a change of the maxillomandibular relationship and therefore in a change in joint position and in the pattern of capsular

stress. . . .''[39] A "pseudomalocclusion" secondary to altered head-neck posture may also lead to capsular stress. This concept of pseudomalocclusion secondary to altered head-neck posture is discussed in Chapter 12. Habits place a strain on the TMJ capsule, which can result in microtrauma to the capsule. Such habits as chewing gum, biting on pencils, and leaning the jaw on the hands should be avoided.

III. Degenerative Arthrosis
IV. Rheumatoid Arthritis
 V. Infectious Arthritis

Joint effusion can cause capsular tightness due to distension of the joint capsule. Parts of the capsule normally lax, allowing a certain ROM, are no longer lax because of capsular distension. Conditions causing a restriction and deviation in movement due to joint effusion are related to inflammatory processes such as rheumatoid arthritis, infectious arthritis, gout, synovitis, and retrodiscal inflammation. Direct trauma to the joint capsule also involves joint effusion, especially if the joint capsule is torn or stretched. Inflammatory conditions causing distension of the joint capsule and restrictions in joint movement must be recognized. Stretching the joint capsule in these inflammatory conditions by the use of intraoral techniques or exercises is contraindicated. Instead, the clinician should assist in resolution of the acute intracapsular inflammatory process. Once the inflammation is controlled, examining and treating for capsular tightness by intraoral techniques may be necessary.

Examining for Capsular Tightness

Relevant history, restricted mandibular osteokinematic movements, and restricted joint play movements will determine if capsular tightness exists. When the "total" capsule is tight, mandibular deflections and restrictions will manifest as a capsular pattern.

The capsular pattern has already been discussed in the osteokinematics section. Whenever translation is restricted, as in a total capsular tightness, the condyle is still able to rotate but not translate. Rotation will allow 20 to 25 mm of mandibular opening.[40,41] During opening, the mandible will deflect to the side of capsular tightness. Spin, like rotation, does not require extensibility of the joint capsule. Normal range of active lateral excursion of the mandible toward the side of capsular tightness occurs because the ipsilateral condyle spins. Active lateral excursion to the contralateral side of the capsular tightness is restricted. Protrusion, which involves translation, is also restricted, resulting in deflection to the side of capsular tightness. Pain, muscle guarding, and/or inflammation, if involved, influences the overall amount of opening, protrusive, and lateral excursions.

Clinically, the active accessory movement primarily limited by capsular tightness is translation. Distraction, translation, and "lateral glide" will be the joint play movements that are limited.[42] Lateral glide is an additional joint play movement to those joint play movements covered in the arthrokinematic section. Lateral glide should not be confused with lateral excursion of the mandible. The active accessory movement of translation, when restricted by capsular tightness, is restored by treating any combination of distraction, translation, and lateral glide joint play movements.

Without a capsular pattern, certain aspects of the capsule can still be tight. A clinical challenge then occurs. No obvious osteokinematic restrictions/deflections may be observed during mandibular dynamic testing when only partial capsular tightness is present. Minor or major symptoms may still result if portions of the capsule are tight. To determine if certain areas of the capsule are tight, the clinician examines for joint play movements (distraction, translation, and lateral glide) by using intraoral techniques.

Hand placement, direction of force, and stabilization of the patient for the application of these joint play examination techniques is covered in the treatment section (p. 150). Obvious modifications in techniques will apply when examining rather than treating for the loss of joint play movements. For evaluation of joint play, the force is a slow, steady, deliberate pressure that allows the clinician to feel a "give" at the end of the expected range. Whenever possible, placing a finger of the stabilizing hand over the lateral pole to palpate

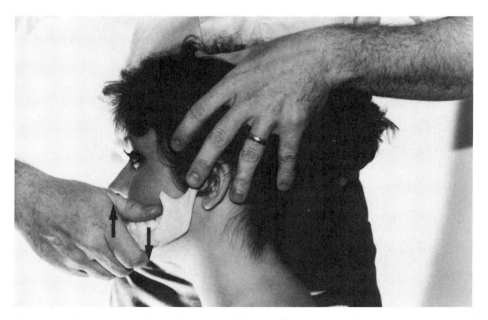

Fig. 6-1. Distraction indicated for examining and/or treating joint play movement of distraction; recapturing an anterior disc dislocation that does not reduce (see Chapter 3); unloading the joint to help in differentiation of a capsulitis or retrodiskitis (see Chapter 4). Direction of force: The thumb presses down on molars as the rest of the hand pulls up slightly on the front of the mandible (force couple).

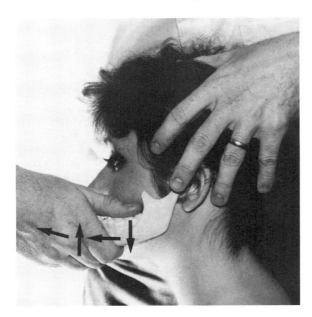

Fig. 6-2. Translation with distraction indicated for examining and treating joint play movement of translation and distraction; recapturing an anterior disc dislocation that does not reduce, with emphasis on translation; relocating a dislocated condyle: Translation would be in the posterior direction. Direction of force: Distraction is the same as in Fig. 6-1. The rest of the hand pulls mandible forward and slightly across midline.

for the expected movement will help in the examination (Figs. 6-1 through 6-3). A capsular restriction is determined by the clinician's concept of "normal" for the movement tested. A "gummy" end feel may best describe what is felt at the end of the pathological range caused by a tight capsule. If possible, the state of the dysfunctional joint can be compared with the noninvolved contralateral joint. The patient's subjective response as to the degree of irritability or a therapeutic feeling is to be considered. The clinician's knowledge of anatomy and mechanics and experience, expertise, application of force, and stabilization of the patient will aid in making a clinical judgment regarding any limitation in joint play movements.

Treatment for Capsular Tightness

When capsular tightness exists, the patient should be considered as having TMJ dysfunction, a category of TMJ disorders. There are, indeed, other causes for TMJ dysfunction. The primary treatment for capsular tightness is application of intraoral joint mobilization techniques. These joint mobilization techniques should be directed at the area or areas of capsular tightness.

Joint mobilization is a very general term that can be applied to any active or passive attempt to increase movement of a joint. The term mobilization, as used in this chapter, refers to specific mobilization techniques applied to areas of capsular tightness that are restricting distraction, translation, and lateral glide joint play movements.

Restoring normal arthrokinematics of a joint will allow full, pain-free os-

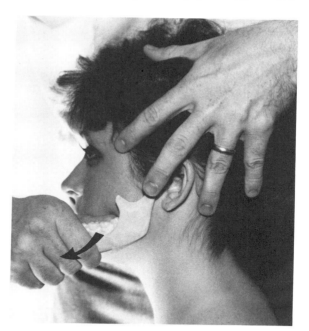

Fig. 6-3. Lateral glide indicated for examining and treating joint play movement of lateral glide. Direction of force: The thumb on the inside of the molars is pressing out, slightly down and forward. The rest of the hand is pulling the tip of the mandible slightly across midline, in the opposite direction of the joint being mobilized.

teokinematic movements to occur. Using intraoral techniques rather than forcing osteokinematic movements results in less risk of damaging the joint by compressing isolated portions of the articular cartilage or overstretching isolated capsular ligamentous structures. In the initial treatment phase, the use of force between the anterior central incisors by the use of separating arms of a mouth prop and/or by having the patients themselves pry with their fingers anteriorly is discouraged. The rationale for the use of joint mobilization techniques is to restore specific arthrokinematic movement limited secondary to capsular tightness.

The involvement of joint tissues, including the tissues of the TMJ, rarely occurs singly but usually in combination with other tissues. The clinician must recognize when to examine for joint play movements and then apply joint mobilization techniques. Such intraoral examining and treatment techniques often need to be used in sequence or in combination with other forms of treatments. The following are a few examples of situations in which a tight capsule may exist but, because of the very nature of the situation, joint play intraoral examining and treatment techniques will either have to be applied later or omitted.

1. Joint effusion, capsulitis, and or muscle guarding.
2. TMJ surgery: Waiting 2 to 3 weeks after surgery will usually be satisfactory. This may vary from surgeon to surgeon and according to the type of TMJ surgery performed. If the surgery was a posterior and/or lateral disc plication and/or graft repair, use of the joint play lateral glide technique initially is discouraged because it may place undue stress at the surgical repair sight. Satisfactory improvement in mobility after TMJ plication and graft surgery is

achieved by using distraction and translation intraoral techniques. In surgery involving discectomies replaced by an implant, all intraoral techniques are safe and effective.

3. A symptomatic anterior disc dislocation that reduces, being treated by an interocclusal appliance: No examination or treatment using intraoral joint mobilization techniques should be applied until "healing" of the disc attachments occurs.

Joint Mobilization Techniques

Distraction. Distraction is application of a force parallel to the longitudinal axis of the bone that one wishes to move, in this case, the mandible. Distraction is the preferred intraoral technique because of the safety, ease, and effectiveness of its application. The clinician's thumb is placed on the patient's molars, on the side of capsular involvement, with the remaining fingers wrapping comfortably around the patient's chin (Fig. 6-1). The clinician's other hand stabilizes the patient's cranium, the middle or index finger palpating the lateral pole to monitor movement. If a limitation of jaw opening prevents placement of the thumb on top of the molars, the clinician can begin in the premolar area, progressing with the thumb into the molar areas as more opening occurs. Caution should be taken because premolar contact will tend to induce osteokinematic rather than arthrokinematic movement unless the clinician is alert to the forces being placed on the mandible.

All intraoral techniques are done with the clinician standing on the opposite side of the involved capsule. Preferably, the techniques are done with the patient lying supine with the cervical spine supported appropriately. Patients can be sitting for these techniques, but relaxation by the patient is sometimes more difficult (all intraoral techniques have been demonstrated in the sitting position for clarity).

Distraction has three stages:[43]

Stage I: Piccolo—movement so small that only the compression effect on the joint is released as the joint pressure is neutralized. The joint surfaces are not separated from each other.

Stage II: Taking up the slack, using little force, moving the joint partner only as far as the soft tissues allow.

Stage III: A continuation and an extension of stage II, but using more force.

Translation. Anterior translation follows distraction (Fig. 6-2). Anterior translation is always performed in either stage I, II, or III distraction to avoid any jamming effect of the disc-condyle-articular eminence relationship. Hand placement for translation is the same as for distraction. Anterior translation is done not only by pulling the condyle straight forward, but also by pulling forward and slightly across midline.

Lateral Glide. Lateral glide hand contact places the thumb on the inside of the molars. The fingers wrap around the mandible comfortably. The other hand stabilizes the cranium, with the middle or index finger palpating the lateral pole to monitor movement (Fig. 6-3). Lateral glide is done by pressing laterally with the thumb, at the same time directing the force slightly downward and forward. Using this direction of force avoids discomfort on the contralateral side, which may occur if a lateral glide is done only in the horizontal plane.

While distraction, translation, and lateral glide joint play techniques are applied, graded rhythmic oscillatory movements may also be applied. Rhythmic oscillatory movements are graded 1 through 5.[44] The grades of oscillations refer to location of occurrence in the range and the amplitude of the oscillations rendered.

Grade I: Small-amplitude motion performed at the beginning of the available range.

Grade II: Large-amplitude motion performed within the available range.

Grade III: Larger-amplitude motion performed up to the limit of range available.

Grade IV: Small-amplitude motion performed at the limit of range.

Grade V: Manipulation, which is a high-velocity, low-amplitude thrust, is performed at the limits of the available range. Clinically, I have never found it necessary to apply a thrust to the TMJ and would not advise it.

These grades are related to the pathologic limits of the joint play movements and are not related to the normal limits of the joint. The rationale for applying joint play mobilization techniques (distraction, translation, and lateral glide) with oscillatory techniques is to achieve neurophysiologic and mechanical effects.

Distractional techniques of stages I and II and oscillatory techniques of grades I and II primarily influence the mechanoreceptors, since these techniques are done well within the available pathological range. The neurophysiologic effects of a decrease in pain, reflex inhibition of muscles, and promotion of relaxation will result, followed by an increase in ROM.[45–47]

The effects of mobilization techniques using stage III distraction and grades III and IV oscillatory techniques and the grade V thrust technique are mechanical. The range of restriction is reached with the force used moving into the area of elastic deformation of the collagen. If a tissue is stretched within the elastic range, no permanent structural change will occur. When the tissue (capsule) is stretched into the plastic range, permanent structural changes will occur.[48,49] If tissue is stretched beyond the plastic range to the fatigue point, damage may result; thus, the clinician needs to develop a sixth sense for the proper therapeutic amount, direction, and duration of forces applied.

To enhance mobilization techniques, active participation by the patient is encouraged e.g., while performing the distractional technique, have the patient actively open or close on command using minimal muscle contraction. When the patient relaxes, additional force of distraction can be achieved. Performing the distractional technique during active participation of the patient not only deals directly with a tight capsule, but the joint is also actively moved through the available range in a nonstressful, nonpainful manner. Active intermittent participation by the patient allows better proprioception by the patient of what should be perceived as a pain-free movement of the joint.

General rules for applying joint play intraoral techniques to the TMJ are:

1. Patient and clinician must be properly positioned and relaxed.
2. The patient should be stabilized firmly.
3. The clinician must be willing to modify the technique based on the tissue's response and needs. The clinician must be able to "think" through his or her fingers. This is known as "tissue" tension sense.
4. The minimum force consistent with achieving the objective should always be used: restoring capsular extensibility.

If mobilization techniques are used when not indicated or, if indicated, are used out of sequence, or if the direction or amount of force is improperly applied, resulting symptoms and signs may be: (1) increase in pain, (2) increase in swelling and/or muscle guarding, and (3) decrease in mobility.

Patient Preparation Prior to Intraoral Joint Mobilization Techniques

To prepare the articular capsule for the specific joint mobilization techniques, heat is placed on the capsule prior to and during stretching with tongue blades. Tongue blades are placed far back on the molars on the side of the involved joint, placing the capsule on moderate stretch. After heat, ice may be placed on the capsule while maintaining the capsule on stretch with the tongue blades. This use of the combination of heat/ice while the tongue blades stretches the joint capsule appears to achieve better results in tight periarticular tissue.[50,51]

Forcing a stretch with tongue blades is not encouraged; instead, the tongue blades are simply used to take up the slack. Tight capsules secondary to post TMJ surgery will not be placed in the stretched position for a long duration at first. No more than one to two minutes of stretching post TMJ surgery is recommended initially. The use of heat and ice while on stretch with the tongue blades will become more effective as the time of use of the tongue blades is increased.

The use of tongue blades serves an additional function of stretching the tight elevator muscles of the mandible that usually accompany a restriction in jaw opening. These muscles (temporalis, masseter, internal pterygoid) are unable to lengthen because of the various factors restricting jaw opening, such as capsular tightness, postorthognathic surgery, post-TMJ surgery, or an anterior disc dislocation that does not reduce.

Animal studies have shown that when a muscle is subjected to changes in length, it undergoes anatomic, biochemical, and physiologic changes that are not immediately obvious or readily considered by the clinician.[52] These length-associated changes occur within a few hours, days, or weeks. Animal studies indicate that muscles that cannot lengthen have a decreased number of sarcomeres in both young and adult animals. In the young, the rate of additional new sarcomeres decreases; in the adult, there is an absolute loss of sarcomeres.[53] Biochemical changes that occur to a muscle that cannot lengthen include increased catabolism and a concomitant loss of weight.[54] Physiologically, the amount of passive and active tension developed by a shortened muscle is less than that of normal muscles.[55] Studies indicate[52] that termination of immobilization results in full recovery from the anatomic, biochemical, and physiologic changes. Recovery is time-dependent and may occur within a few days to up to 60 days after termination of immobilization of the muscle.

This brief overview of length-associated changes emphasizes the need to regain normal mandibular dynamics as soon as possible. Careful use of tongue blades intraorally to take up the slack will aid not only in regaining capsular extensibility but also muscle length. Muscle length will also be increased by neuromuscular exercises done by the patient (these are discussed later in the chapter).

The reader is cautioned not to confuse a tight muscle undergoing length-associated changes with a tight muscle having an increase in muscle tone secondary to an increase in γ motor neuron activity. An increase in motor neuron activity occurs in response to, but not limited to, peripheral (occlusion/cervical spine) and/or cortical (emotions/pain) aberrant afferent input influencing cranial V motor neuron activity. Stretching with tongue blades may be done to avoid secondary length changes within the muscle. The clinician takes a degree of risk of actually facilitating further increase in tone by placing the muscle and the associated shortened muscle spindles on stretch, especially if it is done too rapidly.[56] As a priority, the clinician should address those areas (occlusion, cervical spine, and emotions) contributing to aberrant afferent input, causing the altered γ motor neuron activity of those muscles innervated by cranial nerve V. Understanding of why a muscle is tight (length-associated changes vs altered γ motor neuron activity) is important before a tight muscle is placed on stretch.

Home Exercise Program for the Patient with a Tight Capsule

To improve mandibular opening, the patient is instructed to use heat/ice to the involved joint while tongue blades are placed intraorally on the molars of the involved side. The tongue blades are used to take up the slack of the available range and more, but never by forcing. How long the tongue blades are kept in is based on the etiology of the tight capsule. Progressing duration

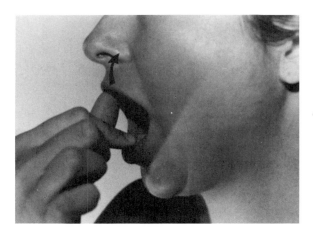

Fig. 6-4. Active/passive exercise for increasing mandibular opening. Patient actively opens and then relaxes; the thumb and index fingers then apply a force of depression to mandible.

of stretch up to ten minutes is satisfactory. The patient first places heat on the involved joint for 5 minutes, then inserts the tongue blades while continuing to apply heat for the designated time. For the remaining minutes, the heat is removed and ice is applied as tolerated by the patient while still on stretch with the tongue blades. The stretching program ideally is repeated four to six times a day.

Patients can be instructed on using the index and thumb fingers between the anterior central incisors (Fig. 6-4). The patient actively opens and then relaxes, then applies force with the index and thumb fingers to encourage more mandibular depression. Another way to encourage mandibular depression is to have the patient place an index finger on the lower anterior central incisors (Fig. 6-5). The patient actively closes gently, resisting the movement with the index finger. After the active closure, the patient relaxes, and with the index finger applies force to encourage mandibular depression. The amount of muscle contraction and the force used by the finger(s) in either of the preceding ex-

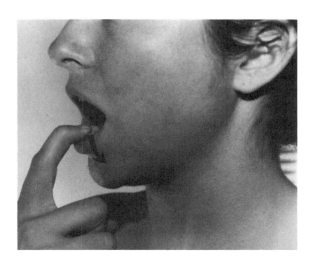

Fig. 6-5. Active/passive exercise for increasing mandibular opening. Patient actively closes against index finger, which is resisting such motion. Patient then relaxes; the index finger then applies a force of depression to mandible.

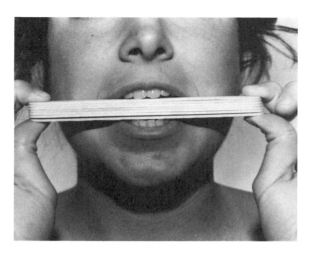

Fig. 6-6. Active exercise for increasing mandibular protrusion. Patient is supported at 11 mm of opening by tongue blades. Patient then protrudes mandible to improve translation. Patient can selectively work on translation on one side by protruding mandible forward and to the opposite side of involved joint.

ercises is kept to a minimum. More force to encourage mandibular depression may be used if such restriction is secondary to muscle length changes. These active-passive exercises can be done easily often throughout the day.

Improving translation is accomplished by having the patient place six to seven tongue blades horizontally between the anterior incisors. This will open the mandible approximately 11 mm. During normal mandibular opening, translation begins beyond 11 mm. The patient can work on protrusive and lateral excursions but avoid any jamming effects that might occur if translation is done within the first 11 mm of opening (Fig. 6-6). These exercises can be done often throughout the day. Caution should be used if this exercise is done soon after disc plication or graft.

As mandibular dynamics improve, the patient is instructed on neuromuscular reeducational exercises (discussed later in the chapter). Neuromuscular reeducational exercises will help to maintain proper motor control within the available range of mandibular opening and closing in the sagital plane. Neuromuscular reeducational exercises can be used safely within the first 2 weeks after TMJ surgery to encourage muscle relaxation and mandibular mobility.

Other Indications for Intraoral Techniques

Intraoral techniques can be applied for other TMJ disorders, such as (1) anterior disc dislocation that does not reduce; (2) symptomatic or asymptomatic anterior disc dislocation that does not and will not reduce with conservative treatment; (3) joint effusion, retrodiscal inflammation, or excessive loading of the joint as with bruxism; and (4) muscle guarding (increase in γ activity) of muscles innervated by cranial nerve V.

Anterior Disc Dislocation That Does Not Reduce

Intraoral techniques of distraction or distraction with translation may help in recapturing the disc (Fig. 6-1 and 6-2). Minimal muscle guarding, sufficient elastic properties in the superior lamina, and proper application of the technique may recapture the disc. Successful relocation of the disc can be confirmed usually by a pop/snap with full restoration of mandibular dynamics. The patient must be told not to bring the back teeth together. The physical therapist places cotton rolls between the patient's back teeth to prevent the disc from dislocating again and refers the patient to a dentist knowledgeable in application of interocclusal appliances and management of this condition.

Symptomatic or Asymptomatic Anterior Disc Dislocation That Does Not and Will Not Reduce With Conservative Treatments

The morbidity of the disc functioning off the condyle is not entirely pathological.[57-60] A treatment choice may be to allow the disc to stay anteriorly dislocated; the clinician works instead on restoring mandibular dynamics. After all advantages and disadvantages have been discussed with the patient, physical therapist, and oral surgeon concerning the condition of the disc-condyle derrangment with or without surgery, all parties may agree to use intraoral techniques simply to push the disc further anteriorly to allow better translation. Mandibular dynamics can be restored by using all intraoral techniques and placing the patient on a home exercise program such as that previously described. A patient having a wide range of adaptability apparently can function with the condyle on the retrodiscal tissue. Scarring of the retrodiscal tissue has likely occurred, allowing this condition to exist without pain. If pain and limitation of function persist with an anterior disc disclocation that does not reduce, an oral surgery consultation is indicated.

Joint Effusion, Retrodiscal Inflammation, and Excessive Loading of Joint as With Bruxism

Applying distractional techniques of stages I and II with oscillatory techniques of grades I and II may allow a temporary decrease in pain associated with the previously listed conditions. Maintaining distraction with or without oscillations for several minutes within the patient's tolerance can achieve temporary pain reduction by modulating type IV receptor activity. Other treatments for the etiologies of the conditions are also given.

Muscle Guarding (Increase in γ Activity) of Muscles Innervated by Cranial Nerve V

Rhythmic, passive, and oscillatory movements of the capsule done with intraoral techniques may enhance muscle relaxation of the muscles innervated by cranial nerve V. Other ways to normalize muscle activity, discussed throughout this text, are considered in addition to the use of these techniques.

NEUROMUSCULAR CONTROL ON MANDIBULAR POSITIONS AT REST AND DURING MOVEMENT

Muscle hyperactivity plays a predisposing, precipitating, and/or perpetuating role in the management of TM disorders. The various therapies used in management of TM disorders focus on the need to gain neuromuscular relaxation. Neuromuscular reeducational exercises should be instituted at the initial evaluation and treatment session for all patients.

Neuromuscular reeducational exercises are used as a means of initiating cortical awareness and control of what is "normal" for a specific area at rest and during movement. When properly understood and used frequently by the patient, this conscious awareness and control then occurs subconsciously.

To be optimally effective, the clinician must have the ability to demonstrate and communicate to the patient the importance of such exercises. When performing the exercises, the patient must put forth a cortical effort of awareness that an exercise is being experienced rather than merely go through the motions. Patients who have been instructed on what is normal (mandibular positions at rest and during movement) have a means to check and verify if the proprioceptive and kinesthetic afferent information they are receiving is correct; if the information is not correct, patients can take action to correct it. Such neuromuscular reeducational exercises aid the patient in changing a "bad" behavioral response into a "good" behavioral response when stress/pain is experienced.

TTBS

The following neuromuscular reeducational exercises are used to initiate steps toward achieving a rest position of the mandible. These neuromuscular reeducational exercises are called the TTBS awareness exercises:

T—Tongue position at rest
T—Teeth apart
B—Breathing: nasal-diaphragmatic
S—Swallowing

The basic fundamental importance of the rest position (upright posture) of the mandible is that most of our time is spent with our mandible in a rest position. The total time the teeth are together during chewing, talking, and swallowing activities do not amount to much more than 20 minutes in 24 hours. The mandible essentially exists in a rest position.

Tongue Position at Rest

The tongue is active during most oral-mandibular functions. The tongue assists in mixing food and in delivery of food into the posterior part of the mouth for swallowing, and plays an important role in swallowing. The tongue not only has numerous sensory functions, but also acts efficiently in discriminating the characteristics of food and contributes to speech. We seldom bite our tongues during normal oral functioning because of the highly developed, skillfully coordinated neurofunctions operating between the tongue and the mandibular muscles. The functional coordination between the tongue and mandibular muscles depends on the jaw-tongue reflex.[61,62]

The tongue is composed of various intrinsic and extrinsic muscles. The genioglossus is the main muscle responsible for positioning the tongue in the oral cavity and also is primarily responsible for establishing and maintaining the rest position and the actions of elevation and protrusion of the tongue. The rest position of the tongue, often referred to as the "postural position," is up against the palate of the mouth.[63] The most anteriosuperior tip of the tongue lies in an area against the palate just posteriorly to the back side of the upper central incisors. The remaining portion of the tongue, at least the first half of the tongue, also lies against the palate. The most posterior part of the tongue forms the anterior wall of the pharynx.

The rest position of the tongue, by way of neuroreflexes (jaw-tongue reflex), provides a foundation for the resting muscle tone of the elevator muscles of the mandible (temporalis, masseter, internal pterygoid) and for the resting activity of the tongue muscles themselves.[64] The patient is instructed on the position of the tongue when at rest. Unless the patient is chewing, talking, coughing, licking the lips, or swallowing, the tongue should be in the rest position at all times.

Teeth Apart

When the patient maintains the back teeth together during functional and parafunctional activities, muscle activity increases. Many factors can cause an increase in activity of the elevator muscles of the mandible. Informing the patient of the simple fact that back teeth should be apart is therapeutic. To help in the patient's awareness of the teeth being apart, the correct rest position of the tongue must be established. When the tongue is in the correct rest position and patients brings the back teeth together, they will either have to pull the tongue back or bite it. For most patients who have an overbite relationship of the anterior central incisors, maintaining the rest position of the tongue will enhance awareness of the back teeth being apart.

Breathing Nasal-Diaphragmatic

Nasal breathing is essential to the normal well-being of the body.[65] Nasal breathing permits air to be warmed, moistened, and cleansed before it reaches the lungs. Nasal breathing will make more ideal use of the diaphragm, the principle driver of respiration. Proper use of the diaphragm allows ideal ventilation of the lungs.

Diaphragmatic breathing occurs more easily when one breathes through the nose. Having a correct rest position of the tongue will force the patient to be a nasal-diaphragmatic breather. Nasal-diaphragmatic breathing occurs more easily if there is no resistance in the upper airway cavity.

Breathing through the mouth decreases the effects of diaphragmatic breathing and increases use of accessory muscles of breathing. The accessory muscles are the scalenes and the sternocleidomastoid.[66] The therapist may need to apply various techniques to enhance proper use of the diaphragm and encourage rib cage and thoracic spine mobility.

Swallowing Sequence

Altered sequence of swallowing is called a tongue thrust. Tongue thrust has no single name or definition.[67] The most frequently cited signs of tongue thrust activity during swallowing include protrusion of the tongue against or between the anterior teeth and excessive circumoral muscle activity.[68] There is considerable debate as to whether a tongue thrust is pathological. A strong relationship however, does appear to exist between a tongue thrust and pediatric anterior open bites.[69] In the absence of a pediatric tongue thrust and the frequently associated dental and skeletal changes, I observe that adults can acquire a tongue thrust I term "an acquired adult anterior tongue thrust."

This acquired adult anterior tongue thrust occurs secondary to the forward head posture (FHP). Symptoms frequently associated with an acquired tongue thrust are: difficulty in swallowing, scratching sensations in the throat that do not become a sore throat, and shortness of breath. The literature is not clear in stating whether humans swallow with the teeth together or apart. I observe that in normal swallowing, if head-neck environment is normal, our teeth do not come into contact. With the acquired adult anterior tongue thrust, not only are the muscles that function during swallowing used incorrectly, duration of tooth to tooth contact is likely to increase, at the expense of increased muscle activity. This relationship between a change in the anterior and posterior head posture and altered tongue activity during swallowing (genioglossus) has not been scientifically addressed in the literature until recently.[70]

The evaluation used by Barrett and Hanson[71] to determine the presence of a pediatric anterior tongue thrust may not be helpful in determining if an adult has an anterior tongue thrust that was acquired later in life. Their evaluation appears to rely on existing dental and skeletal changes to determine whether a tongue thrust exists. The following is the evaluation I recommend to help in determining the presence of an acquired adult anterior tongue thrust (Fig. 6-7).

1. Have the patient swallow water two to four times, pausing between each swallow. During each swallow, palpate the hyoid bone. A quick up and down movement of the hyoid bone, (like a flicker) should normally be felt.

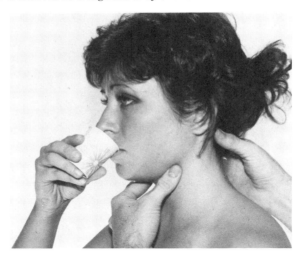

Fig. 6-7. Examining for "an acquired adult anterior tongue thrust." The following are signs indicating an altered sequence of swallowing, believed to be secondary to the forward head posture: slow movement of the hyoid bone; contraction of the suboccipital muscles; extension of head on neck (so as to crane the neck); excessive lip activity; patient perceives the tongue pressing forward against the teeth. A combination of these movements are needed to confirm the clinical impression of an altered sequence of swallowing.

With an acquired anterior adult tongue thrust, a slow up and down movement of the hyoid bone is felt.

2.   During swallowing, palpate the suboccipital muscles. Normally, minimal if any muscle contractions should be felt. With an adult tongue thrust, suboccipital muscle contractions are felt.

3.   During swallowing, no head movement should be observed. With an adult tongue thrust, extension of the head on the neck and, in more severe cases, an actual forward movement of the entire head and neck, as if to crane the head on the neck, is observed.

4.   During normal swallowing, no excessive lip activity should be observed. Lip activity will be seen with the adult tongue thrust. Excessive lip activity is the least observable activity with the adult tongue thrust.

5.   While the patient swallows, have the patient become aware of tongue movement and position during swallowing, especially the anterior tip of the tongue. During normal swallowing, the patient should not be aware of the tip of the tongue pressing forward. With an adult tongue thrust, the patient will typically state that the tip of the tongue presses against the back side of their upper front teeth or straight forward or down against the back of the bottom front teeth.

An acquired anterior adult tongue thrust is treated by correcting head-neck position and instructing the patient in the normal sequence of swallowing, which is as follows:

1. Instruct the patient on the proper position of the tongue at rest.
2. When water enters the oral cavity, the tongue will have dropped down from the rest position.
3. The initial phase of swallowing occurs when the tip of the tongue returns to its rest position. From that point on, no pressure should be felt with the tip of the tongue pressing against the teeth.
4. The main force of swallowing occurs with the middle one-third of the tongue. The tongue should be perceived as moving like a wave that starts at the tip of the tongue with the main force occurring with the middle one-third of the tongue.

Instructing the patient on the correct sequence of swallowing and correcting cervical spine dysfunction will begin to decrease altered muscle activity in the masticatory-cervical areas.

If patients achieve a good understanding of application of the TTBS awareness exercises, the exercises can help patients change poor behavioral responses to pain, physical, environmental and emotional stresses to good behavioral responses. Patients then become active participants in management of TMJ dysfunction and muscle imbalances.

NEUROMUSCULAR CONTROL OF MANDIBULAR MOVEMENT

Periarticular tissue restricting arthrokinematic movements was the main emphasis in part I of this chapter. Evaluation and treatment of excessive arthrokinematic movement is also of clinical importance. Translation is usually the excessive arthrokinematic movement. Excessive translation occurs with both of the following categories: too much translation (subluxation), and translation occurring too soon within the initial phase of opening. Excessive translation is considered to be due to muscular imbalances.[72,73] Instructing the patient in neuromuscular reeducational exercises to control excessive translation is the suggested treatment.

Subluxation

The literature describes various ways of defining subluxation. The word subluxation has been interchanged with dislocation and has been used in reference to an abnormal position of the condyle and/or the disc. Subluxation is defined operationally as a condylar position outside the physiologic range but within the anatomic range. The condyle can return to the physiologic range by neuromuscular effort.

Anatomically, subluxation of the condyle(s) occurs when the condyle(s) is in front of the crest of the articular eminence.[74] Seventy percent of the condyles in normal persons sublux by this definition.[75]

With subluxation occurring so readily in normal persons, how important is subluxation clinically? Because subluxation occurs at the end of opening, tension/stress is placed not only on the ligamentous and capsular tissues but also on the retrodiscal tissue and the disc–condyle relationship.[76] The length and degree of slope of the articular eminence, the size and shape of the head of the condyle, and the frequency and duration of such subluxation are all factors contributing to the tension/stress on the interarticular and periarticular tissues.

A patient who has symptomatic TMJ dysfunction usually has a preexisting subluxation. Subluxation needs to be evaluated and, if present, controlled. Otherwise, the subluxation can perpetuate the patient's TMJ dysfunction. Subluxation may have been the sole cause of the patient's TMJ dysfunction.

The following are guidelines used in determining the presence of subluxation and are listed in the order of most to least significant. All tests are done by palpating the lateral poles of the condyle bilaterally during jaw opening, except for number 4:

1.   Instruct the patient to open as wide as possible. If subluxation exists, there will be a depression between the lateral pole and the tragus of the ear because the condyle is translating too far anteriorly. The lateral poles during normal translation should not be felt to move anteriorly. Biomechanically, this occurs because the lateral pole lies in front of the transverse condylar rotational axis. During mandibular depression, the lateral pole actually moves downward and backward.[77]

2.   With a unilateral subluxation, the mandible deflects abruptly to the opposite side at the end of the opening. On closing, an abrupt movement of the mandible back to midline is seen.

3.   Joint noises (crepitus), if present, may be felt and/or heard at the end of the opening. There may be crepitus at the beginning of closing; the closing noise is generally the loudest.

4.   Mandibular opening will be more than 40 mm.

Of the four criteria used to determine if subluxation is present, the least significant is the amount of opening. The clinician should not assume that all patients who sublux will measure more than 40 mm. Clinically, subluxation has been observed in less than 40 mm of opening. Subluxation prior to 40 mm of opening usually is related to the individual's osseous joint structures. Radiograph evaluation is usually not done, because a good clinical examination will tell the clinician if the patient subluxes. Radiographs taken only to determine whether subluxation exists are not indicated.

The reader should be alert not to confuse the reciprocal joint noises occurring with subluxation and the reciprocal joint noises occurring with an anterior disc dislocation that reduces. Joint noises occurring with a subluxation and joint noises occurring with an anterior disc dislocation that reduces have several different distinguishing characteristics. The opening click related to a subluxation occurs at the end of opening and is usually a softer noise. The closing click occurs at the beginning of closing and is typically louder. A reciprocal click related to the disc will usually have an early to intermediate abrupt opening click. The closing click related to the disc usually occurs just before tooth-to-tooth contact and is a softer noise.

If the above characteristics are not helpful as a differential diagnosis, the clinician should have the patient open wide enough to get the opening joint noise and then have the patient close to an edge-to-edge position with the maxillary and mandibular incisors. From this anterior central incisor position, the clinician should have the patient open wide. The patient returning to an edge-to-edge position while opening and closing will usually cease making the joint noises that occur with an anterior disc dislocation that reduces, but the joint noises that occur with a subluxation will not stop. A false negative may occur if the clinician does not encourage the patient to open as wide as possible during the entire testing procedure.

The only definitive treatment for subluxation suggested in the literature is surgical alteration of the morphology of the joint itself, (i.e., eminectomy).[78] Another treatment suggested is extraarticular injections of sclerosing solutions.[79] Such suggested treatments are far too extensive for the condition and the symptoms experienced by the patient unless other forms of conservative care have been exhausted.

When the condyle subluxes, the disc is fully rotated posteriorly on the condyle.[78] If the disc and condyle are unable to return to within their physiologic range, a dislocation is present. In a dislocation the condyle and disc are both outside their physiologic and anatomic range and cannot return under neuromuscular effort. The disc and condyle can only be returned by an outside force. The outside force, in this case, is a distractional technique very similar to the distractional technique used to recapture an anterior disc dislocation that does not reduce (Fig. 6-1). Instead of moving the condyle forward during distraction to "recapture" the disc, the condyle and disc are moved backward onto the articular eminence from their anteriorly dislocated position.

Translation Occurring Too Soon Within the Initial Phase of Opening

The first 11 mm of opening involves rotation. Thereafter, anterior translation of the condyle occurs with continued rotation.[80,81] It is incorrect to observe translation occurring within the first 11 mm of opening. Frequent early translation occurring causes stress on the disc, collateral ligaments, and retrodiscal tissue. Early translation may hinder ideal management of TMJ dysfunction and/or may cause a TMJ dysfunction. Readers may appreciate how this condition may cause local discomfort by simply protruding the jaw repeatedly for several minutes with the teeth apart just enough to clear the upper central incisors. This form of translation occurring too soon is an expression of muscular imbalances.

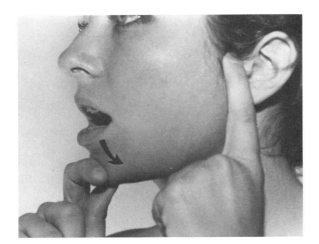

Fig. 6-8. Neuromuscular reeducational exercise to control for excessive translation: Tongue is placed up against palate. Patient touches tip of chin *lightly* with index finger and thumb. Index finger touches lateral pole of TMJ.

Translation occurring too soon is evaluated by palpating for excessive translation of the lateral poles of the condyle bilaterally. The fingers lightly touching can easily monitor the movement of the lateral poles. What is felt in this condition is the lateral poles moving forward at the onset of opening. The patient may also be observed to protrude the mandible during the initial phase of opening.

Treatment for Excessive Translation

Instructing the patient in performing a neuromuscular reeducational exercise, is the simplest and most effective treatment to gain immediate control of translation. The exercise consists of having the patient touch the lateral pole of the condyle on the most involved side with the middle or index finger. The patient very lightly touches the chin with the other hand. The patient then places the tongue flat against the palate of the mouth. The patient is asked to open the mouth, keeping the tongue against the palate, while palpating the lateral pole (Fig. 6-8). Proprioceptive feedback of the tongue against the palate and the fingers contacting the mandible will cause the condyles to rotate during opening. The progression of this exercise is to have the patient drop the tongue away from the palate and finally to remove the fingers that are touching the chin (Fig. 6-9). Normal translation will now be allowed to occur but is controlled by the proprioceptive feedback of the palpating finger over the lateral pole.[42] As with any exercise, repetition and the patient's conscious effort will determine the success of this form of treatment.

In addition to the neuromuscular exercise, patients may be instructed in doing traditional isometric exercises to the mandible. These isometric exercises classically involve resisting opening, closing, lateral, protrusive, and retrusive movements of the mandible.[82] The resistance is usually offered by the patient's hand or fingers. Isometric exercises have been prescribed to help in: "mini-

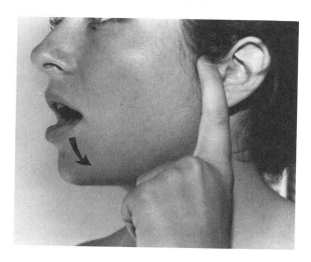

Fig. 6-9. Neuromuscular reeducational exercise to control for excessive translation. To provide the least amount of assistance, patient controls translation with index finger touching lateral pole of TMJ only (this is a progression from Fig. 6-8).

mizing clicking, retraining muscles to contract symmetrically, overcoming zigzag opening patterns, and increasing mouth opening when it is restricted by muscle spasm."[83]

Isometric exercises for the previously mentioned indications lack some important clarifications the clinician must be aware of:

Isometric exercises for reciprocal clicks: Isometric exercises for reciprocal clicks related to an anterior disc dislocation that reduces should be done with the disc in proper position. This can be accomplished by instructing patients to open the mouth until they get the opening click and then close until they just feel that the closing click might occur. At this point of jaw closure, with the disc in place, isometric exercises to the mandible may be performed. If the patient does not first relocate the disc, isometric exercises will not help to resolve the problem. Often, the patient and the clinician think the exercises are helping because the patient is not experiencing any joint noises. The reciprocal click is not present because the patient's condyle is only rotating and not translating to expose the opening click. If the reciprocal click is significant enough to warrant treatment, the isometric exercises will be done to supplement the treatment of an interocclusal appliance.

Isometric exercises for "zigzag" opening-closing pattern: Asymmetries of mandibular movement are frequently seen during mandibular opening and closing. When all other findings of the TMJ evaluation are negative, the asymmetries may be normal and do not require any form of treatment. Bony anomalies with regard to shape of the condyle, and slope of the articular eminence can exist with any asymptomatic and symptomatic TMJ. Instructing the patient on doing isometric exercises to correct this type of zigzag opening–closing pattern related to bony anomalies would be unproductive.

Isometric exercises for weak jaw muscles: Weakness of jaw muscles is the exception rather than the rule. Isolating a jaw muscle to test whether the muscle is weak is very difficult. False-positive muscle testing can occur because of: (1) the patient's unwillingness to contract, (2) pain limiting such a contraction, and (3) pseudoweakness secondary to reflex inhibition. Isometric exercises recommended for jaw muscle weakness need to be reevaluated.

Isometric exercises for inhibition of muscles: Contracting the depressor muscles of the mandible to cause a reciprocal inhibition to the elevator (antagonist) muscles is an isometric exercise frequently taught to patients. This form of isometric exercise for the depressor muscles is often applied too quickly without consideration of the various segmental, intersegmental, and cortical-spinal reflexes influencing the reciprocal inhibition circuits. The various peripheral and cortical afferent influences operating in a normal state are not fully understood, far less the various afferent influences occurring in dysfunctional (physical and emotional) states. How long and what amount of resistance is needed to initiate, if at all, inhibition of the antagonist muscles in a dysfunctional state is still unknown.[84,85]

Isometric exercises may be more beneficial when contracting the muscle(s) one is trying to inhibit (i.e., elevator muscles of the mandible). To inhibit the elevator muscles effectively, the elevator muscles should be in a position of slight stretch (mouth opened). The patient is then asked to contract the elevator muscles maximally against an unyielding force (patient's fingers holding the mandible from moving). With the muscles in a lengthened range, a great amount of tension is needed to stimulate the golgi tendon organs of the elevator muscles, causing them to relax reflexly. No physiological information is available, however, as to how long this inhibition persists.[86] Application of this form of maximum isometric contraction to symptomatic muscles with secondary loading to a possible symptomatic TMJ needs to be reevaluated.

Of the varying amounts of muscle contractions a patient can achieve, minimal contractions of the mandibular muscles often produce the best results. Minimal isometric contraction may give the patient cortical awareness of the muscle contracting and then relaxing. Over time, this contraction may provide relaxation if done in conjunction with other forms of treatment.

Isometric exercises of minimal contractions may be used to treat subluxations and translations that occur too soon. Contracting the muscles may help to reflexly coordinate a very detailed neuromuscular system. The patient is instructed to place the tongue in the rest position, teeth apart, and to place each index finger against the side of the jaw (Fig. 6-10). The patient commands herself or himself: "Hold, do not let me move my jaw," thereby making the exercise a hold–relax technique vs. a contract–relax technique. A hold–relax technique gives the patient more finesse in controlling the amount of pressure applied to their jaw. The force of the isometric exercises is very slight. The direction of force to the mandible will be in various planes of movements (sagittal, horizontal, frontal, oblique) to work with all the various muscles playing a part in positioning and movement of the mandible. The duration of such muscle contraction may be short.

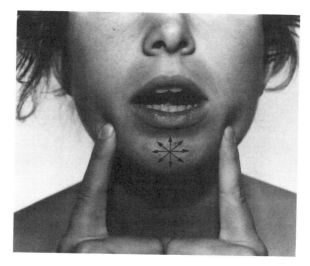

Fig. 6-10. Isometric exercise to control for excessive translation. Tongue is placed up against palate. Patient's index fingers press in all directions on the mandible, using light pressure only.

In summary, *conclusions on doing isometric exercises to the elevator and depressor muscles of the mandible have been repeated so often in the literature and in clinical practice that their repetition has inferred a validity on the data that has not yet been earned.* Isometric exercises with minimal contraction in conjunction with the neuromuscular reeducational exercises allows better symmetry of condylar movement and positioning with the least amount of muscular effort.

CLOSING REMARKS

The purpose of this chapter was to cover the basic sciences and sequelae of capsular tightness and steps to gain neuromuscular control on mandibular movement and position at rest. Capsular tightness is an area of TMJ dysfunction often overlooked by clinicians and clinical researchers. Examination and treatment of capsular tightness of the TMJ has been covered. To initiate immediate control over muscle imbalances, the TTBS exercises and their application were discussed. To gain control over muscle imbalances contributing to subluxation and translation occurring too soon, neuromuscular reeducational and isometric exercises, and their application were discussed. Clinical understanding of treatment for capsular tightness and the use of neuromuscular exercises will enhance the clinician's management of TMJ dysfunction.

REFERENCES

1. Wyke B: Neuromuscular mechanisms influencing mandibular posture. J Dent 2:111, 1973
2. Ogus HD, Toller PA: Common Disorders of the Temporomandibular Joint. 2nd Ed.

John Wright & Sons Ltd, Bristol, England, 1981
3. Dorland's Illustrated Medical Dictionary. 24th Ed. WB Saunders, Philadelphia, 1965
4. Burkhart S: The rationale for joint mobilization. p. 153. In Kent B (ed): Proceedings of the International Federation of Orthopaedic Manipulative Therapists. Third international seminar, International Federation of Orthopaedic Manipulative Therapists, Hayward, California 1977
5. Peacock E Jr: Some biochemical and biophysical aspects of joint stiffness. Ann Surg 164:1, 1968
6. Salter R, Simmonds D, et al: The biological effect of continous passive motion on the healing of full-thickness defects in articular cartilage. J Bone Joint Surg 62:1232, 1980
7. Ilyinsky OB, Krasnikova TL, Akoev GN, et al: Functional organization of mechanoreceptors. Prog Brain Res 43:195, 1976
8. McCloskey DI: Kinesthetic sensibility. Physiol Rev 58:763, 1978
9. Wyke B: The neurology of joints. Ann Coll Surg Engl 41:25, 1967
10. Griffin CJ, Hawthorn R, Harris R: Anatomy and histology of the human temporomandibular joint. Monogr Oral Sci 4:1, 1975
11. Gray's Anatomy. 35th Br Ed. WB Saunders, Philadelphia, 1973
12. MacConaill MA: Studies in the mechanics of synovial joints II. Ir J Med Sc 6:223, 1946
13. MacConaill MA, Basmajian JV: Muscles and movements: a basis for human kinesiology. Williams & Wilkins, Baltimore, 1969
14. Moss M: The functional matrix concept and its relationship to temporomandibular joint dysfunction and treatment. Dent Clin North Am 27:445, 1983
15. MacConaill MA: The movements of bones and joints. Bone Joint Surg [Br] 35:290, 1953
16. MacConaill MA: The geometry and algebra of articular kinematics. Biomed Eng 1:205, 1966
17. MacConaill MA: Joint movement. Physiotherapy 359, 1964
18. Mennell J: Joint pain: Diagnosis and Treatment Using Manipulative Techniques. Little, Brown, Boston, 1964
19. Zohn DA, Mennell JM: Musculoskeletal Pain: Diagnosis and Physical Treatment. Little, Brown, Boston, 1976
20. Cotta H, Puhl W: The pathophysiology of damage to articular cartilage. Prog Orthop Surg 3:20, 1978
21. Radin EL, Paul IL: Response of joints to impact loading. Arthritis Rheum 14:356, 1971
22. Radin EL, Paul IL: Does cartilage compliance reduce skeletal impact loads? Arthritis Rheum 13:139, 1970
23. Glineburg RW, Laskin DM, Blaustein DI: The effects of immobilization on the primate temporomandibular joint: a histologic and histochemical study. J Oral Maxillofac Surg 40:3, 1982
24. Thilander B: Innervation of the temporomandibular joint capsule in man. Trans R School Dent Stockholm 7:1, 1961
25. Clark RKF, Wyke BD: Contributions of temporomandibular articular mechanoreceptors to the control of mandibular posture: an experimental study. J Dent 2:121, 1974
26. Harris R, Griffin CJ: Neuromuscular mechanisms and the masticatory apparatus. Monogr Oral Sci 4:45, 1975

27. Klineberg IJ, Greenfield BE, Wyke BD: Contributions to the reflex control of mastication from mechanoreceptors in the temporomandibular joint capsule. Dent Pract Dent Rec 21:73, 1970
28. Wyke BD: Articular neurology—a review. Physiotherapy 58:94, 1972
29. Wyke BD: Neurology of the cervical spinal joints. Physiotherapy 65:72, 1979
30. Bell WE: Orofacial pains differential diagnosis. 2nd Ed Year Book Medical, Chicago, 1980
31. Clark R: Neurology of the temporomandibular joints: an experimental study. Ann R Coll Surg Engl 58:43, 1976
32. DeAndrade J, Grant C, Dixon A: Joint distention and reflex muscle inhibition in the knee. J Bone Joint Surg [Am] 47:313, 1965
33. Larsson L, Thilander B: Mandibular positioning, the effect of pressure on joint capsule. Acta Neurol Scand 40:131, 1964
34. Akeson WH: An experimental study of joint stiffness. J Bone Joint Surg [Am] 43:1022, 1961
35. Akeson WH, Amiel D, LaViolette D, et al: The connective tissue response to immobility: an accelerated ageing response. Exp Gerontol 3:289, 1968
36. Akeson WH, Amiel D, Woo S: Immobility effects of synovial joints: the pathomechanics of joint contracture. Biorheology 17:95, 1980
37. Donatelli R, Owens-Burkhart H: Effects of immobilization on the extensibility of periarticular connective tissue. J Orthopaedic and Sports Physical Therapy 3:67, 1981
38. Rheumatoid Arthritis, Section 7. (supplement) Hussey HH (ed): In J Am Med Assoc, Suppl., 224:687, 1973
39. Clark RKF, Wyke BD: Temporomandibular arthrokinetic reflex control of the mandibular musculature. Br J Oral Surg 13:196, 1975
40. Posselt U: Hinge opening axis of the mandible. Acta Odontol Scand 14:61, 1956
41. Osborn JW: The disc of the human temporomandibular joint: design, function and failure. J Oral Rehabil 12:279, 1985
42. Kraus S: Temporomandibular joint. p. 171. In Saunders D: Evaluation, Treatment and Prevention of Musculoskeletal Disorders. Saunders, Minneapolis, 1985
43. Kaltenborn FM: Manual Therapy for the Extremity Joints. 2nd Ed. Olaf Norlis Bokhandel, Oslo, 1976
44. Maitland GD: Vertebral Manipulation. Butterworths, London, 1981
45. Newton R: Joint receptor contributions to reflexive and kinesthetic responses. Phys Ther 62:22, 1982
46. Freeman M, Wyke B: The innervation of the knee joint: an anatomical and histological study in the cat. J Anat 101:505, 1967
47. Paris SV, Kraus S: Advanced evaluation and manipulation of the craniofacial, cervical, and upper thoracic spines (course notes). Institute of Graduate Health Sciences, Atlanta, Georgia, 1986
48. Stromberg D, Wiederhielm CA: Viscoelastic description of a collagenous tissue in simple elongation. J Appl Physiol 26:857, 1969
49. LeBan MM: Collagen tissue: implications of its response to stress in vitro. Arch Phys Med Rehabil 43:461, 1962
50. Sapega A, Quedenfield T, Butler R: Biophysical factors in range of motion exercises. Phys Sports Med 9:57, 1981
51. Prentice W Jr: An electromyographic analysis of the effectiveness of heat or cold and stretching for inducing relaxation in injured muscles. J Orthop Sports Phys Ther 3:133, 1982

52. Gossman MR, Sharmann SA, Rose SJ: Review of length-associated changes in muscle. Phys Ther 62:1799, 1979

53. Tabary JC, Tabary C, Tardieu G, et al: Physiological and structural changes in the cat's soleus muscle due to immobilization at different lengths by plaster casts. J Physiol (Lond) 224:231, 1972

54. Schár I, Takacs O, Guba F: The influence of immobilization on soluble proteins in muscle. Acta Biol Med Germanica 36:1621, 1977

55. Goldspink G, Williams PE: The nature of the increased passive resistance in muscle following immobilization of the mouse soleus muscle. Phys Soc 00:55, 1978

56. Jacobs M: Neurophysiological implications of slow active stretching. Am Corr Ther J 30:151, 1976

57. Toller P: Non-surgical treatment of the temporomandibular joint. Oral Sci Rev 7:70, 1976

58. Rasmussen OC: Description of population and progress of symptoms in a longitudinal study of temporomandibular arthropathy. Scand J Dent Res 89:196, 1981

59. Clark GT, Mulligan RA: A review of the prevalence of temporomandibular dysfunction. J Gerodontol 3:231, 1986

60. Greene CS, Turner C, Laskin DM: Long-term outcome of TMJ clicking in 100 MPD patients. J Dent Res 61:218, 1982

61. Schoen R: Der Kieferzungenreflex und andre proriozeptive reflexe der zunge und der Kiefermuskulatur. Arch Exp Pathol Pharmacol 160:29, 1931

62. Morimoto T, Kawamura Y: Properties of tongue and jaw movements elicited by stimulation of the orbital gyrus of cat. Arch Oral Biol 18:361, 1973

63. Fish F: The functional anatomy of the rest position of the mandible. Dent Pract 11:178, 1961

64. Atwood DA: A critique of research of the rest position of the mandible. J Prosthet Dent 16:848, 1966

65. Emslie RD, Massler M, Zwemer JD: Mouthbreathing: I. Etiology and effects. J Am Dent Assoc 44:506, 1952

66. Sharp J, Druz W, Danon J, et al: Respiratory muscle function and the use of respiratory muscle electromyography in the evaluation of respiratory regulation. Chest suppl. 70:150, 1976

67. Manson R: Tongue thrust. p. 32. In Bryant P, Gale E, Rugh J (eds): Oral Motor Behavior: Impact on Oral Conditions and Dental Treatment. Workshop Proceedings. US HEW, Washington, DC, 1979

68. Weinberg B: Deglutition: a review of selected topics. In Proceedings of the Workshop, Speech and the Dentofacial Complex: The State of the Art. ASHA Rep 5. American Speech and Hearing Association, Washington DC, 1970

69. Kelly J, Sanchez M, Van Kirk L: An assessment of the occlusion of teeth of children. National center for health statistics, US Public Health Service, Washington, DC, 1973

70. Milidonis M, Kraus SL, Segal R, et al: Suprahyoid muscle activity in response to changes in anterior/posterior head posture. (submitted for publication)

71. Barrett R, Hanson M: Oral myofunctional disorders. CV Mosby, St. Louis, 1978

72. Landa JS: A scientific approach to the study of the temporomandibular joint and its relation to occlusal disharmonies. J Prosthet Dent 7:170, 1957

73. Landa JS: Preliminary survey and a new approach to the study of the temporomandibular joint syndromes. Ann Dent 9:5, 1950

74. Sheppard IM, Sheppard SM: Range of condylar movement during mandibular opening. J Prosthet Dent 15:263, 1965

75. Nevakari K: Elapsio praearticularis' of the temporomandibular joint. A panto-mographic study of the so-called physiological subluxation. Acta Odontol Scand 18:123, 1960

76. Okeson J: Diagnosis of temporomandibular disorders. p. 252. In Okeson J (ed): Fundamentals of Occlusion and Temporomandibular Disorders. CV Mosby, St. Louis, 1985

77. DuBrul EL: The craniomandibular articulation. In Sicher's Oral Anatomy. 7th Ed. CV Mosby, St. Louis, 1980

78. Okeson J: Treatment of acute muscle disorders. p. 304. In Okeson J (ed): Fundamentals of Occlusion and Temporomandibular Disorders. CV Mosby, St. Louis, 1985

79. Poswillo D: Surgery of the temporomandibular joint, p. 413. In Zarb G, Garlsson G (eds): Temporomandibular Joint, Function and Dysfunction. CV Mosby, St. Louis, 1979

80. Posselt U: Hinge opening axis of the mandible. Acta Odontol Scand 14:61, 1956

81. Osborn JW: The disc of the human temporomandibular joint: design, function and failure. J Oral Rehabil 12:279, 1985

82. Schwartz L: Therapeutic exercises. p. 223. In Schwartz L (ed): Disorders of the Temporomandibular Joint. WB Saunders, Philadelphia, 1959

83. Zarb G, Speck J: The treatment of mandibular dysfunction. p. 382. In Zarb G, Carlsson G (eds): Temporomandibular Joint, Function and Dysfunction. CV Mosby, St. Louis, 1979

84. Smith AM: The coactivation of antagonist muscles. Can J Physiol Pharmacol 59:733, 1981

85. Burke D: Critical examination of the case for or against fusimotor involvement in disorders of muscle tone. p. 133. In Desmedt JE (ed): Motor Control Mechanisms in Health and Disease. Raven Press, New York, 1983

86. Tanigawa MC: Comparison of the hold-relax procedure and passive mobilization on increasing muscle length. Phys Ther 52:725, 1972

7 | TMJ and Orthognathic Surgery

Robert A. Bays

The use of physical therapy in oral and maxillofacial surgery falls into two categories: (1) management of myofascial pain dysfunction (MPD) of the mandible and cervical spine areas before and after TMJ surgery, and (2) restoration of mandibular dynamics following intracapsular TMJ surgery or orthognathic surgery on the mandible. The management of MPD has, in general, been covered elsewhere in this book; therefore, this chapter focuses on preoperative MPD management as it relates to intracapsular TMJ surgery and mobilization of the mandible following intracapsular TMJ surgery and orthognathic surgery. These subjects are covered separately.

INTRACAPSULAR TMJ SURGERY

Opinion varies widely among oral and maxillofacial surgeons regarding indications for various TMJ surgical techniques. A complete review of this subject is beyond the scope of this chapter and is unnecessary in this context. Brief discussions of the various types of intracapsular surgery will be included, however, so that the physical therapy needs can be more clearly delineated.

Internal Derangement of the TMJ Discs

The most common surgical problem of the TMJ is a derangement of the disc. This may take many forms and is often oversimplified. Disc derangement is considered a surgical problem only when stringent criteria are met. Signs and symptoms of disc derangement have been discussed in other chapters and are not reiterated here.

To be considered for surgery, the patient should meet the following criteria:

1. Pain in the TMJ, especially with function (i.e., chewing, opening, talking, yawning, etc.). Absence of pain is almost always a contraindication to surgery.

2. Evidence of mechanical disc dislocation such as decreased opening and reciprocal clicking or the history of either. This is very important because pain in the TMJ can exist even though the disc–condyle relationship is normal. MPD or referred pain from the cervical spine is a frequent cause for such pain. The exact mechanism is not fully understood, but various joint noises may occur as a result of MPD without the existence of a true disc dislocation. Considerable clinical experience and skill are required to determine disc dislocation in patients with concomitant MPD.

Clicking and reciprocal clicking of the TMJ are found in up to 40 percent of the population; only 2 to 3 percent of these dislocations are painful.[1] Arthrographic or other evaluation of individuals with such clicking to confirm disc dislocation has not been done. Many of these, however, may reasonably be assumed to represent nonpainful disc dislocations. With this in mind, one must be careful about overtreating painless disc dislocations.

If a disc–condyle derangement causes a reciprocal click but is not painful, does not limit function, and is not bothersome to the patient, I believe that the therapist should make the patient aware of but not alarmed about the condition. If the therapist is treating the patient for cervical or headache pains, it would be most appropriate to treat the patient and reevaluate the TMJ. If the clicking becomes painful or changes in nature, referral of the patient to an appropriate clinician is in order.

A physical therapist whose patient has an anteriorly dislocated disc without reduction that cannot be reduced by the distraction techniques described in Chapter 6 may decide to allow the disc to remain anteriorly dislocated without any further attempts at relocation. This depends greatly on whether the patient has pain or limitation of function or is in some other way inhibited by the dislocation. It is also heavily influenced by any further treatment that may be contemplated, especially orthodontic, major dental restoration, or orthognathic repositioning of the jaws. All these treatments have a profound influence on the occlusion. Even if treatment by such means is anticipated, the therapist and/or patient may decide not to attempt surgical relocation of the discs. The patient must be made fully aware of the condition, however, and must also be warned that pain or increase in dysfunction may result from the major changes in occlusion produced by orthodontics, major restorative dentistry, or orthognathic surgery. Whether to treat a nonpainful dislocated disc with or without reduction is always a difficult clinical judgment and must be made on the basis of other procedures contemplated in the patient's overall care.

The most conclusive evidence of disc dislocation is the arthrogram.[2] (Arthrography is a dynamic study that is done so that disc position can be evaluated during function). Computerized axial tomography (CT scan) has been advocated as a replacement for arthrography. Several studies, however, have shown that other soft tissue structures can be confused with the disc on CAT scans.[3-5] Magnetic resonance imaging (MRI) shows great promise for future diagnosis of internal derangements.[6] MRI has not yet been perfected for this purpose, however, and standardization has not been achieved.

Arthrography should be considered whenever temporomandibular surgery is contemplated. In some cases, the disc dislocation may be so obvious clinically that arthrography is omitted. Arthrography is often performed after conservative TMJ treatment (i.e., splint therapy) has failed. Although arthrographic identification of a disc dislocation might be helpful prior to any treatment, arthrography is usually not performed because of its invasive nature and the satisfactory success rate of conservative therapy when performed by qualified clinicians.

Arthrographic Technique

Arthrography is performed in the fluoroscopy room of a hospital radiology department. The patient is placed on one side so that a transcranial view of the TMJ can be achieved. Local anesthetic is injected over the TMJ to anesthetize the soft tissues and capsule surrounding the joint. In experienced hands, this should be a relatively pain-free procedure. Following the achievement of complete local anesthesia, a radiopaque medium is injected into the inferior joint space, using only enough volume so that it can be detected on the fluoroscopy monitors. This procedure is videotaped while the patient is asked to open, close, and go into lateral and protrusive excursions of the mandible. In some cases, the patient may be asked to attempt to cause clicking if it is not readily apparent. It is sometimes helpful to inject the radiopaque medium into the superior joint space, especially for delineation of the anteriorly dislocated disc without reduction.

In more than 200 arthrograms, I have seen no complications beyond occasional postarthrogram tenderness. This occurs when entering the inferior joint space is difficult. Most arthrograms leave the patient with no more soreness than any other soft tissue injection.

Arthrograms may be performed by oral surgeons, radiologists, or any other trained clinician. I believe, however, that the clinician caring for the patient will often be the one who is most gentle in performing arthrography, although most trained clinicians can do this with a minimum amount of discomfort and a maximum amount of effectiveness.

Clearly, the most common cause for inaccurate arthrography is operator error. Experience has shown that the most common false positive is the movement of the dye from the inferior to the superior joint space, indicating a possible perforation. Indeed, the dye may escape around the needle due to excessive manipulation at the time of injection and possibly no perforation exists.

False negatives occur if the inferior joint space is overfilled with dye and effectively "washes out" the click, causing a normal disc–condyle relationship to appear on an arthrogram when the disc is actually anteriorly dislocated.

Disc Dislocations and MPD

Once the patient has been determined to have a disc dislocation that is painful and cannot be corrected without surgery, an assessment is made of MPD as a contributing factor. Many patients with disc dislocations have a large amount of MPD of both the masticatory and cervical spine musculature, either secondary to or preceding disc dislocation. The sequence of symptoms is important to ascertain. If MPD is secondary to disc dislocation, it is reasonable to assume that correction of the disc position, proper occlusal management of jaw position, and physical therapy to the cervical spine and jaw as indicated should lead to a great reduction or to elimination of MPD postoperatively. If MPD has preceded disc dislocation, however, and actually may have caused it by the constant forces delivered to the TMJ by parafunctional activity, disc repair may have little affect on pain experienced by the patient unless MPD can be decreased postoperatively. A complete history of the patient's pain complaints and considerable clinical skill are often required to make this differentiation.

Important historical facts include the timing of clicking and reciprocal clicking relative to pain and limitation of opening. Often, clicking and reciprocal clicking have occurred for several years during the patient's teen years, after which clicking will cease and a limitation of opening is noticed. Years later, opening and range of motion (ROM) improve and crepitus ensues. This is typical of an anteriorly dislocated disc with reduction proceeding to an anteriorly located disc without reduction and ending with a perforation and degenerative changes in the joint.

A history of atypical migraines, neck and shoulder pain, or other vague types of facial and neck pain may indicate that myofascial involvement of the jaw and neck preceded internal joint pathology. Known psychosomatic illnesses (gastrointestinal disturbances such as frequent indigestion, peptic ulcer disease, Crohn's disease, ulcerative colitis, or chronic diarrhea, psoriasis, lower back pain, neurogenic bladder, certain types of asthma associated with stress, palpitations of the heart) that have been ascertained by appropriate medical experts and either left untreated or treated with medicines such as tranquilizers, antidepressants, mood elevators, B-blockers, or hynotics indicate that heavy emotional input may contribute to a patient's complaints. Emotional and psychosomatic influences play a large role in myofascial pain and should affect internal joint pathology only secondarily.[7]

Finally, an additional piece of information is the effect of local anesthesia injected into and around the joint capsule either diagnostically or for the purpose of arthrography. In patients with myofascial pain, the pre-auricular pain usually radiates into the temple or neck and increases in intensity after adequate anesthesia of the joint has been achieved. This is a clear indication that most of the pain does not originate in the capsular or intracapsular structures.

Preoperative MPD Management

In cases of painful internal derangement of the TMJ, nonsurgical therapy should almost always be attempted prior to consideration of surgery. Physical therapy and occlusal appliances have been generally successful in maintaining the disc in the proper relationship.[8] If a painful disc is being treated conservatively by physical therapy, 6 to 8 weeks would probably be an adequate period of time to use this mode of therapy before proceeding to more aggressive techniques.

Interocclusal splint therapy is somewhat more complex. In some cases, anterior dislocation of the disc can be reduced with an anterior repositioning splint. The mandible is generally maintained anterior to the habitual occlusion for 2 to 4 months. If the disc cannot be reduced with the anterior repositioning appliance and if the patient continues to have pain in the forward position, early surgical intervention may be indicated (as early as 1 to 2 months after initiation of anterior repositioning splint therapy). The primary source of pain, however, may not be the joint; if it is not, anterior relocation of the joint with the appliance will not be successful. The overall evaluation of the patient and patient's history together with the signs and symptoms of other causes of pain must be addressed.

After successful reduction of the disc with an anterior repositioning appliance, the splint is changed to a centric relation splint, also known as a superior repositioning or muscle relaxation splint. Regardless of the name, the objective is to allow the muscles of mastication to position the mandibular condyles in the most comfortable position without interdigitation or malocclusion of the teeth playing a role.

The subject of condylar positioning is another area of great controversy. I believe that there is no perfect or ideal position for the condyles. Instead, there is a range of positions in which an individual can function in relative comfort. In some persons, the range is very wide, and any position of the condyle will satisfy them functionally. Other individuals have a very narrow range and any positioning of the condyles outside that range will precipitate intracapsular or myofascial discomfort and dysfunction. Thus, the concept of allowing the muscles of mastication to seat the condyles upward and forward against the articular eminence with the disc interposed has been developed.[9,10] This appears to be a position that is reproducible and comfortable in most patients. This also eliminates clinician's judgment dictating condylar position and allows the patient's own masticatory musculature to seat the condyles appropriately.

An anteriorly dislocated disc may be reduced and maintained pain-free for a period of 2 to 4 months, but on relocation of condyle–disc complex into the fossa with use of the centric relation splint, dislocation of the disc may recur.

The dentist who is treating the patient with splints must use clinical judgment in deciding whether to reattempt an anterior repositioning therapy or to evaluate the patient for surgery. Such patients tend to be excellent surgical candidates because the anterior repositioning appliance and resultant good condyle–disc relationship has provided symptomatic relief. Positioning the patient into the seated condyle position with the centric relation splint does not maintain the disc in the appropriate position, however, and the symptoms return. In my clinical experience, such patients have the highest incidence of success from surgical repositioning of the disc.

Patients who have successful anterior repositioning and centric relation splint therapy resulting in a satisfactory relocation of the condyle–disc complex but have residual muscular pain are not candidates for intracapsular TMJ surgery. Their MPD symptoms should be treated conservatively as outlined elsewhere in this text.

Finally, in splint management, as in any other mode of therapy, it is extremely important that the individual clinician treating the patient with splints is well versed not only in the technical aspects but also in the theoretical and pathophysiologic considerations underlying the splint therapy. Any dentist or dental specialist can achieve a level of expertise through study and experience. One may also place a splint in a patient's mouth, however, without having a full and complete understanding of the basic principles of this therapy. This may lead to failures in conservative therapy that are operator dependent rather than technique dependent.

Once one decides that intracapsular surgery is to be performed to correct a disc dislocation, all efforts should be made to decrease MPD preoperatively, if it exists. Most of the physical therapy techniques described elsewhere in this book should be considered depending on the patient's specific complaints. Specifically, the muscles of mastication and the various cervical muscles should be treated for 3 to 6 weeks prior to surgery. This should not only reduce preoperative MPD but also familiarize the patient with the therapist and techniques so that postoperative physical therapy will be facilitated.

Intracapsular TMJ Surgery

Surgical procedures are performed on the TMJ to relocate and/or repair dislocated or perforated discs, correct bony aberrations in the joints, overcome bony or fibrous ankylosis and, occasionally, to reduce fracture dislocations of the entire condyle. These various problems are discussed separately.

Most intracapsular surgery performed today is done to relocate a disc that is dislocated. Sometimes the disc may have suffered severe wear and even perforation. Surgical treatment of perforation is described later. Most authors advocate some sort of disc plication when the disk is dislocated but not severely damaged.[11] Plication is used to designate a procedure in which a structure, in

Fig. 7-1. Modified facelift incision is made in the pre-auricular area. Intrameatal extension to include the skin over the tragus in the anterior flap results in two separated visible portions of the incision which lie in the preauricular fold. Optimal postoperative esthetics and adequate surgical exposure are provided by this approach.

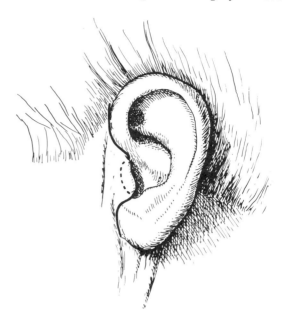

Fig. 7-2. Lateral capsule is incised (arrow), and superior joint space is entered just below the zygomatic arch. Distraction of the condyle inferiorly will allow visualization of the superior surface of the disc.

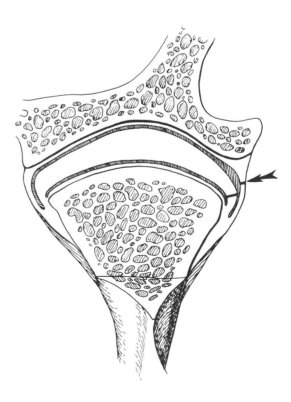

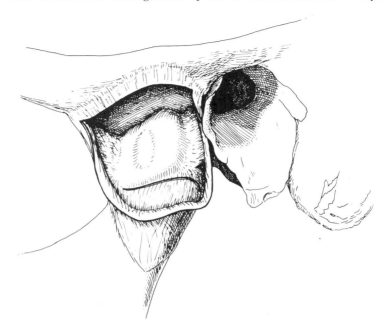

Fig. 7-3.   Inferior joint space is entered, and the condyle is visualized through the illustrated incision of the lateral collateral ligament of the disc.

this case the TMJ disc, is secured or tacked down so that it is either less mobile or is held in place. The dissection I use is as follows.

Conservative TMJ Surgical Technique

A modified facelift incision is made in the preauricular area, allowing an esthetic, functional exposure of the TMJ (Fig. 7-1). The dissection is carried under the superficial temporalis fascia down to the level of the zygomatic arch. The TMJ capsule is cleaned off but not divided until it is exposed from the lateral aspect of the glenoid fossa to the neck of the condyle. An incision is made into the superior joint space through the lateral capsule (Fig. 7-2). The lateral collateral ligament of the disc is divided so that the inferior joint is entered and the head of the mandibular condyle is visualized (Fig. 7-3). An assessment is then made of the disc position and its health. If the disc is significantly displaced anteriorly or medially, the surgeon must determine if excessive tissue exists in the bilaminar zone. If so, a wedge of tissue is removed at the junction of the disc and the bilaminar zone (Fig. 7-4A and B) and is sutured with a long-lasting but resorbable suture (Fig. 7-5A). In such cases, one would expect a longer healing period when this wedge of tissue is removed because the support of the posterior attachment, the bilaminar zone, has been weakened by the surgical removal of this wedge of tissue. Whether or not a

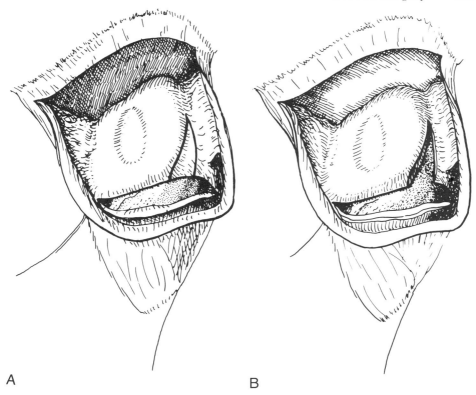

A   B

Fig. 7-4. (**A**) If present, amount of excess posterior tissue is estimated and outlined at the disc–bilaminar junction. (**B**) A wedge of posterolateral tissue is removed to facilitate posterolateral disc repositioning. The size of the excised tissue wedge is designed to provide correct postoperative disc position as well as primary closure with minimal tension.

wedge is removed and plicated posteriorly, a lateral plication should be performed. This is done by placing a mattress suture, using a long-lasting but resorbable material, to shorten and laterally reposition the lateral collateral ligament (Fig. 7-5B). The capsule is sutured (Fig. 7-6), the wound is closed in layers, and a pressure dressing is placed over the skin.

Because patients are asked to use no chewing force for at least 3 weeks following surgery, a soft diet is necessary. Generally, no exercises are given for this 3-week period; however, mild active mobility is encouraged.

Intracapsular TMJ Surgery for Correction of Perforated and Degenerative Discs

Much more controversy exists as to the treatment of cases in which the disc is either perforated or severely altered in shape. This is usually due to chronic dislocation or parafunctional stresses such as clenching or bruxism.

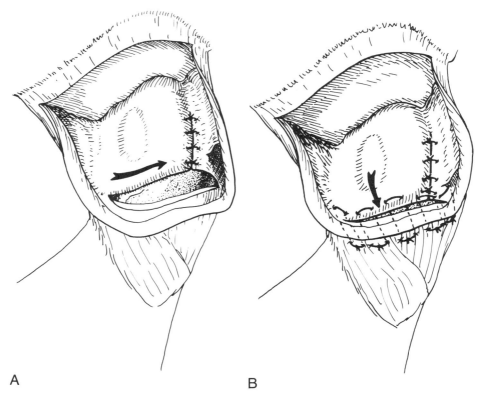

A   B

Fig. 7-5. (A) Primary closure of posterior band and attachment is accomplished using slowly resorbable suture. Arrow shows predominant posterior movement of the disc that results from posterolateral plication. (B) Similar suture is used in mattress fashion to close and plicate lateral colateral ligament, thus repositioning medially displaced disc laterally (arrow). Completed disc repositioning will allow coordinated disc–condyle complex function.

Surgeons agree on surgical repair of dislocated discs when the discs are healthy, as those just described. When perforations exist in severely degenerated discs, however, treatment preferences vary widely. Alternatives have included menisectomy (removal of the disc),[12] menisectomy with replacement by an autologous graft (dermis or skin harvested from the same individual),[13] menisectomy with replacement by alloplastic material (silastic or Teflon proplast implants),[14] eminectomy,[15] condylectomy,[16] condylotomy,[17] and total joint replacement.[18]

Our studies[19] indicated that an experimentally induced perforation in the posterior lateral aspect of the TMJ disc of a Macaque monkey generally lead to degenerative changes, including proliferation of the superior surface of the condylar head and proliferation on the articular surface of the fossa. These proliferations appear to be the first stages of degeneration and resorption. The

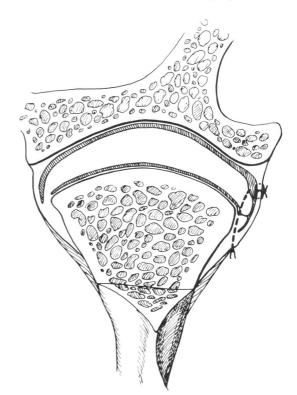

Fig. 7-6. Superior and inferior capsular flaps are primarily closed using interrupted sutures.

disc perforations tended to become larger mediolaterally in the postsurgical period. In 2 of 10 joints, however, perforations healed spontaneously without any treatment.

In a subsequent study,[20] a double-layered synovial membrane flap was used to close surgically induced experimental perforations in the discs of monkeys, and repair of disc perforations was extremely successful. Continuity of the discs was reestablished, thus preventing proliferative and degenerative changes of the articular surfaces of the condyle and glenoid fossa. Therefore, we devised a procedure inside the joint that uses tissue available and that has been used in more than 25 persons with large TMJ perforations. The superior and inferior lamina of the bilaminar zone together with the covering of synovial membrane and its subintimal vasculature is used to repair and reconstitute discal structures. Obviously, a badly perforated or degenerated disc will never be completely normal again. Cadaver studies[21] have indicated, however, that perforation and degenerative changes inside the human TMJ are relatively common. Therefore, a completely normal structure may not be necessary to facilitate adequate TMJ function. I believe that restoring the integrity of the joint internally using structures available locally (i.e., synovial membrane and its vasculature) is vastly superior to the introduction of either alloplastic or autogenic materials from other areas.

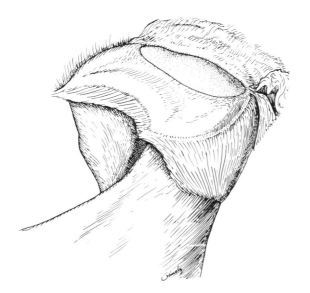

Fig. 7-7. Large perforation that may be identified after entrance into superior joint space. Extensive defect in the disc prohibits its inclusion in a conservative plication procedure. Perforations may occur in the disc (as shown), the bilaminar region, or at the junctional area.

Our stereoscopic and histologic studies have indicated that the double-layered synovial membrane flap used to close large perforations in the discs of monkeys has led to a relatively normal reconstitution of the disc and maintenance of articular surfaces. These studies were performed in the short-term animal studies, and long-term studies are obviously necessary. A description follows of the technique for closure of large perforations using the synovial membrane flap and remobilization of the remaining elements of the discs.

TMJ Surgical Repair of Large Perforations

The surgical approach to the TMJ is exactly the same as described above to the point of identifying a large perforation somewhere in the discs or retrodiscal tissues (Fig. 7-7). When the perforation is identified, the superior and inferior joint spaces are fully opened and the extent of the perforation is observed. An incision (Fig. 7-8A) is made through the lateral collateral ligament to expose the perforation laterally so that the entire borders of the perforation can be seen from the lateral aspect. The bilaminar zone is then divided carefully with the small dissecting scissors into two distinct lamina all the way back to their origins. (Fig. 7-8B). The superior lamina originates from the tympanic plate of the temporal bone. The inferior lamina originates in the neck of the condyle. The two lamina should be divided with a fine scalpel blade where they join on the medial aspect of the perforation. The anterior margin of the perforation is usually in the cartilaginous discal tissue. This is divided very carefully in a filet manner so that an incision approximately 1-mm deep is made in the middle of this discal tissue and brought around all the way to the lateral aspect at the junction of the condylomeniscal ligament. (This permits closure

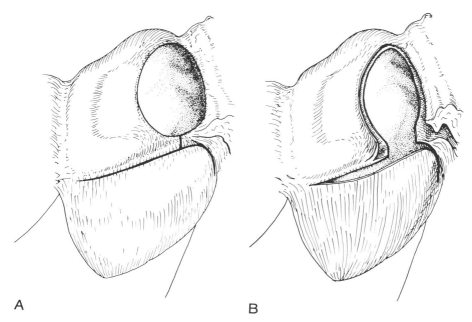

A   B

Fig. 7-8. **(A)** Inverted T-shaped incision is made lateral to perforation. Horizontal arm enters the inferior joint space through the lateral colateral ligament. Vertical arm connects previous incision with the perforation, allowing complete visualization of the edge of the defect. **(B)** With a fine scissors and blade, the entire perforation and vertical incision periphery is divided into superior and inferior layers. Extensive anterior dissection is accomplished to provide freedom for posterior repositioning of anterior disc segment.

of the wound in a double-layered fashion, much as an oronasal or oroantral fistula would be closed.) The inferior aspect of the disc is often convex in these cases and does not fit well over the head of the condyle. If this is so, the surgeon may need to recontour slightly with a scalpel blade the inferior convexity of the disc so that it is somewhat more concave and fits the head of the condyle. Condyle or fossa that have irregularities should be extremely conservatively removed, with every intention of maintaining articular surface in its best integrity. The two lamina of the bilaminar zone should be mobilized maximally until the disc and the bilaminar attachments can be approximated without tension. The anterior dissection must be extensive enough to mobilize the remaining portion of the disc so that it can be moved in a posterior direction.

The inferior lamina is sutured (Fig. 7-9A) to the lower filet of the discal tissue from medial to lateral using a 5/0 vicryl resorbable suture with the knots tied on the superior side. When this has been completed, the superior lamina is sutured (Fig. 7-9B) to the superior aspect of the discal filet with the knots on the inferior side. Some dead space (Fig. 7-10) between the superior and inferior laminae will exist and is allowed to remain. It will fill with blood, clot,

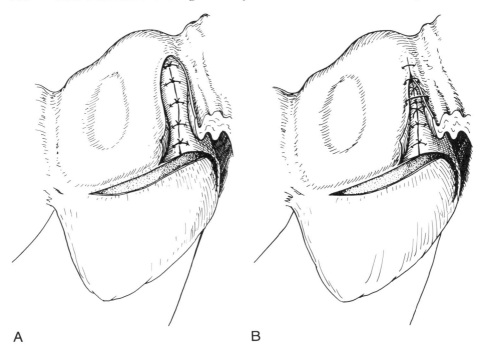

A   B

Fig. 7-9. (**A**) A double-layered closure is performed. First, inferior lamina and lower filet of disc are advanced and closed primarily. (**B**) Superior lamina and upper disc tissue are then opposed and sutured. Interrupted resorbable sutures with knots directed toward the center are used.

and ultimately organize into a scar of fibrous connective tissue. Often, the superior lamina may be sutured first due to access.

The remaining lateral incised tissue is plicated using horizontal mattress sutures as described above, thus securing the posterior lateral disc to the lateral portion of the condyle.

The rest of the surgical closure is then performed in a manner identical to the procedure described for intracapsular TMJ surgery (p. 183).

When large perforations have been repaired, a more gentle postoperative protocol must be adhered to because of the delicateness of the repair. Certain splint alternatives are also used in these cases.

No general formula can be given for postoperative physical therapy following these procedures. A close communication between the surgeon and the physical therapist is required to insure proper postoperative management. Generally, the more tenuous the repair, the more cautious the approach must be to physical therapy in the early stages. Following surgery, the surgeon should have some feel for the strength of his repair and should communicate this to the physical therapist so that a reasonable physical therapy program can be designed.

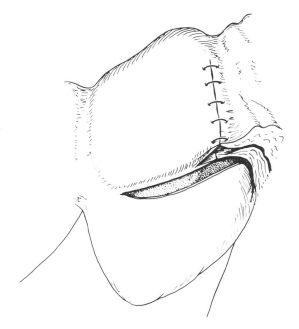

Fig. 7-10. Completed posterior repair and resultant dead space. This space will be obliterated by fibrous connective tissue formed during healing.

Autologous and Alloplastic Versus Natural Repair

An area of intense disagreement and controversy regarding surgical repair of the TMJ centers around the use of implant and alloplastic materials. It is important to divide TMJ disorders into two categories. The first category involves dislocated discs without gross perforations or degenerations. The general consensus among surgeons is that a conservative relocation and plication of the disc into its most anatomical position is necessary for this group.[11] Some surgeons, however, advocate more radical measures such as menisectomy[12] with or without alloplastic or autologous implant.[13,14] An autologous implant is a material harvested from the same individual and reimplanted without its own original blood supply. A good example of this is a skin graft taken from the hip and placed on the face in reconstruction of a burn injury. In such an implant system, the graft is intended to be placed on a vascularized bed that will rapidly revascularize the implant, rendering it essentially functioning as a normal part of the recipient site. Autologous graft survival following TMJ menisectomy is uncertain.

The second category, alloplastic implants, refers to substances that are artificially produced, such as silicone rubber (Silastic, Dow Corning, Midland, MI) or Proplast/Teflon (Vitek, Houston, TX). Animal studies[22] and our own clinical observations indicate that use of alloplastic materials causes a degenerative process in the joint. The bone of the fossa and condylar head resorb and remodel even when the implant is placed without harming the articular surfaces. Several investigators[23] have reported fraying and disintegration of the implants, with distant migration of small alloplastic particles as a result of their inability to withstand the trauma of constant occlusal forces. Giant cell inflammatory reactions have been observed around these particles, indicating a foreign body response.

Because most patients receiving TMJ surgery are in their late twenties and early thirties, use of materials that in the short term appear to cause degenerative, destructive changes would appear to be contraindicated when a normal life span is anticipated for these persons. Unlike hip prostheses that are generally placed in persons in their sixth and seventh decades of life, a TMJ implant or prosthesis may be required to function for 40 to 50 years. Therefore, I believe that in patients who have normal continuity to the disc, there is no indication for removal of the disc and replacement with an autologous or alloplastic implant material.

Autologous and Alloplastic for Repairing Large Perforations

In cases with large perforations or degeneration of the disc, the same choices for treatment are available; however, several pertinent factors should be mentioned.

Patients with perforations tend to be approximately 10 years older on the average, having parafunctional habits such as bruxism (grinding of the teeth) and often extreme emotional involvement regarding their facial pain.[24] The significance is that these patients may continue their parafunctional and emotional targeting of the TMJ after the surgical procedure. The accompanying microtrauma that occurs in the joint will also continue over the postoperative period. Many surgeons[25,26] believe that the TMJ lacks the capability for healing and that one should therefore be much more aggressive in treating these patients.

The TMJ has a considerable capability for healing.[19,20,27] The cartilage in the joint is not hyaline cartilage, but fibrocartilage, and undifferentiated mesenchymal tissue in the joint does have a potential for remodeling and healing. Synovial membrane with its vasculature has a tremendous potential for repair. Therefore, much of the controversy about handling of the severely damaged TMJ centers around the opinion of the surgeon as to the healing capabilities of the joint. Alloplastic implant materials have a consistent experimental record of causing degenerative and resorptive changes in the bones and articular surfaces of the TMJ. I believe, therefore, that these substances should be avoided, since it is highly unlikely that anything resembling a normal TMJ can be achieved using these materials.

Regarding the use of autogenous graft materials, dermis[13] and fascia harvested from any fascia surface (personal experience) have been used and may serve to "patch" perforations in the TMJ disc and bilaminar zone. These materials do not function as a true graft, however, in that they are not placed in a vascularized bed where one would expect them to "take" in classical fashion. These materials will act as a matrix for the ingrowth of fibrous connective tissue, synovial membrane, and scar formation that may function as a replacement disc.

For a 3-year period following studies on monkeys, we have treated more than 40 human TMJs with large perforations using a flap from the retrodiscal tissue lined with synovial membrane.[20] Rather than harvesting autologous graft materials from distance sites, we believe that a more physiologic method is to mobilize the two layers of the retrodiscal tissue and reapproximate them with the disc allowing for healing, scar formation, and remodeling of the disc and retrodiscal tissues. In conjunction with carefully planned centric relation splint and physical therapy, this technique can render most of these patients vastly improved over their preoperative situation without risking increased degenerative changes and further degeneration of the joint. Over this 3-year period, these patients have scored nearly as highly as the patients with routine joint plications in terms of resolution of postoperative pain. In our experience, ROM is more limited. Although why this is so is not entirely clear, two reasons probably explain this phenomenon. First, many of these patients have had severe limitation of motion for many years prior to their surgery; therefore, a number of muscular and tendonous structures act as limiters of mandibular ROM. Second, the double-layer flap closure does decrease the overall size of the joint, causing more tension and tightness in the joint. One would therefore expect ROM to return more slowly and also some permanent ROM loss.

Whatever the reason, the decrease in ROM may not be any greater than the decrease in ROM of patients who have other types of procedures for gross disc perforation. This specific group of patients has not been fully studied, however.

Postoperative Physical Therapy

Postoperative physical therapy can be divided into two general categories: MPD management and mobilization.

MPD Management.

MPD management is similar to that used for nonsurgical patients or for preoperative management of surgical cases. This treatment can begin within 2 to 3 weeks postoperatively depending on patient comfort. Assuming that no major stress is placed on the TMJ, any technique designed to reduce muscle pain or tension is acceptable.

Mobilization.

Mobilization of the TMJ after intracapsular surgery is a different matter entirely. Much depends on how much mobility existed prior to surgery and how long the decreased mobility existed. If the patient had limited mobility for a short time only or not at all, after surgery only simple stretching exercises, opening against resistance, and active lateral movement are necessary. Opening against resistance and lateral movements must be performed with caution early after surgery. How soon and to what degree will often depend on the extent of the repair and the ability of the surgeon to establish a strong reconstruction. Often this can be taught to the patient by the surgeon and may not require formal physical therapy.

If decreased mobility has existed for several months or longer preoperatively, shortening of the muscles of mastication and capsular tightness should also be expected. In addition, in many cases, more severe internal damage and thus more extensive surgery and scarring exists in the joint. Therefore, the obstacles to overcome in hypomobility are both chronic muscle shortening and loss of extensibility of the TMJ capsule and ligaments. Pain is also a factor since these patients tend to have longer, more painful postoperative courses than do the simpler cases.

The dilemma faced in these severe cases is that the sooner mobilization procedures are begun, the better the chance of overcoming capsular tightness and muscle shortening. Conversely, if a large perforation has been repaired, a longer healing period is ideal before the repair is stressed. Clinical judgment is our only guideline in deciding when to begin postoperative physical therapy.

Capsular tightness and muscle shortening that may occur after surgery should not be confused with that which exists prior to surgery. Any capsular tightness that occurs prior to surgery should simply be the result of chronic lack of mobility. After surgery, since incisions are made through the superior aspect of the capsule into the superior joint space and through the lateral collateral ligament into the inferior joint space, the resuturing and healing of these structures will undoubtedly cause scarring, contracture, and some loss of extensibility in the TMJ capsule. Muscle shortening that exists in these patients should be only a result of decreased ROM prior to surgery which has an affect on the overall muscle length and muscle flexibility. Nothing occurs during the TMJ surgery to shorten or change muscle length.

Muscular pain (i.e., myofascial pain) may very much limit joint mobility following surgery. In my experience in many cases, as the postoperative swelling declines, the mandible changes position. If the centric relation splint is not adjusted frequently, the muscles of mastication may become extremely tender, causing limitation of opening, deviation of opening, and various other muscular influences on the position of the mandible. Sometimes this can be deceiving to the clinician as the occlusion and opening are evaluated. Persistent muscle hyperactivity and dysfunction following surgery can make it very difficult to determine normal seated condylar position and to achieve increased ROM. Often the repair is more tenuous, requiring a longer healing period before stress can be placed on the joint. Again, a close communication between surgeon and physical therapist is essential to facilitate proper timing of mobilization procedures. Mobilization techniques must obviously be continued much longer in such patients, and gains will be more gradual. In the most severe cases, the mobility attained after surgery may be greater than preoperative mobility; however, it may remain less than that of the normal population. Therefore, persistence over the long term will usually provide satisfactory results.

No good clinical and basic research has been done on postoperative adhesions. We have observed postoperative adhesions between the articular surfaces of joints following trauma or surgery. This is supposed to result from bleeding into the joint which, due to a lack of mobility, permits organization of the clot as opposed to lysis. Studies[28] show that constant mobility after joint trauma or surgery generally causes lysis of blood clots rather than organizationn into connective tissue. If this organization is permitted to progress, however, adhesions may occur in which strands of fibrous connective tissue exist between the disc and the fossa or condyle. In the first 3 to 4 weeks after surgery, patients commonly experience tightness on opening and during some sort of mild forced opening such as yawning, laughing, or opening for tooth brushing; patients hear a snap in an operated joint that may deliver a sharp pain but also gives them a feeling of somewhat greater ROM. This may represent the breaking of an adhesion and even though patients may feel some discomfort, it probably represents a favorable occurrence in the mobilization and return to normal function of the joints.

Cervical spine MPD that exists pre- or postoperatively must be addressed in the postoperative phase. Range of motion exercises, splint management, pain control, and head posture management to minimize myofascial pain of the cervical and shoulder musculature are in essential part of managing MPD of the masticatory system.

Postoperative Splint Therapy

Postoperative splint therapy plays an important role in recovery from TMJ surgery.[11,24] Malocclusion plays a role in both disc dislocations of the TMJ and MPD of the muscles of mastication.[29] If dental occlusion plays any role in the etiology or perpetuation of TMJ dysfunction, a postoperative splint is probably necessary in most cases. Even when a satisfactory occlusion is ultimately reached, it is unrealistic to expect that this occlusion will occur in the first or second week after surgery, because pain, swelling of the joints, and altered muscular activity will continue. In certain cases, after a 6- to 8-week healing period, splints are removed and a satisfactory occlusion has occurred; in such cases, no further occlusional adjustments need be made. Frequently, however, a significant malocclusion exists following completion of TMJ surgical and nonsurgical management.

Recently, a tremendous increase in orthognathic surgery has occurred for several reasons. In the early years of orthognathic surgery, this type of facial correction was performed primarily for esthetic considerations. As the orthodontic and gnathological specialties have grown, however, the awareness of both the professional (dental and medical) and lay communities, and the criteria on which a satisfactory bite is based, have become more demanding. We are now capable of positioning teeth, jaws, and TMJs in almost ideal positions, both functionally and esthetically. Therefore, postoperative splints are designed to compensate for any malocclusion that may exist after surgery.

The centric relation splint is placed in the mouth the day after surgery and is adjusted to a position comfortable for the patient. It is adjusted again at 1 week postoperatively because the mandibular position changes as swelling diminishes. This procedure is continued until a stable mandibular position is achieved. In patients with minimal MPD, this stable position is usually reached in 3 to 6 weeks. In the most severe cases, 3 to 4 months may be necessary, especially when MPD is a major factor.

Once the stable mandibular position is achieved, measures must be taken to change the occlusion of the teeth so that this mandibular condylar position can be maintained in the muscle-dictated position achieved with the postoperative splint. The methods used to alter the occlusion depend on the extent of malocclusion. In minor cases, grinding of the teeth (equilibration) or minor orthodontic tooth movement may be all that is necessary. Severe cases may require major orthodontic tooth movement, major dental reconstruction, or orthognathic surgery to reposition the entire lower and/or upper jaws depending on the type of the malocclusion.

When large perforations have been repaired, splint management postoperatively is somewhat different. In large perforation repairs, the suture line may be directly superior to the head of the condyle. Therefore, an anterior repositioning splint that moves the condyle slightly forward for a period of 6 to 8 weeks after surgery probably provides the best possibility for healing of the bilaminar attachment to the disc. After 6 to 8 weeks of anterior repositioning just sufficient to prohibit pressure from the condyle on the suture line, the splint is changed to a centric relation splint and the same method as described above is followed for seating the condyles and muscle relaxation.

Bony and Fibrous Ankylosis

Intracapsular surgery to correct ankylosis is different from other types of TMJ surgery. Ankylosis indicates that the joint is "frozen" either by a direct bony connection between the condyle and the glenoid fossa of the temporal bone or by dense fibrous connective tissue. If this condition has existed for more than a few months, severe muscle shortening will have occurred in the muscles of mastication, especially the temporalis, as well as capsular tightness.

Surgical correction of this situation usually involves removal of the bony or fibrous connections and interposition of some material such as silicone to prevent reankylosis.[30] Often this will achieve only partial mobility, so removal of the coronoid process of the mandible, which is the temporalis muscle insertion, will be neceeessary. Because reattachment of these muscles to the mandible occurs rapidly after surgical removal of the coronoid process, intense mobilization must be undertaken immediately after surgery.

The immediacy of mobilization after ankylosis surgery is a major difference between this type of surgery and other TMJ surgeries. Mobilization exercises, complete with strong active stretching using tongue blades or other mechanical devices, should begin the day after surgery and should continue at frequent intervals for 6 to 12 months. It is almost impossible to be too rigorous in the attempt to prevent reankylosis. The major deterrent to proper postoperative mobilization in these patients is pain. Strong analgesics may be necessary in the early postoperative period to achieve adequate mobility. These should be decreased as soon as possible, however, to prevent drug dependence. In these cases, the obstacles to mobility are dense scar tissue and chronically shortened muscles. Short of loosening the teeth, little harm can be done by vigorous, frequent stretching of mandibular opening. Strengthening of the depressors of the mandible (suprahyoid muscles) is also helpful in increasing mandibular opening.

Orthognathic surgery refers to surgical repositioning of the jaws in the most normal position possible to optimize function and esthetics. The primary functions of the jaws are speech, mastication, swallowing, and respiration. The jaws and mouth play a major role in personal appearance and thus in interpersonal relationships, self-image, and confidence. One cannot separate functional and esthetic considerations in orthognathic surgery because regardless of the motivation for treatment, both must be addressed to achieve a satisfactory result.

Of patients who elect TMJ treatment, many have a class II (retrognathic) dental skeletal relationship.[31] Why this facial deformity exists most frequently in TMJ patients is not completely clear. Habitual protrusion of the mandible is believed to be performed to achieve a more appropriate incisor relationship in order to improve breathing and airway management or to facilitate speech or simply for esthetic reasons. This constant protrusion of the mandible may introduce a laxity into the stabilization ligaments of the TMJ disc, permitting a frequent dislocation. Whatever the reason, correlation between class II malocclusions and disc dislocations is quite high. Therefore, a significant portion of patients who have been treated successfully for TMJ internal derangement are left with a class II malocclusion following successful treatment, with or without surgery on the joints. Often, the only possibility for correcting a class II dental skeletal relationship is not only orthodontic management but surgical advancement of the mandible.

In patients with craniomandibular deformities, orthognathic surgery is often performed to correct a malocclusion that prevents proper TMJ function. Many patients with TMJ complaints have major malocclusions that are due to deformities of the jaws that can be corrected only by altering the jaw position surgically. TMJ patients include both intracapsular problems and MPD complaints. The role of orthognathic surgery is to correct jaw malpositioning whenever it contributes to either of these maladies.

Many MPD patients are treated successfully with the centric relation splint. Often this reveals that their teeth do not fit together properly when the muscles of mastication place the condyles in their most comfortable position. Wide clinical experience demonstrates that if a centric relation splint renders the patient comfortable, surgical repositioning of the jaws can be expected to achieve the same comfort.

Orthognathic surgery is indicated whenever nonsurgical means cannot properly position the occlusion. Orthognathic surgery may involve surgical repositioning of the maxilla, mandible, or both. Surgical repositioning of the maxilla alone has very little effect on mandibular mobility.[32] Mandibular surgery, however, especially sagittal-split osteotomy of the mandible, does contribute to decreased mobility of the mandible.[32]

Sagittal-split osteotomy of the mandible is most often performed to advance the retrognathic mandible; however, mandibular setback and corrections of asymmetry are also performed. The technique involves an intraoral incision along the anterior border of the ramus so that the entire external oblique ridge is exposed. A subperiosteal dissection is performed along the medial aspect of the mandibular ramus inside the medial pterygoid muscle. A subperiosteal dissection is also performed on the lateral aspect of the mandible where the mandibular ramus and the mandibular body meet. This is deep to the more anterior aspect of the masseter muscle insertion. A horizontal osteotomy (Fig. 7-11A) is made on the medial aspect of the mandible just above the entrance of the inferior alveolar neurovascular bundle into the ramus. This osteotomy penetrates approximately halfway through the medial ramus cortical plate. A vertical osteotomy (Fig. 7-11B) is made on the lateral cortex of the mandible at the junction of the mandibular ramus and mandibular body. This osteotomy penetrates only the lateral cortical plate. A connecting cut is then made between the two so that the mandible can then be split (Fig. 7-12A through C) into a proximal and distal segment. Following completion of this procedure bilaterally, the mandible is repositioned into a predetermined occlusion, and the teeth are wired together. The proximal and distal segments on each side are then wired (Fig. 7-13 A and B) or fixed rigidly with screws, with the condyles of the mandible unchanged from their preoperative position. Probably the most frequent complication in sagittal-split surgery of the mandible is failure to place the condyles in their preoperative position. This is especially true if a rigid fixation system is used.[33]

To understand this inability to place the condyles in their preoperative position, one must understand the situation that exists at the time of surgery. Following completion of the sagittal-split operation, one essentially has the mandible in three pieces. The distal segment includes all the teeth, the body of the mandible, and the chin. The two proximal segments include the condyles, coronoid processes, and mandibular rami bilaterally. All three segments are independent of one another. At this point in the surgery, the surgeon wires the distal segment into the desired postoperative occlusion by fitting the teeth together, using a preformed occlusal template, and wiring the teeth together. This establishes the postoperative position of the distal segment. How then can one establish the desired positioning of the proximal segments so that the condyles will be in exactly the same position they were in prior to surgery after they have been appropriately seated using one of the methods already described? This particular issue is the subject of much controversy among surgeons. An

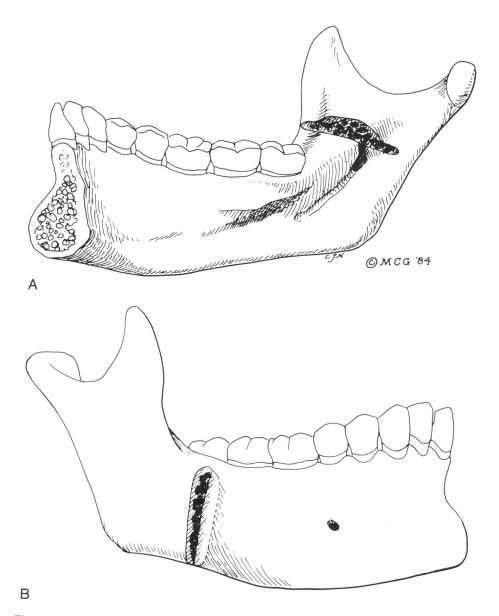

Fig. 7-11. **(A)** Initial long cut made during sagittal split osteotomy of the mandible is a medial horizontal osteotomy through the medial cortex. It extends from the anterior border of the ramus to just posterior and above the mandibular lingula and inferior alveolar neurovascular bundle. **(B)** Vertical osteotomy is then made through the lateral cortex in the posterior body of the mandible. An access bevel is placed on the anterior lip of the osteotomy.

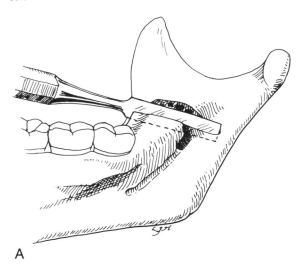

Fig. 7-12. After lateral vertical and medial horizontal cuts are connected by an osteotomy along the anterior border of ramus and external oblique line of the mandible, the distal and proximal segments are separated (split) with chisels introduced into the medial, anterior ramus, and lateral osteotomy sites. **(A)** medial site (*Figure continues*).

A

extensive review is beyond the scope of this chapter; however, positioning of this segment can best be achieved by carefully studying the plaster model of the proposed surgery prior to the actual surgery and radiographic evaluation of the cephalometric head films. The surgeon should go into surgery with a precise knowledge of the defect that will be created between the proximal and distal segments on each side (Fig. 7-13 A and B) as the mandible is advanced into its new position. If simple bony wiring and intermaxillary fixation for 8 weeks are to be used, this will be sufficient to permit proper positioning of the proximal segments at the time of surgery.[34] If a rigid system of fixation is to be used between the proximal and distal segments, such as bone screws, however, it is safe to assume that some mediolateral discrepancies will exist in condylar positioning following the technique.[35] I am now working on a system for a more accurate positioning of the condyles at the time of surgery; results will be reported in a later article.

In the creation of mandibular hypomobility following sagittal-split osteotomy it is important that the temporalis muscle is detached from the retromolar area to the anterior aspect of the coronoid process. In addition, the medial and lateral periosteum is elevated from the mandibular ramus, and most of these patients are wired into intermaxillary fixation for 8 to 12 weeks. Studies[32] show that of all the orthognathic procedures used today, this operation results in the greatest decrease in mandibular mobility.

Following release of intermaxillary fixation, mobilization procedures should begin immediately and continue for at least 4 to 6 months. The probable cause for decreased mobility is scarring and contracture of the temporalis tendon. Moreover, the TMJ has been immobile causing some decreased extensibility of the capsule and supporting ligaments. Studies[36] show that with proper postoperative exercises performed long enough, mandibular mobility can be regained after sagittal-split osteotomy of the mandible.

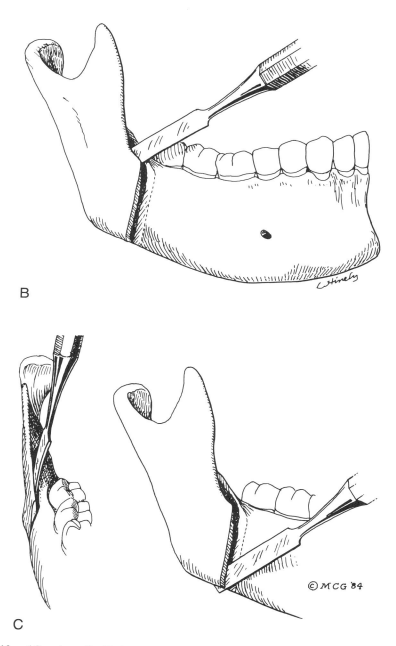

B

C

Fig. 7-12. (*Continued*). (**B,C**) anterior ramus and lateral ostemysites. Gentle prying and incising movements complete sagittal splitting.

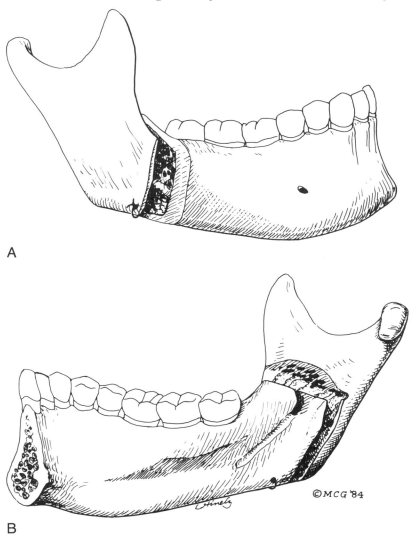

Fig. 7-13. Tooth-bearing distal segment is advanced, and the condyle of the proximal segment is postured in its preoperative position. When the resulting cortical defect is as predicted from preoperative planning, an inferior border wire may be placed for stabilization of segments: **(A)** lateral; and **(B)** medial views.

Relapse following surgical advancement of the mandible has been reported[37] by authors over the years and is believed to be due to several factors. Clearly, previous studies[37] and my own experience show that one of the primary factors has been improper positioning of the proximal segment at the time of surgery. For instance, chronic shortening of the lateral pterygoid muscles may have occurred prior to surgery owing to a patient's constant forward posturing of the mandible. This may not be detected in the surgical workup or at the time of surgery. The shortened lateral pterygoid muscles will not permit full intra-operative seating of the condyles. Therefore, if the patient is wired or fixed with rigid screw fixation in this position with the condyle slightly out of the glenoid fossa, the amount of actual bony advancement of the mandible will be insufficient. Later, once the patient is released from intermaxillary fixation or from training elastics, functional factors influencing jaw position may permit relaxation of the lateral pterygoid muscles, which would seat the condyles and lead to "immediate" surgical relapse. I believe that this is the overwhelming major cause for "relapse" in mandibular advancement surgery. Other factors that obviously play a role are the muscular attachments to the mandible, such as the suprahyoid musculature, that resist advancement. This is especially true when the mandible is advanced and rotated to close an open bite.[38] Devices and techniques have been developed to contour these soft tissue restraints on the advanced mandible; however, no consensus has been reached on successful treatment. Rigid fixation techniques may overcome much of this problem if condylar positioning during surgery can be achieved with a higher degree of accuracy than is now available.

My experience with several patients who have had surgery elsewhere has been that a restriction of mandibular opening occurred either immediately after surgery or later, when screws were used to fix segments rigidly in the sagittal-split osteotomy. This may have been due to rotation or torquing of the condyles that mechanically locked the opening. Moreover, discs may be dislocated by this technique or others, which can also obstruct opening. Prior to treatment of mandibular hypomobility, a diagnosis must be made. Chronic muscle short-ening, muscle or tendon scarring and contracture, fibrosis of TMJ capsule, fibrous or bony ankylosis, and pain all contribute to mandibular hypomobility. Methods to improve mobility should be aimed at overcoming the etiology while protecting vulnerable or recently operated structures.

SUMMARY

Physical therapy is an integral component of management of mandibular and cervical spine myofascial pain prior to and following TMJ surgery and of restoration of mandibular dynamics after intracapsular TMJ or orthognathic surgery on the mandible. The specific therapy regimen and goals are dependent on the preoperative diagnosis, the preexisting muscular and osseous anatomic limitations, the patients' emotional status, the type and success of the surgical intervention and adjunctive therapy, and patient cooperation. The frequent and free interchange of information between surgeon and physical therapist is of paramount importance for the successful management of the oral and maxil-lofacial surgical patient.

REFERENCES

1. Agerberg G, Carlsson GE: The symptoms of functional disturbances of the masticatory system: a comparison of frequencies in population sample and in a group of patients. Acta Odontol Scand 33:183, 1975
2. Omnell KA: Historical review of temporomandibular joint arthrography, p. 1. In Moffett BC, Westesson PL (eds): Diagnosis of Internal Derangements of the Temporomandibular Joint. Vol. 1: Double Contrast Arthrography and Clinical Correlation. University of Washington, Seattle, 1984
3. Roberts D, Pettigrew J, Lewis B et al: Differentiation of the TMJ meniscus in CT sections. J Dent Res (special issue) 63:228, 1984
4. Wilkinson T, Maryniuk G: The correlation between sagittal anatomic sections and computerized tomography of the TMJ. J Craniomandibular Practice 1:37, 1983
5. Helmy E, Bays R, Devkota J, Sharawy M: Correlation of TMJ true planes and reconstructed planes of computed tomography (CT) to anatomical sections (abstr.). American Association of Oral and Maxillofacial Surgery annual meeting, Washington DC, 1985
6. Harms SE, Wilk RM, Wolford LM, et al: The temporomandibular joint: magnetic resonance imaging using surface coils. Radiology 157:133, 1985
7. Travell JG, Simons DG: Myofascial Pain and Dysfunction: The Trigger Point Manual, p. 177. Williams & Wilkins, Baltimore, 1983
8. McNeill C: Nonsurgical management, p. 193. In Helms CA, Katzberg RW, Dolwick MF (eds): Internal Derangements of the Temporomandibular Joint. Radiology Research and Education Foundation. San Francisco, 1983
9. Roth RH: Temporomandibular pain dysfunction and occlusal relationships. Angle Orthod 43:136, 1973
10. Williamson EH, Steinke RN, Morse TK, Swift TR: Centric relation: a comparison of muscle determined position and operator guidance. Am J Orthod 77:133, 1980
11. Dolwick MS, et al: 1984 criteria for TMJ meniscus surgery. Am Assoc Oral Maxillofac Surg, 1984
12. Bowman K: Temporomandibular joint arthrosis and its treatment by extirpation of the disc. Acta Chir Scand, suppl. 95:118, 1947
13. Georgiade N: The surgical correction of temporomandibular joint dysfunction by means of autogonous dermal grafts. Plast Reconstr Surg 30:68, 1962
14. Gordon S: Surgery of the temporomandibular joint. Am J Surg 95:263, 1958
15. Myrhaug H: New method of operation for habitual dislocation of the mandible. Acta Odontol Scand 9:247, 1951
16. Henny FA, Baldridge OL: Condylectomy for the persistently painful temporomandibular joint. J Oral Surg 15:214, 1957
17. Ward TG: Surgery of the mandibular joint. Ann R Coll Surg Engl 18:139, 1961
18. Kent GN, Misiek DJ, Akin RK, et al: TMJ condylar prosthesis, a 10 year report. J Oral Maxillofac Surg 41:245, 1983
19. Helmy E, Bays RA, Sharawy M: Microscopic alterations in the TMJ of the adult monkey (abstr.). American Association of Oral and Maxillofacial Surgery, annual meeting, New York, 1984
20. Bays RA, Helmy E, Sharawy M: The synovial membrane flap for the repair of TMJ disc perforations in *Macaca* fascicularis: a stereometric study (abstr.). American Association of Oral and Maxillofacial Surgery, annual meeting, Washington D.C., 1985

21. Oberg T, Carlsson GE, Fajers C: Temporomandibular joint, a morphological study on human autopsy material. Acta Odontol Scand 29:349, 1971

22. Stewart LR: Histology of host response to alloplastic condylar implants in *Macaca fascicularis* (abstr.). American Association of Oral and Maxillofacial Surgery, annual meeting, New York, 1984

23. Timmis D, Aragon SB, VanSickels JE, Aufdemorte TB: A compared study of alloplastic TMJ meniscal replacements in rabbits (abstr.). American Association of Oral and Maxillofacial Surgery, annual meeting, Washington, 1985

24. Bays RA: Temporomandibular joint meniscus repair surgery: a follow-up study. Fac Orthop Temporomandib Arthrol 2:11, 1985

25. Wilkes CH: Structural and functional alterations of the temporomandibular joint. North West Dentistry 57:287, 1978

26. Silver CN, Simon SD: Meniscus injuries of the temporomandibular joint. J Bone Joint Surg 38:541, 1956

27. Wallace D, Laskin DM: Healing of surgical defects in retrodiscal tissue of rabbit temporomandibular joint. J Dent Res (special issue) 866, 1984

28. Salter RB: Regeneration of articular cartilage through continuous passive motion. Past, present and future. p. 101. In Staub R, Wilson PD (eds): Clinical Trends in Orthopedics. Thieme Stratton, New York, 1982

29. Krough-Poulsen W: The significance of occlusion in temporomandibular function and dysfunction. In Solburg WK, Clark GT (eds): Temporomandibular Joint Problems: Biologic Diagnosis and Treatment. Quintessence, Publishers Chicago, 1980

30. Henny FA: The temporomandibular joint. p. 428. In Kruger G. (ed): Textbook of Oral and Maxillofacial Surgery. 5th Ed. CV Mosby, St. Louis, 1979

31. Dibbets JM, van der Weele LT, Uildriks AK: Symptoms of TMJ dysfunction: indicators of growth patterns? J Pedodontics 9(4):265, 1985

32. Aragon SB, VanSickels JE, Dolwick MF, Flanary CM: The effects of orthognathic surgery on mandibular range of motion. J Oral Maxillofac Surg 43:938, 1985

33. Kundert M, Hadjianghelou O: Condylar displacement after sagittal splitting of the mandibular rami. J Maxillofac Surg 8:278, 1980

34. Singer RS, Bays RA: A comparison between superior and inferior border wiring techniques in sagittal split ramus osteotomy. J Oral Maxillofacial Surg 43:448, 1985

35. Spitzer W, Rettinger G, Sitzmann F: Computerized tomography examination for the detection of positional changes in the temporomandibular joint after ramus osteotomies with screw fixation. J Maxillofacial Surg 12:139, 1984

36. Bell WH, Gonyea W, Finn RA, et al: Muscular rehabilitation after orthognathic surgery. Oral Surg 56:229, 1983

37. Schendel FA, Epker BN: Results after mandibular advancement surgery: analysis of the 87 cases. J Oral Surg 38:265, 1980

38. Proffit WR, Bell WH: Openbite. p. 1075. In Bell WH, Proffit WR, White RP (eds): Surgical Correction of Dentofacial Deformities. WB Saunders, Philadelphia, 1980

8 | Stabilizing the Occlusion: Finishing Procedures

Duane Grummons

In the past decade, our understanding and capability to manage cranio-mandibular and craniocervical dysfunction patients properly and differentially have advanced immeasurably. Better patient management and predictable treatment response can occur when comprehensive clinical findings and factors are integrated into an approach based on scientifically based fundamentals.

Once therapeutic procedures have been properly integrated with whole-person treatment approaches, TMJ components have been stabilized, and dysfunction issues have been optimally managed, dental colleagues are called on to correct and optimize occlusal factors definitively. Of critical importance is the understanding of relationships between facial orthopedics and occlusion as they influence the craniomandibular and cervical regions. The concept has too often been to abandon TMJ splints while providing subsequent dental care. Also vitally important is provision of continued management of the cervical spine issues in conjunction with splint maintenance as dental factors are corrected and occlusal stability is established.

Dentistry and allied professions continue to provide solutions for these difficult TMJ patients during the definitive occlusal corrective phase. Only biologically sensible and practical treatment alternatives should be considered. Progressive treatment is provided in a caring manner with a coordinated team approach.[1]

PHASE I AND PHASE II CONCEPTS

Phase I management refers to pain/dysfunction management implementing the specific modalities subscribed to in a team approach as covered in other chapters. Phase II care refers to the definitive jaw and occlusal corrective procedures that are generally intended to permit patients to withdraw from stabilization/repositional splints while providing optimal mandibular and cervical musculoskeletal relationships. Optimized TMJ function, harmonized jaw (skeletal) and bite interrelationships are a priority now. Functional relationships and mitigating occlusal factors are corrected definitively in phase II, once phase I pain/dysfunction priorities have been resolved optimally.

Phase II occlusal-related procedures may be considered for patients having pain associated with functional jaw movements. When pain exists without movement (resting pain), phase II definitive dental-related procedures may be neither helpful nor required in the pursuit of wellness. Be suspicious of other possible etiologies for such pain.[2-4] A key is whether any pain or restriction occurs with movement, with loading of the jaws, and/or whether full functional range of motion (ROM) exists. If factors confirm a muscle dysfunction and/or internal derangement finding, their management becomes a requirement prior to and in conjunction with any orthodontic procedures.

Often, patients have malocclusion discrepancies that would benefit from corrective procedures. Yet such procedures may not be the priority. The patient's primary complaint typically is pain related, for which bite correction may provide no predictable improvement.

Frequently, patients and/or physical therapists are aware of some facial pain, mandibular dysfunction, or TMJ disorder/symptoms, while the dental clinician is not. The best approach for the physical therapist is to make appropriate, honest, and unbiased suggestions to patient/clinician. In this way, patients remain appropriately appraised of their problems and needs while, it is hoped, the understanding of all clinicians is elevated.

Patients fluctuate between disease and health status. When their adaptive capacity is exceeded (as in distress, facial or whiplash trauma, poor posture, hormonal changes, jaw or bite disharmonies), previously tolerable conditions become intolerable (e.g., signs/symptoms may become evident after extensive dental procedures, with revision of one's orthotic appliance, with tension of orthodontic elastics, after removal of wisdom teeth, and/or after intubation for surgery.) These clinical and mandibular hyperextension examples frequently trigger patient complaints and changes in comfort and stability. Friable patients need to be approached with gradual changes and slow introduction of new treatment procedures in the process of managing/correcting the problems at hand.

I contend that TMJ patients are generally "managed" and only selectively "cured",[5] an orthopedic concept that must apply for craniomandibular, craniocervical pain, and dysfunction patients. These patients have unique treatment and management requirements that can perplex the typical dental office.

GUIDELINES PRIOR TO PHASE II TREATMENT

Comprehensive assessment is important in the initial phases of treatment from a diagnostic, treatment, and communication standpoint. Comments made to patients at the beginning of treatment are considered part of the evaluation and are generally well accepted and respected. Explanations not adequately provided until later in treatment may be questioned or considered excuses by patients. In the course of treatment, doctor and therapist must assume the status of a director and a helper. Moreover, it is vitally important that the patient share responsibility for problems, conditions, and achieving wellness.

We understand that patients in pain often fail to listen effectively to comprehensive information diligently provided to them at the onset of treatment. Thus, review of treatment plans and limitations must be provided again for these patients before beginning phase II care to avoid misunderstandings and unrealistic patient expectations. We must not promise what we cannot deliver. Information should be summarized in written form for patients and clinicians alike, using available computerized communication systems.[6]

There cannot be one treatment for all patients. We must be adept at helping patients understand when occlusal adjustment might be more appropriate than comprehensive orthodontics and/or orthognathic (jaw) surgery. Not all patients require "ideal" treatment, but certainly any treatment provided must be efficacious and comprehensive enough to attend to the patient's primary concerns and needs. Altering the occlusal scheme affects the functional mechanics of the TMJ.[6–9] Such treatment may not reverse unfavorable dysfunctional effects that have already occurred. Instead, treatment must provide for best whole-patient rehabilitation and stabilization, while applying scientifically valid approaches as understood today.

Many issues influence ongoing comfort and stability.[10] Giving fullest cooperation with postural and parafunctional behavioral modifications, while following prescribed physical therapy programs for mandibular and cervical spine concerns are musts. Doing so helps provide for best patient resilience and phase II results. Keeping the patient motivated requires proper support and praise from the doctor and staff, focusing on improvements and change rather than on the remaining problems. The integration of counseling, relaxation therapy, distress reduction, structured exercise, long-term selective use of medications [i.e., nonsteroidal antiinflammatory (NSAIDs), analgesics, muscle relaxants, mood elevators, sleep inducers, etc.] with chronic pain management is appropriate as well. The intraoral orthotic (splint) remains part of this corrective program as phase II occlusotherapy is contemplated.

Patients often require support from the physical therapist to maintain proper mobility and positioning of their cervical spine. Modalities for the mandibular muscles and TMJ are beneficial if flare-ups occur during orthodontic/dental procedures. Physical therapists must understand the complexities involved in stabilizing the occlusion while realizing that frequent exacerbations can plague the more chronic patient. Communication and continued coordination between physical therapist and dental clinician/orthodontist remain most important so that best patient care and understanding prevails.

Often orthodontists and restorative clinicians must treat patients with an asymptomatic click. Whether this click requires specific management with splints prior to such definitive care, or whether the click can simply be brought to the attention of the patient without any specific treatment is controversial. On one hand, not every click requires treatment, yet we do not wish to ignore a possible disc dislocation/luxation that may progress[11-14] to greater dysfunctional problems in the future. Sufficient clinical experience and increasing specific information[1] exist today to identify situations that should be treated vs. those better left alone. In persons in whom a painless click exists, I recommend no treatment unless progression toward problems and/or movement restriction/disability exist. Other chapters in this text explain factors influencing decisions about splint use. Stabilization splint therapy is usually followed by reassessment once functional conditions have been improved as much as possible.

CLASSIFICATION OF FACE AND OCCLUSION

Prior to phase II treatment, one must determine the facial type and class of occlusion exhibited by the patient. The straight profile (Fig. 8-1) of class I occlusion typifies a harmonious maxillomandibular relationship.[15] The convex profile associated with a class II malocclusion is due to the protracted maxillae (midface) and/or retrognathic mandible. A prognathic mandible and/or retracted maxillae produces a concave profile as in a class III malocclusion.

A class I malocclusion (Fig. 8-1) is usually associated with a balanced maxillomandibular skeletal (jaw) relationship. All ideal occlusions are class I; however, all class I occlusions are not ideal. In a class I ideal occlusion, the mesiobuccal cusps of the maxillary first permanent molars occlude in the buccal grooves of the mandibular first permanent molars. The lips and soft-tissue profile should be in a harmonious relationship as well. A class II malocclusion exists when the mandibular arch is distal (behind) its maxillary counterpart (Fig. 8-1). This may be the result of a retrognathic mandible, protracted or vertically excessive maxillae, or a combination of these. Typically, upper teeth protrude and/or lower teeth recede in conjunction with class II patterns. In a class III malocclusion, (Fig. 8-1) the mandibular arch is mesial (anterior) to the maxillary dentition. Often crossbites are evident. The profile typically appears prognathic at the chin or flat in the midface, or a combination of both.

PHASE II REEVALUATION

The clinical exam is repeated as phase II procedures are contemplated (see Chapter 4 and 11). This evaluation includes dynamic TMJ evaluation (loading the joints) during functional movements, bimanual palpation of jaw and cervical muscles; ROM assessment; facial proportions analysis of asymmetry;

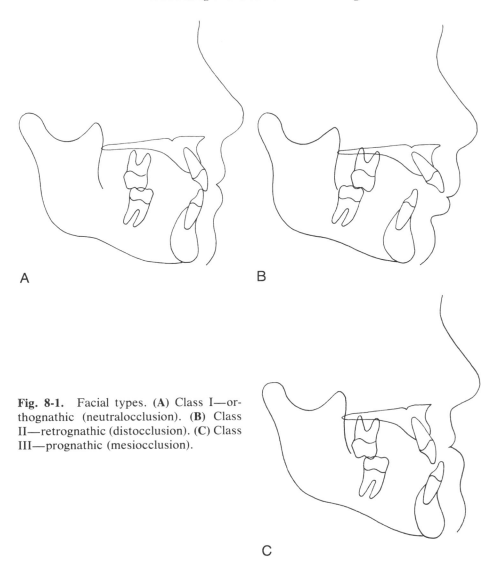

Fig. 8-1. Facial types. (**A**) Class I—orthognathic (neutralocclusion). (**B**) Class II—retrognathic (distocclusion). (**C**) Class III—prognathic (mesiocclusion).

occlusal analysis and articulated mounted models; and progress radiographs including those with phase I splint in. Special laboratory tests (i.e., blood studies, arthrograms, magnetic resonance imaging [MRI], computed tomography [CT] scans, etc.) may be selectively prescribed.

Pain and dysfunction of the joints and muscles should have been optimally managed with phase I care. There are, however, patients for whom one may need to consider phase II treatment, despite varying degrees of continuing pain and dysfunction. The key is to distinguish those patients with absence of masticatory problems (related to jaw use) from those with continuing cervical spine dysfunction or other medical problems. Those who are comfortable and stable from facial pain and mandibular function aspects are candidates for definitive occlusal therapy, even though treatment may be continuing for cervical spine, systemic, and/or psychogenic components. Hence, occlusotherapy, orthodontics, and/or splint withdrawal may be appropriate while pain/dysfunction care continues for problems not directly related to jaw use.

No universal condylar position (Fig. 8-2) is unequivocally correct for all patients. Posterior condylar displacement appears to be the one most associated with TMJ pain/dysfunction (Fig. 8-2A) as reported by Ricketts,[16] Weinberg,[17] Mikhail and Rosen,[18] Weinberg,[19] and Dumas.[20,21] Farrar and McCarty[22-25] have shown that distally displaced condyles frequently progress to TMJ internal derangement, especially anterior disc displacement with degenerative changes.

The concentric position should be the practitioner's goal (Fig. 8-2B and E), but a slight anterior repositioning is acceptable when needed to stabilize anterior disc displacement (Fig. 8-2C). Excessive prolonged anterior condylar placement from a neutral position appears, however, to exceed the physiological limitations for the TMJ. The condyle position that is more comfortable and physiological for patients with posterior condylar displacement combined with anterior disc dislocation is often slightly anterior to concentric. Gelb[26] suggests that an anterior and inferior position is the preferred condyle position (Fig. 8-2D).

Long-term anterior mandibular displacement in adults can lead to pathologic remodeling of the condyle and TMJ components, as shown by Ricketts,[16,27-31] Grummons,[1,4] and other authors.[32-35]

Gianelly[36] described anterior repositioning of the condyles during class II treatments with functional jaw orthopedic (FJO) appliances, stating that condyles should not be left in an excessively anteriorly displaced position. McNamara, Hinton, Hoffman,[37] and other researchers[38-40] showed that such hyperpropulsion can promote a histologic response on the condyle, but that care should be exercised when using FJO treatment for class II cases after growth has been completed.

Various condylar positions are considered optimal by respected clinicians. The more chronic and unstable the disc and ligament tissues, the more the stabilized condylar position may require slightly forward posturing to sustain patient comfort and stability. Thus, the final condylar position becomes the most physiologic, sensible, comfortable and stable for patients, after all factors are considered (e.g., the condylar position may have to be compensated forward[4,26] or mildly distracted so that patient comfort and stability prevail in chronic inflammatory conditions, disc disease, disc shape alterations dyscrasias, loose collateral ligaments, and/or muscle dysfunction conditions).

In the physiologic condylar position established for patients, the disc–condyle assembly is stabilized (to the degree clinically possible) and functioning against the posterior superior slopes of the articular eminentia, in accordance with anatomic arrangement and muscle action across the joints (Sicher's law).[41] As the mandible functions, the teeth should come together with the condyles

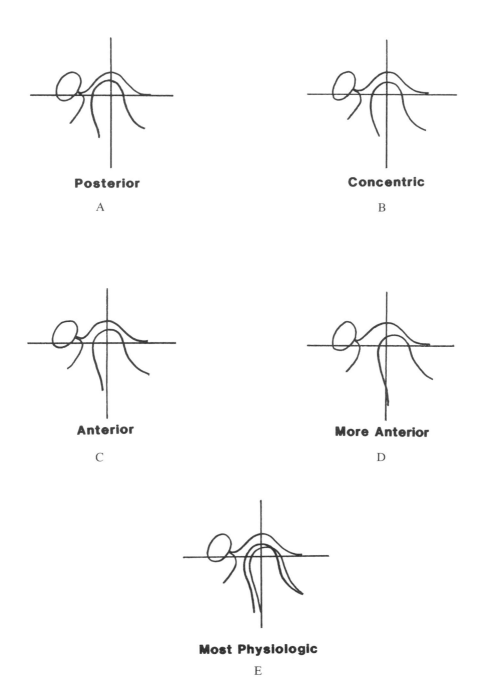

Posterior

A

Concentric

B

Anterior

C

More Anterior

D

Most Physiologic

E

Fig. 8-2. Condylar positions (**A**) Retrusive condylar position, unfavorable compression and loading. (**B**) Concentric position, physiologic and biologic. Ricketts, Grummons, McNeill, Williamson, Slavicek, Owen, Weinberg and others. (**C**) Slightly forward as therapeutic position or in chronic cases. Farrar and others. (**D**) Moderately forward, less favorable position long-term. Gelb and others. (**E**) Condylar positions vary with chronic conditions of TMJ components.

and discs centered within the fossae from all dimensions, including the transverse, while neuromuscular components function optimally.

To reposition a patient abruptly from an anterior condylar position to one that is concentric is generally discouraged since many chronic disc patients cannot tolerate this immediate increase in loading and joint compression. If any intolerance and/or return of pain/problems is reported, many clinicians decide to proceed with intracapsular surgical procedures. With our conservative therapy today, we should be able to promote noninflammatory pseudoarthrosis status with gradual treatment changes, though longer term splinting and eventual final treatment without disc recapture (disc off the condyle) may be necessary. Intracapsular surgical considerations remain appropriate for those chronic inflammatory, painful, restrictive situations, as described in Chapter 7.

ORTHODONTICS AND TMJ FACTORS

The percentage of nonorthodontically treated patients (including children) exhibiting craniomandibular (TMJ) disorders is far greater than most clinicians realize. Routinely, patients who have never received orthodontic treatment come to the orthodontic office with unrecognized and potentially damaging TMJ signs/symptoms. Prior to and/or during orthodontics, signs or symptoms indicative of mandibular dysfunction (i.e., clicking/locking episodes, inflammatory response, loose supportive ligaments, muscle hyperactivity in the elevator muscles of the mandible, parafunction, distress) require appraisal.

Subjective symptoms of jaw disorder in youth have been reported in epidemiologic studies by Solberg,[42] Nilner,[43,44] Egermark-Erikson, Carlsson and Ingervall[45] and Solberg et al.[46] Many nonorthodontic patients with mandibular pain/dysfunction findings (typically TMJ sounds and/or muscle tenderness) were studied by Nilner,[43] Solberg,[46] Helkimo,[47,48] Bush et al[49] and Green and Marbach.[50]

Malocclusion has been implicated in TMJ disorders by Johnston,[51] Perry,[52] Ricketts,[53] Thompson,[54] Roberts,[55] Grummons,[1] Owen,[56,57] Funt,[58] and Williamson.[59] Higher percentages were found in adults studied by Thompson (50%),[54] Owen (76%),[56,57] and Grummons (62%).[1]

Rieder[60] evaluated 1,000 noncomplaining "healthy" dental patients, and discovered that many of these patients demonstrated TMJ clicking, chronic headaches, and neckaches. Gross and Gale[61] reported that one-third of 1,000 dental patients had mandibular dysfunction disorders. Such preorthodontic TMJ disorders require careful screening, documentation, and clinical management before and/or during orthodontic treatment. Lack of attention and understanding has caused the dentist/orthodontist to be held responsible for creating problems that may have preexisted. Patient comfort and stability before, during and after dental procedures remains a priority.

In the assessment[1] of 800 "new" patients (400 TMJ and 400 orthodontic),

Table 8-1. Common Findings Coexistent With Class II Malocclusions[a]

Class II, Division I Malocclusion
Manidibular deficiency
Often vertically long face types
TMJ osteoarthritis
Forward head posture
Myofascial factors

Class II, Division II Malocclusion
TMJ clicking frequent
Distal condylar displacement
Skeletal and dental overclosure
Parafunctional habits
Myofascial factors

[a] The findings listed may exist in either division I or division II categories; neither are they limited to class II malocclusion types only.

Grummons[1] discovered that only 12% of those presenting as TMJ patients had previous orthodontics. True TMJ dysfunction correlated with (1) facial trauma, (2) TMJ hyperextension insults, (3) laxity (loose ligament) conditions, and/or (4) loss of posterior dental support, more than with any history of previous orthodontics.

Ricketts[53] reported TMJ disorders to vary with facial skeletal types (i.e. class II, III types). Inconsistent condyle–eminence relationships in opening with a predominance of distal condylar displacements in closing were observed in mandibular dysfunction patients. J. Howard (personal communication, July 1983) reported class II and class III malocclusion patients demonstrated much higher incidence of related temporomandibular disorders.

Electromyographic (Ingervall and Thilander,[62] Moller and Troelstrup,[63]) and kinesiologic studies of mandibular movement patterns (Moller,[7] Hamerling[9]) confirm that malocclusions (cross-bites, class II, division I, and deep-bite cases) cause neuromuscular dysfunction and reflex mandibular positioning (Hamerling[9]). Observable disharmonies in chewing patterns (Gibbs and Lundeen[64]) occur when these dysfunctions are sufficient to produce ischemic circulatory effects. Malocclusions may be a significant factor predisposing to temporomandibular disorders (Moller[7]).

My concern with any studies is whether cervical spine factors were adequately considered or ruled out. In addition to clicking of the TMJ, the cervical spine can be a cause of many symptoms that may be believed to be related to the TMJ (i.e., headache, ear, throat, swallowing, etc.), and which really are not TMJ problems (see Chapter 12).

Wright[65] and Grummons did a long-term study of 83 patients who had definitive phase I therapeutic approaches followed by definitive phase II care. Of these patients, 94% reported that they were pain-free 18 months after completion of treatment. Residual problems were primarily of cervical spine origin, with 68% resolution of craniocervical issues (Table 8-1). These patients were

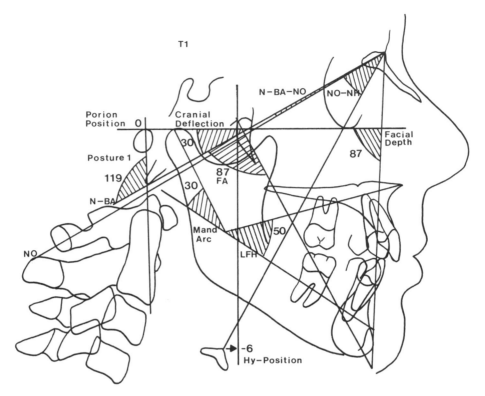

Fig. 8-3. Grummons craniocervical (GCC) analysis from RMO Diagnostic Services. (Courtesy of RMO Diagnostic Services, Calabasas, CA.[109])

seen primarily by physical therapists, although some patients saw chiropractors, osteopaths, massage therapists, acupuncture/acupressure and/or biofeedback therapists. These results moderate our clinical promises since postural problems tend to leave patients with a lesser extent of pain relief and clinical response. Thus, functional limitations are not necessarily cured, but rather are managed. Older patients were more recalcitrant, irrespective of type of therapy applied. Long-standing problems demonstrated a lesser percentage of clinical resolution.

In realizing that occlusal therapy is not the primary solution for cervical issues, dental clinicians are subject to certain limitations. Clinicians must be careful with promises and predictions when definitive occlusal procedures are provided in conjunction with TMJ procedures. If cervical spine dysfunction is suspected (see Chapters 10, 11, 12), the dentist should make appropriate referral.

When cervical myofascial injury is sustained, the patient generally alters head posture to avoid painful positions. This compensation induces increased muscular activity elsewhere; The compensating mandibular postural change and altered occlusal contacts [through central nervous system (CNS) proprioceptive input] cause a protective muscle splinting reflex. Stomatognathic myospasm typically ensues for the patient with myofascial problems. The entire kinetic chain tends to become affected, and integrated team management is a requirement.

The postural position of the head and neck affects the rest position of the mandible. Physical therapy designed to improve the posture of the head and neck increases the vertical dimension at rest. Darling et al.[66] found that an increase in vertical dimension at rest occurs with an increase in the angle of habitual head posture. Alterations of anteroposterior head and neck posture have an immediate effect on the trajectory of mandibulaar closure in a normal population.[67] Thus, the influence of the cervical spine should be considered when optimal results are sought in dental and orthodontic procedures (Fig. 8-3) (see Chapter 12.)

MAINTAINING JOINT AND MUSCLE STABILITY DURING ORTHODONTICS

Once craniomandibular and cervical spine pain/dysfunction has been managed (phase I treatment) and patients are rehabilitated toward optimal capabilities, the orthodontist is, or should be, one of the most important members of the dental rehabilitation team. Because occlusal compensations commonly accompany craniomandibular disorders, occlusal rehabilitative measures are needed and can include orthodontics, restorative procedures (bonding, crowns, bridges), overlay splint restorations, comprehensive equilibration (bite adjustment), orthognathic surgery, and often a combination of these approaches.

A major rehabilitative advantage provided by the orthodontist (to the patient's benefit) is that corrective changes occur over an extended period of time. Because orthodontics is a gradual process, TMJ remodeling and adaptive changes can occur with minimal periodic mandibular functional position changes. Muscular compensations should be achieved with moderate splint adjustments from month to month as orthodontic treatment is rendered. Many patients with chronic instability of the disc component, or muscle hyperactivity, demonstrate abilities to remain comfortable and stable when such minimal changes are introduced.

Splints should not be abandoned as orthodontics begins. Transitional splints or certain removable orthodontic appliances are useful stabilizers while permitting sections of the dental arch to become aligned. Various and specific splint designs should be prescribed to fit the needs of the patient and circumstances. No one splint design can be applied for all patients. The clinician must be effective and knowledgable in management of multiple appliance designs to minimize mitigating factors.

Many splint (orthotic) designs exist for either phase I or phase II care. A specific concept and treatment objective are in mind as a specific design is prescribed for a patient. The splint should fit the needs of patients, rather than all patients being expected to fit one splint design or one splint therapy approach. There cannot be one treatment for all, as many splint therapy approaches would imply.

Neither can we insist on a technique of having an upper splint always or a lower splint always since individual occlusal schemes and stabilization requirements dictate whether upper rather than lower arches should be splinted. Usually, the clinician can accomplish optimal functional relationships with a physiologic basis, using a splint in either arch depending on one's clinical preference, training, and objectives. Approaches should not be empiric. Splint designs cannot be the same for all patients/problems.

Any malocclusion (bad bite) or even a beautifully aligned occlusion with the TMJ components not appropriately related leaves a patient with an unstable status and represents incomplete treatment. The era of limiting orthodontic concepts and treatment to the teeth and supporting tissues without necessary regard for TMJ and cervical factors is fast becoming a thing of the past.

Intermediary (transitional or sectional) splints should be used so that stabilized TMJ components are maintained to the extent possible throughout the corrective orthodontic phase. It is inappropriate to introduce orthodontic movements and forces when an occlusal splint is needed to maintain corrected jaw and disc positions, stabilized neuromuscular, ligamentous, and craniocervical relationships. The therapeutic splint can be modified so that certain segments of teeth can be removed from confinement within the splint, and then moved by orthodontic techniques. The more crooked teeth are moved, while the straighter teeth are splinted as support areas. Selective teeth should remain in contact with the splint as areas of support, whereas more crooked teeth are aligned in the early stages of orthodontics. Eventually, the functional occlusion and tooth relationships should fit well enough to provide the support that splint(s) may have provided.

Segmental Splints During Orthodontic Treatment

I have used various transitional (intermediary) splint designs successfully to maintain stabilization of the musculoskeletal, TMJ, and/or cervical spine components. These splints stabilize the mandibular complex with coverage over some teeth while other dental segments remain unaffected. Individual teeth are then free to be restored or aligned. Ultimately, all the teeth should be optimally positioned so that reliance on various splint appliances can be discontinued whenever possible.

Transition from one splint to another (i.e., upper to lower, full coverage to segmental) can occur with maintenance of the stabilized mandibular relationships. A bite registration (wax, bite paste, polyether) records this jaw position and can be used for appliance fabrication or for mounted models of teeth.

When orthodontic segmental movements are in progress, three areas should remain in contact to stabilize the jaw position and temporomandibular

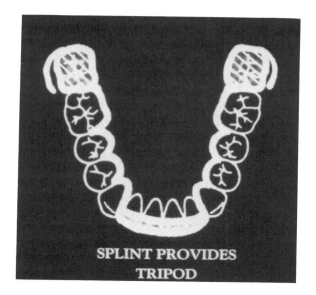

Fig. 8-4. Tripod splint (upper or lower arch).

components; hence, I coined the descriptive term to "tripod the mandible" (Fig. 8-4). Examples of this tripodization with splints are demonstrated.

The tripod effect provides balanced support in three areas of splint or tooth contact (anterior region and each side posteriorly). Some teeth are maintained within the splint, while others can be orthodontically moved. This tripod effect is usually accomplished with a splint indexing the incisor region and also the posteriormost molars, usually the second molars.

The tripod can be established by a combination of segmental splints with either tooth contact, or areas of tooth bonding (e.g., a splint with two posterior molar support areas (dipod) (Fig. 8-5A) can be placed if front teeth already contact, with a tripod effect. Similarly, a molar tooth on each side can be bonded, establishing the tripod effect when anterior teeth also touch. Establishing a vertical stop with the splint or by plastic bonding will tripod the mandible (Fig. 8-5C). Tripoding is especially helpful when deficient posterior occlusal support leads to recurrence of reciprocal clicking, muscle dysfunction, collateral ligament loading, auricular symptoms, etc.[1,68,69]

Segmental splints such as the dipod or unipod allow significant numbers of teeth to be free of the splint for orthodontic movement and/or restorative procedures while maintaining minimal splint contact with stabilized mandibular functional relationships. The unipod splint is often used as treatment nears completion and the occlusion is nearly corrected (Fig. 8-5B). The unipod splint can be used to assist in asymmetry resolution as one side of the occlusion is separated. Teeth on that side are then erupted into better occlusal contact while leveling the occlusal plane. A unipod or occlusal bond is helpful when a joint needs to be decompressed and remodeled to increase joint space on the affected side.

When a patient with asymptomatic or early opening reduction clicking is

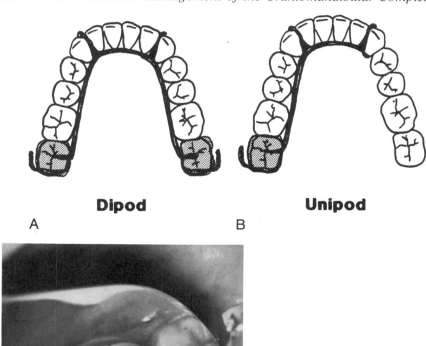

Dipod   **Unipod**

A   B

Fig. 8-5. Teeth contact on each side and in front (tripod effect). TMJ decompression with dipod/unipod splints or bonding. **(A)** Dipod splint; **(B)** unipod splint; **(C)** occlusal bonding.

C

advised to have orthodontics, appliances such as the tripod, Grumzat, dipod, anterior repositioning splint, or molar bonds help provide a stabilized mandibular position with condyle–disc coordination. These patients typically can tolerate orthodontics from the onset, provided that stabilizing splints are maintained during orthodontics in conjunction with craniomandibular cervical spine management. At times, tooth contact may already exist and a smaller splint may suffice.

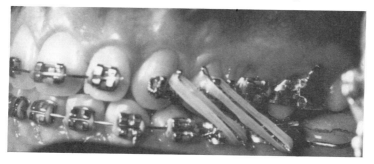

Fig. 8-6.   Class II elastics.

Segmental Splints with Elastics.

Orthodontic mechanotherapy with various elastics (rubber bands) can be difficult for patients to tolerate. With supportive splints in place, the mandibular position is stable, with muscle problems better controlled so that elastics can

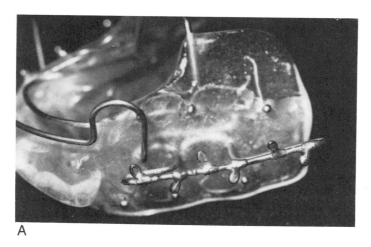

A

Fig. 8-7. Functional appliance. (**A**) Bionator type; (**B**) with eruption elastics.

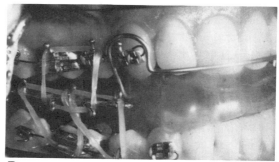

B

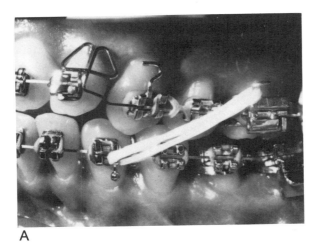

A

Fig. 8-8. Class III elastics with dipod decompression splint. **(A)** Elastics move teeth; **(B)** splint supports TMJ.

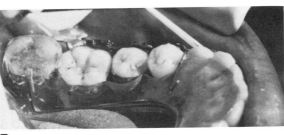

B

be tolerable. Treatment can then proceed on schedule, with predictable response and, generally, excellent results.

Class II elastics are often needed during orthodontics (Fig. 8-6). These may trigger unfavorable and uncomfortable muscle hyperactivity and joint loading, which interrupts the ability of patients to wear elastics. Class II or any vertical elastics are better tolerated with a tripod, dipod, or an anterior repositioning splint as desired tooth movement is achieved.

Elastics also assist in elevating (erupting) teeth as segmental splints provide the biting index with jaw stabilization. Active molar/bicuspid eruption can usually be accomplished at 1 mm a month in children, and 1 mm every 6 weeks in adults, measured at the first molar. The amount of eruption varied up to 5.5 mm. I found that 34 percent of vertical overeruption was required to maintain bite stability. Incisor intrusion to align teeth varied from 0.5 to 4.5 mm and was 80 percent stable. Significant tooth movements can be achieved,[1] unless gum or bone problems exist, altering eruption capabilty.

A Bionator-type appliance (Fig. 8-7) is useful in children and adults for mandibular position control and tooth eruption capabilities. The posterior teeth can be selectively erupted with elastics while supporting the disc–condyle assembly to avoid unfavorable compressive TMJ loading.

Class III elastics applied without a supportive splint can produce unfa-

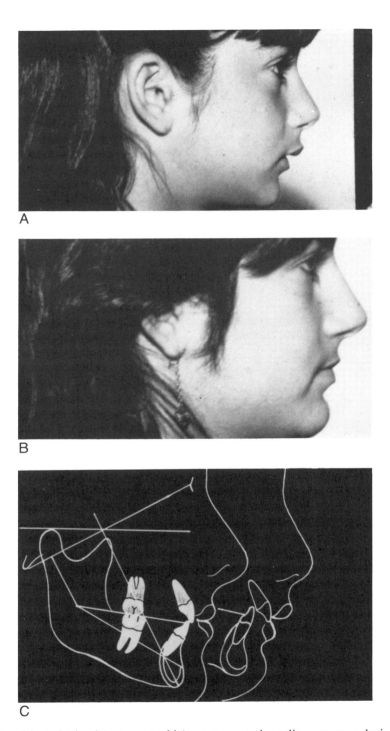

Fig. 8-9. Ligated tripod (not removable) promotes orthopedic responses during mandibular deficiency correction. **(A)** Before; **(B)** after; **(C)** amount of movement achieved for correction.

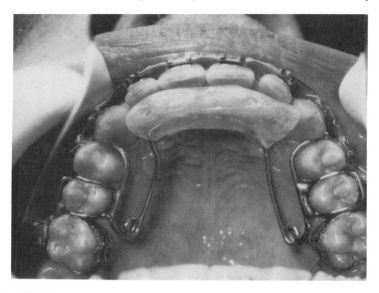

Fig. 8-10.   The Grumzat orthopedic/orthodontic appliance with bite ramp provides TMJ stabilization and tooth movement.

vorable distalization of the mandible with TMJ compression. When class III elastics are used with a supportive splint, (Fig. 8-8), orthodontic changes can occur while limiting TMJ effects. As the upper teeth protract (flare) from the class III elastics, the overjet increases, which in turn permits the mandible to be repositioned slightly more forward. This decompresses the TMJs and assists in disc–condyle stabilization.

The fixed tripod (Grummons) appliance (Fig. 8-9) is effective in children with mandibular skeletal deficiency and/or when disc disorders exist in combination with the need for jaw orthopedics/orthodontics. The posterior occlusal areas provide balanced splint support and desired disc recapture. Thus, the appliance can have multiple advantages for class II skeletal and bite problems as well as clicking (intracapsular) complaints.

Functional appliance therapy following TMJ trauma can be helpful to promote favorable condylar regeneration changes.[1,70–73] Significant improvement in condylar form is demonstrated using the fixed tripod design to accomplish occlusal and orthopedic correction while maintaining facial symmetry for such posttraumatic patients. Other functional appliances (i.e., Bionator, Herbst, Activator, Frankel, etc.) are also effective in this situation.

The Grumzat[74] appliance (Fig. 8-10) improves TMJ relationships, jaw symmetry, and tooth alignment. The appliance provides corrected physiologic jaw position, with the disc–condyle assembly functionally loaded against the superoanterior aspects of the articular eminentia within the glenoid fossae regions. The Grumzat encourages maintenance of optimal contracted muscle lengths[1,54] during functional movements, giving patients continued comfort and

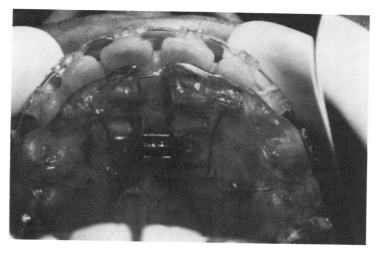

Fig. 8-11.   Anterior advancing screws to achieve functional movements.

stability. Anterior advancing screws (Fig. 8-11) springs assist in changing position and angulation of the upper incisors.

The chronic disc patient (i.e., TMJ laxity, disc instability, inflammatory response) requires definite posterior occlusal support. The Grumzat can include molar occlusion pads, which establish a tripod effect and controlled TMJ loading with jaw closure. Should reciprocal clicking reoccur, the appliance can be adjusted to the previously stable, more forward therapeutic position. Disc recapture or at least improved comfort and stabilization are usually achieved again. Clinical observations of clicking, synovitis, collateral ligament laxity or tenderness, TMJ pain and/or ear stuffiness caution the clinician that chronic problems are evident and that significant posterior occlusal support is a requirement. Hence, molar occlusal pads are recommended to stabilize TMJs by limiting TMJ compression and balancing contacts for best muscular activity.

Extraoral devices can also be helpful in altering tooth positions as mandibular stabilization with orthodontics is accomplished (e.g., the face-mask (Fig. 8-12) can be used with elastics to advance the upper teeth. As this is achieved, the mandible can now remain postured more forward. Another example is to use a headband (Fig. 8-13) design to hold the mandible into the splint during sleep to control mandibular posture while providing disc–condyle stability.

Pitfalls in Appliance Treatment.

Knowing what procedures to avoid in fixed appliance treatment to avoid triggering recurrences of symptomatology is just as important. The overbite should be treated before the overjet so that the front teeth do not collide when

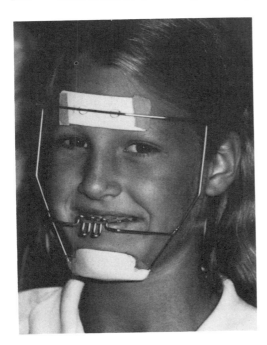

Fig. 8-12.   Face-mask with elastics.

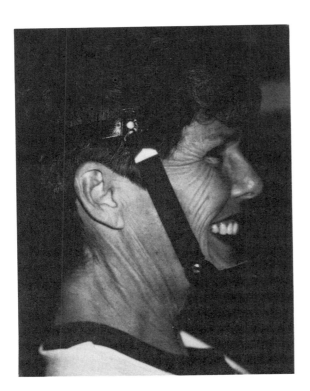

Fig. 8-13.   Elastic stabilizer worn with splint on.

the jaws close. Deep overbite is accomplished by a tendency for the mandible to be thrust backward (distally), thereby compressing the TMJs. Moreover, muscular hyperactivity can be triggered, supportive ligaments can be stretched, and disc dislocation can be promoted.

Dental arches must be coordinated or matched for the best functional fit and avoidance of tooth interferences. Satisfactory interincisal angulations with appropriate overcorrection of bite problems are imperative to minimize post-treatment relapse of corrections. Correction and maintenance of transverse (width) concerns are vitally important to help maintain best vertical dimension support. Only judicious and necessary bicuspid tooth extraction treatment approaches can be tolerated by these postdysfunctional patients, especially those with disc disorders. Maintenance of a stabilized condylar position with optimized muscular components must be emphasized.

Dysfunctional patients seem to have decreased resilience and less tolerance for extensive orthodontic mechanotherapy. Hence, nonextraction treatment is favored since it generally lends itself to less elastic usage, less treatment time, and decreased degree and time that teeth contact traumatically in transition from a malocclusion toward the corrected alignment. Traumatic occlusion can be damaging to the TMJ and cervical functional components and interrelationships.

Indiscriminate biscuspid removal seems to correlate with unfavorable TMJ health, lack of esthetic and facial balance and, often, occlusal disharmonies. In TMJ patients who have reduced tolerances to joint loading, excellence of the final occlusion seems to make an even greater difference since these patients tolerate less bite discrepancy than is tolerated by healthy patients. Removal of bicuspids with inadequate completion of the orthodontics correlate with more disorders. Removal of bicuspid teeth usually does not in itself cause patients to have dysfunctional problems later. The detail and expertise of the orthodontic finishing remains most important.

Jansson[75] compared orthodontically treated Angle class II patients with a similar sample of untreated adults. The class II division I, untreated patients exhibited the highest incidence of symptoms, as did those patients treated with bicuspid extractions. Nonextraction cases showed the fewest post-treatment TMJ disorders.

Ahlin[76] reported that the loss of premolars (bicuspids) can reduce vertical dimension and deepen the bite, which may be harmful to the physiologic stability of the TMJs. The condyles may achieve a more distal and superior position in the fossae.[77] This retruded, superior position can direct the disc anteromedially, with stretching of the lateral and posterior ligament attachments along with clicking, grating, and/or related symptoms. Protection of the vertical dimension and the physiologic relationships of the disc-condyle fossae are essential.

Removal of selected teeth may be prescribed with the orthodontic treatment. In conjunction with such tooth removals, space closure may involve use of elastics (rubber bands) with arch-wire designs for closure of extraction spaces. In this closing process, inclines of teeth may inappropriately contact

Table 8-2. Warning Signals During Orthodontic Treatment

1. Pain (arthralgia, myalgia)
2. Limitation of mandibular movement
3. Irregular mandibular movement (dyskinesia)
4. Presence of crepitus, clicking, ligament laxity
5. Excessive tooth tipping and interferences
6. Braces or wire interference that promotes muscle hyperactivity and TMJ leveraging
7. Vertical collapse in extraction cases
8. Elastics (class III, vertical) or chin cup therapy causing TMJ loading and compression
9. Improper incisor angulation, especially lingual (inward) tipping of uppers.
10. Inadequate overbite control resulting in restrictive anterior guidance.
11. Lack of recognition and treatment of skeletal problems with facial orthopedics or orthognathic (jaw) surgery
12. Molar fulcruming (pivotal interferences) with condylar distraction and associated disc/muscular compensations
13. Lack of transverse uprightness in dental arches
14. Loss of posterior support due to: missing teeth, inadequate growth, incomplete tooth eruption, use of an oversized splint, muscle hyperactivity, chronic clenching habit, lateral tongue-thrusting habit, alveolar resorption beneath dentures

until treatment has progressed sufficiently to permit good fit. Such deflective contacts contribute to unfavorable muscle activity, TMJ instability, and frequent episodes of symptom return. The key is to bring these conditions under management and stabilization as quickly as they are discovered by the clinician and/or are reported by the patient. Several problems may occur during orthodontics (Table 8-2).

Cases properly diagnosed and well-treated to optimal orthodontic standards will usually not promote TMJ disorders. What is most important in any bicuspid extraction case is how we manage the vertical dimension, TMJ stabilization, angulation of upper incisors, and transverse control of the arches without undesireable narrowing or constriction. Excellence in the finished result with optimal functioning conditions for the health and well-being of the individual is most important.

ORTHOGNATHIC SURGERY CONSIDERATIONS

Adults necessarily required modified, individually specific treatment approaches. Many TMJ/cervical spine patients should consider benefits of orthognathic (jaw) surgery subsequent to pain and dysfunction management. Although minimal skeletal imbalances can be nicely improved by applying orthopedic and orthodontic procedures in the growing patient, such options are very limited in the nongrowing, adult patient.

Some of the reasons why orthognathic surgery should be considered in adults[78] as part of their comprehensive treatment are:

1.   Orthodontic problems in adults have existed for many years and are usually more advanced and progressive.

2. Two, three, or more years of fixed appliance mechanotherapy (braces) is often not well tolerated.

3. Extensive restorations, crown and bridgework may be present. With routine orthodontics, this bridework may have to be sectioned or replaced. With surgical procedures, bridgework can often be preserved or modified.

4. Because surgery gives a more ideal result, fabrication of any crowns or other restorations can occur to a more optimal occlusion.

5. Nonextraction orthodontic treatment is more often possible with surgery than without surgery.

6. Time savings with surgery (often 6 to 12 months or more) is of significant importance to adult patients.

7. Long-term elastic use and orthodontic mechanotherapy are reduced with surgical approaches.

8. Because nonsurgical treatment may not result in correction, future periodontal, TMJ and other functional problems may be more likely.

9. Adult patients primarily seek treatment for cosmetic reasons. A balanced and harmonious appearance with a heightened self-esteem is important and is achieved for these patients.

10. Stability of the case result is significantly improved since surgical orthodontics is completed to optimal objectives.

With these concepts and thoughts in mind, clinicians should encourage patients needing orthognathic surgery to follow this route of management. With today's knowledge, research, and technical capabilities, these cases should be well diagnosed and planned, with excellent results (see Chapter 7).

When TMJ and other dysfunctional issues are producing significant pain and limitation, TMJ issues must receive the fullest attention first. Cervical, muscular, psychogenic, systemic and occlusal aspects must be co-managed, as explained in other chapters. TMJ surgery may be an appropriate part of this care in properly selected cases. When such TMJ surgery is accomplished, the patient is reassessed for other orthognathic and malocclusion issues as a part of follow-up phase II care. Provided that TMJ problems can be adequately controlled, the orthognathic surgical correction should be accomplished as early in treatment as feasible, before refined intracapsular surgical procedures are attempted. Generally, patients are able to be more optimally stabilized for mandibular dysfunction problems post-orthognathically once skeletal and dental units have a better functional fit. TMJ surgery may now be unnecessary since more definitive stabilization therapy can be achieved.

Intraoral orthotics continue to be beneficial and are required with patients being prepared for orthognathic surgery. Malocclusions remain, and often worsen, as an expected part of presurgical orthodontic corrections. Unfavorable tooth contacts and TMJ loading must be minimized or avoided by continuing to use a splint until surgery occurs. Even after orthognathic surgery, one-third of patients of 100 orthognathic surgery patients required stabilization splints according to Grummons' research.[1] Such patients typically demonstrated

TMJ x-ray findings prior to jaw surgery (Doyle, 27%,[79] Grummons 78%[1]) Degenerative changes within the TMJs tend to be associated with the pattern of facial morphology.[80,81] Certain patients may need further TMJ and/or mandibular/cervical attention after orthognathic surgery.

As class II skeletal problems are treated toward class I balanced skeletal proportions, forward head posture (FHP) should be uprighted or improved toward a more neutral posture. Physical therapy is vitally helpful for cervical spine problems together with restoration of mandibular dynamics, orthodontics, and orthognathic surgery.

The intraoral orthotic maintains the corrected jaw position and interocclusal distance so that teeth can be repositioned from a deficient vertical dimension to an acceptable, physiologic range (Fig. 8-14). Not every patient should have the vertical dimension of occlusion (VDO) increased; rather, a high proportion of the true class II skeletal and dental patients have vertical deficiencies (overclosure) in the closed jaw position. A modest increase in vertical dimension does not appear to be detrimental to the patient[82–84] Excessive increase into the freeway space, however, can lead to intrusion of the posterior teeth.[85–90]

Vertical dimension for the skeletal and dental components can be determined by phonetic methods. A patient can repeat words such as "Boston," "hiss," "house," "church," "judge," and "zebra" to yield repetitive mandibular reference positions. Instructions such as "Lips together, teeth apart," or "Let your jaw hang" assist patients in assuming a relaxed jaw position. Deliver a squirt or sip of water, instructing the patient to close the lips together and swallow into the bite-registration material. This produces a bite index, capturing the mandibular posture that is functionally optimal. Such procedures must be done with good mobility and positioning of the cervical spine since cervical spine influences on the mandibular posture at rest are significant (see Chapter 12).

Another method for measuring vertical dimension is to place bite registration material around the dental arch (horseshoe shape) without crossing the tongue or encroaching on any of the buccal or lingual space. Phonetic methods with the material between the teeth produces an index that can be used for articulating models for analysis or splints. This bite index can be placed in the mouth while cephalometric x-rays are taken to measure jaw and skeletal relationships in conjunction with restorative, orthodontic, and/or orthognathic surgery planning. Static (closed-jaw) records may show a class III bite and profile, whereas dynamic (phonetic) records in resting jaw posture shows better facial and occlusal balance. Differing conclusions would obviously be drawn if only one set of these records were studied by a clinician. For patients with overclosure of the mandible, whether owing to skeletal or dental reasons, optimal craniocervical and jaw posture is important to establish, followed by alignment of the teeth to the best functional relationships (Fig. 8-15).

These procedures rely on neuromuscular coordination and health. If cervical spine influences are not optimal, appropriate physical therapy treatments need to be reinstituted before any final occlusal treatment is planned or com-

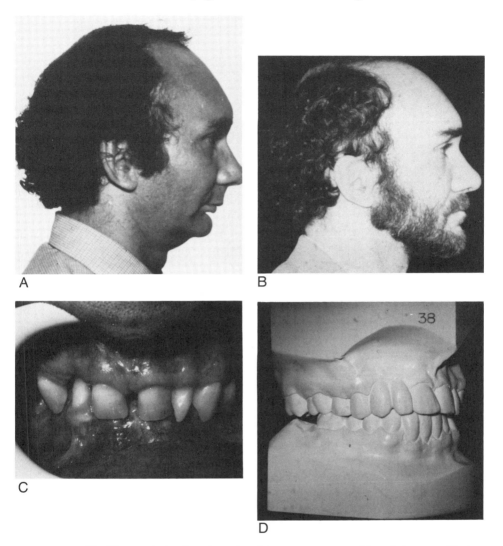

Fig. 8-14. Significant skeletal and occlusal improvements achieved by mandibular splinting with orthodontics and orthognathic surgery. (A)Unfavorable jaw proportions; (**B**) balanced facial features; (**C**) deficient vertical; (**D**) corrected vertical.

pleted. In every patient, the muscle-dictated position must be in harmony with the condyle-dictated position which must also be in harmony with the tooth-dictated position—all this in addition to optimal mobility and positioning of the cervical spine.

Facial asymmetry is the rule rather than an exception. If dental units are to fit and function optimally, the underlying skeletal or jaw components must

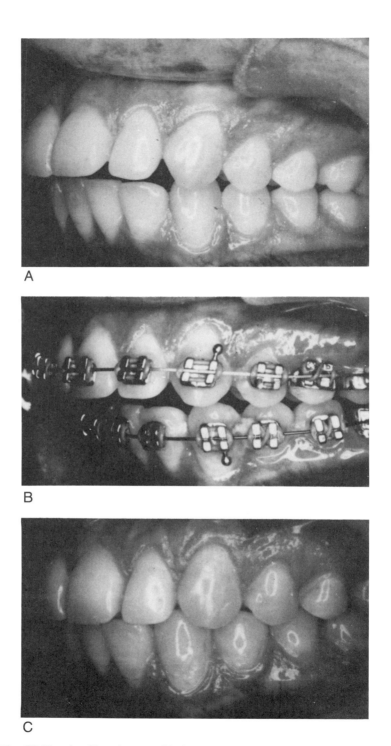

Fig. 8-15. TMJ arthrofibrosis, mandibular deficiency, and class II malocclusion. **(A)** Before; **(B)** during; **(C)** after.

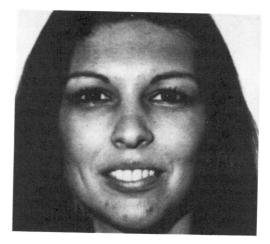

Fig. 8-16. Asymmetric photograph creates two symmetric, but different faces.

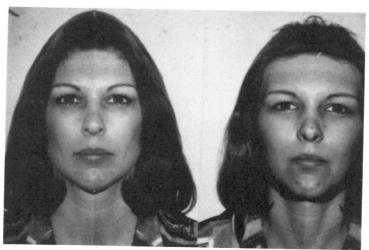

be reasonably well related in size, proportion, and position. Photographs can be printed frontwards and backwards. Then cut in half to create symmetric faces (Fig. 8-16) and permit better asymmetry analysis. The Grummons frontal (posteroanterior) asymmetry analysis[1,109] (Fig. 8-17) depicts skeletal and dental asymmetries.

COMPLETING THE ORTHODONTIC PROCESS

Patients must be closely observed during the retention phase to maintain disc–condyle coordination, neuromuscular comfort, and stability. Functionally balanced occlusal relationships, and all other parameters. When the orthodontic

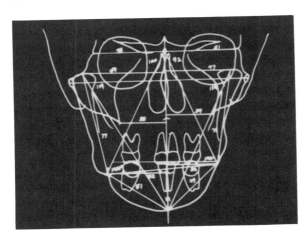

Fig. 8-17. Frontal asymmetry analysis (Grummons).

treatment phase appears to be concluding, the clinician should re-examine functional factors (Chapter 4), reevaluate the cervical spine (Chapter 11), and recheck with models, jaw functional analysis, and x-rays as needed. Patients should be asked to confirm that they are pleased with the results and that functional comfort and stability are as optimal as can be provided.

Orthodontic treatment seems to reduce symptomatology[91–93] and the incidence of TMJ arthralgia.[92,93] The characteristics of ideal occlusal alignment are well accepted.[94,95] Orthodontic treatment resulting in a stable occlusion improves the symmetry of temporalis muscle activity[96,97] and lowers the postural activity levels in the anterior temporalis, posterior temporalis, and masseter muscles.[9,96,97] Orthodontic stabilization should reduce myofascial pain and tenderness.[92,97]

Stability can now be tested and reassessed. Disc–condyle stability without intracapsular inflammation is preferred. Selective occlusal adjustment may be indicated, with comprehensive adjustment to be made when braces are removed or immediately thereafter. Coronoplasty also improves muscular physiology and masticatory reflexes.[97,98] In patients with temporomandibular disorders, however, coronoplasty should be done following orthodontic treatment and not before.[92] Chronic clicking is usually not helped by bite adjustment treatment,[1,54] although symptoms can occur when an incisal or a posterior cuspal guidance is too steep, thereby interfering with the normal muscle resting length[54] or chewing cycles.[64] Simultaneous tooth contacts should exist to ensure optimal muscle activity, especially in the temporalis and masseter muscles.[99–101] Equilibration is difficult to achieve in the presence of pain or dysfunctional issues. Any occlusal bonding or other needs can be assessed and accomplished. Plans for any night appliances, guide ramps in the retainers, and future treatment possibilities can be discussed again.

Certain patients require modification of retention-phase appliances or even require periodic use of a post-orthodontic orthotic coordinated with continuing physical therapy to the cervical spine to maintain the correction achieved. This is not a reflection on the achievement or stability of orthodontic objectives. Patients often have chronic changes and limitations whether or not they have been involved with orthodontics.

Following orthodontics, equilibration to the lingual of the upper incisors permits protrusive freedom.[1,54,102,103] The lower arch can be reproximated (contacts stripped) so that the lower arch can be slightly retracted (moved lingually), allowing freedom of protrusive movements. If greater clearance is necessary, the upper incisors can be torqued or flared forward, with the resulting upper lateral spaces bonded.

Clinicians must be careful not to activate the upper retainer wire to move the upper incisors lingually, since this contributes to mandibular distalization (posterior displacement). Similarly, maintaining the lower anteriors excessively forward can contribute to distalization of the condyles as the overbite deepens (Fig. 8-18).[25]

Positioners can dispose patients to greater incidence of disc dislocation and clicking, again with all related sequelae. Persistence of a clenching pattern while the patient is in a positioner will reintrude posterior teeth, which is unfavorable in cases which required that these teeth be extruded as a part of orthodontic correction. I avoid positioners in post-TMJ cases. A key element is to treat the orthodontic needs well enough so that the positioner is not necessary for the remaining correction.

To maintain stabilization of these TMJ patients further throughout the retention phase, the upper retainer can have a reverse incline placed to encourage mandibular anterior repositioning. Occlusal bonding or a dipod splint can be placed to decompress the joints. Functional appliances (i.e., Mini-Bionator, Herbst, Activator) at night to maintain controlled jaw posture and TMJ stabilization while limiting closure between the posterior teeth, which may have been elevated during orthodontics. Functional appliances used in adult patients for these stabilization reasons are not being applied as growth stimulators. Instead, these appliances assist in holding patients on the disc while limiting side-to-side movement and interrupting parafunctional patterns.

Orthodontic retreatments are necessary for adults who experience dysfunction and/or relapse due primarily to: (1) a treatment approach that may not have been sufficiently complete for the patient's needs; (2) inadequate retention phase follow-through; (3) wrong diagnosis or wrong treatment (e.g., surgical orthodontic approaches were not as common 10 and 20 years ago, nor were our capabilities with TMJ management as expert as today).

Some patients who have received orthodontic treatment subsequently complain of TMJ discomfort/pain/dysfunction and exhibit signs/symptoms consistent with TMJ disorders. Improper orthodontics can contribute and/or be a cause of the incidence of certain categories of TMJ and mandibular pain/dysfunction. Today, TMJ problems in which orthodontics plays a contributing role should be the exception, especially when the patient is treated by an informed orthodontist who understands proper management of TMJ concerns. Actually, orthodontic treatment performed by perceptive and comprehensive orthodontists can and should predictably improve the mandibular function and status of the entire individual.[4,16,69]

Orthodontics, when properly provided for patients who are not predisposed to TMJ disorders does not seem to be a major cause of TMJ (mandibular) pain/dysfunction.[104] Orthodontics usually improves functional capability.[1]

The rigorous long-term study of Sadowsky and Begole[103] concluded that orthodontics appeared to improve the TMJ status of patients. Larsson and Ronnerman[93] examined orthodontic patients 10 years after treatment. Specific headache and cervical analysis were not emphasized. Thirty-one percent of patients exhibited mild joint symptoms. A majority were treated with bicuspid extractions. In this sample, orthodontic therapy helped prevent rather than cause TMJ-related disturbances.

Bucci[105] found no difference in TMJ sounds between postorthodontic patients and untreated subjects. Cohen[106] likewise found no difference between the functional occlusions of orthodontically treated and untreated subjects. Posselt[107] could not identify significant differences between postorthodontic and nonorthodontically treated subjects. Rinchuse and Sassouni,[108] Cohen,[106] and Posselt[107] found no greater occlusal problems in postorthodontic patients as compared with untreated subjects, Grummons[1,60] completed an opinion survey of the orthodontic and TMJ departments of American dental schools. They stated that 40 to 100% of patients having orthodontics developed craniomandibular (TMJ) disorders. The orthodontic departments reported that between 0 and 25% of patients having orthodontics may have had associated mandibular dysfunction, although many situations were improved by such orthodontics. Disparity in these opinions emphasizes the need for better understanding and more study of orthodontic interrelationships with functional disorders. Properly provided orthodontic therapy should be helpful rather than detrimental to craniocervical functional capability.

Successes with treatment are much more predictable and complete today than ever before. Certainly, the percentage of adults who have infused orthodontic practices has provided clinicians with better experience in managing complex adult factors with better long-term results.

REFERENCES

1. Grummons D: Finishing Procedures for the TMJ Patient, Los Angeles, Ed., 10 1986
2. Bell WE: Orofacial Pain: Classification, Diagnosis, Management, 3rd Ed 1985
3. Bell WE: Clinical Management of Temporomandibular Disorders, Year Book Medical Publishers, 1982
4. Travell JG, and Simons DG: Myofascial Pain and Dysfunction: The Trigger Point Manual. Williams & Wilkins, Baltimore, 1983
5. Grummons D: Comprehensive TMJ, Los Angeles, Ed. 10, 1980
6. Patient Communications Systems, Inc., Atlanta, Georgia; 404/381–5051
7. Moller E: The Myogenic Factor in Headache and Facial Pain. In Kawamura, Y, Dubner B. (eds): Oral-Facial Sensory and Motor Function, Quintessence, Tokyo, 1981

8. Enlow DH: Role of the TMJ in facial growth and development. In the President's Conference on the Examination, Diagnosis, and Management of Temporomandibular Disorders. edited by Griffiths. RH. American Dental Association, Chicago, 1983

9. Hamerling J: Mandibular movement patterns: A methodological and clinical investigation of children with lateral forced bite. Ph.D. thesis, University of Amsterdam, 1983

10. Grummons D: TMJ patient goals: comfort and stability. J Craniomandib Pract 3:287, 1985

11. Dolwick ME, Sanders B: TMJ Internal Derangement and Arthrosis, C. V. Mosby, 1985

12. Hansson I, and Oberg I: Arthrosis and deviation in form in the temporomandibular joint. A macroscopic study on human autopsy material. Acta Odontol Scand 37:167, 1977

13. Hansson I, et al: Thickness of the soft tissue layers and the articular disc in the temporomandibular joint. Acta Odontol Scand 37:77, 1977

14. Hansson I, Et al: Anatomic study of the TMJ's of young adults. A pilot investigation. J Prosthet Dent 41:556, 1979

15. Chaconas SJ: Orthodontics. vol. 10, John Wright, Bristol, England, 1982

16. Ricketts RM: Occlusion and the Temporomandibular Joint, Los Angeles, 1974

17. Weinberg LA: Role of condylar position in TMJ dysfunction-pain syndrome. J Prosthet Dent 41:636, 1979

18. Mikhail MG, Rosen H: The validity of temporomandibular joint radiographs using the head positioner. J Prosthet Dent 42:411, 1979

19. Weinberg LA: The role of stress, occlusion, and condyle position in TMJ dysfunction-pain syndrome. J Prosthet Dent 44:642, 1980

20. Dumas AL, et al: A combined tomographic-cephalometric analysis of the TMJ. J Craniomandib Pract 1:24, 1983

21. Dumas AL, Moaddab B, and Homayoun NM: A tomographic study of the condyle/ fossa relationship in patients with TMJ dysfunction. J Craniomandib Pract 2:315, 1984

22. Farrar WB: Differentiation of temporomandibular joint dysfunction to simplify treatment. J Prosthet Dent 28:629, 1972

23. Farrer WB: Diagnosis and treatment of anterior dislocation of the articular disc. NY State Dent J 41:348, 1971

24. Farrar WB, McCarty WL: Inferior joint space arthrography and characteristics of condylar paths in internal derangements of the TMJ. J Prosthet Dent 41:548, 1979

25. Farrar WB, McCarty WL: A clinical outline of temporomandibular joint diagnosis and treatment. Montgomery, Alabama: Normandie Study Group Publications, 1980

26. Gelb H: Clinical Management of Head, Neck and TMJ Pain and Dysfunction, Ed. 2, 1985

27. Ricketts RM: Various conditions of the temporomandibular joint as revealed by cephalometric laminagraphy. Angle Orthod 22:98, 1952

28. Ricketts RM: A study of changes in temporomandibular relations associated with treatment of class II malocclusion. Am J Orthod 38:918, 1952

29. Ricketts RM: Laminagraphy in the diagnosis of temporomandibular disorders. J Am Dent Assoc 46:620, 1953

30. Ricketts RM: Abnormal function of the temporomandibular joint. Am J Orthod 41:435, 1955

31. Ricketts RM: Clinical implications of the temporomandibular joint. Am J Orthod 52:416, 1966

32. Hiniker JJ. Ramfjord SP: Anterior displacement of the mandible in adult Rhesus monkeys. J Prosthet Dent 16:503, 1966
33. Ramfjord SP, Enlow, JJ: Anterior displacement of the mandible in adult rhesus monkeys: long-term observations. J Prosthet Dent 26:517, 1971
34. Weinberg LA: Anterior condylar displacement: its diagnosis and treatment. J Prosthet Dent 34:195, 1975
35. Weinberg LA: The etiology, diagnosis, and treatment of TMJ dysfunction-pain syndrome. Part II: Differential diagnosis. J Prosthet Dent 43:58, 1980
36. Gianelly AG., et al: Mandibular growth, condyle position and Frael appliance therapy. Angle Orthod 53:131, 1983
37. McNamara JA, Hinton RJ, Hoffman DL: Histological analysis of temporomandibular joint adaption to protrusive function in young adult Rhesus monkeys. Am J Orthod 82:288, 1982
38. Stockli PW, Willert HG: Tissue reactions in the temporomandibular joint resulting from anterior displacement in the mandible in the monkey. Am J Orthod 62:469, 1971
39. Petrovic A, Stutzman JJ, Oudet CL: Control process in the postnatal growth of the condylar cartilage in the mandible. In JA McNamara (ed): Determinants of mandibular form and growth. Craniofacial Growth Series, Monograph No. 5. Center for Human Growth and Development, Ann Arbor, Michigan, 1975
40. McNamara JA, Jr, Carlson DS: Quantitative analysis of temporomandibular joint adaptions of protrusive function. Am J Orthod 76:593, 1979
41. Sicher H, DeBrul EL: Oral Anatomy. Ed. 6. CV Mosby. St. Louis, 1975
42. Solberg WK: Epidemiology, incidence and prevalence of temporomandibular disorders: A review, p. 30. in Griffiths, RH (ed): The President's Conference on the Examination, Diagnosis, and Management of Temporomandibular Disorders. American Dental Association, Chicago, 1983A
43. Nilner M. Prevalence of functional disturbances and diseases of the stomatognathic system in 7- to 14-year-olds. Swed Dent J 5:173, 1981
44. Nilner M: Prevalence of functional disturbances and diseases of the stomatognathic system in 15- to 18-year-olds. Swed Dent J 5:189, 1981
45. Egermark-Eriksson I, Carlsson G, and Ingervall B: Prevalence of mandibular dysfunction and orofacial parafunction in 7-, 11-, and 15-year-old Swedish children. Eur J Orthod 3:163, 1981
46. Solberg WK, Woo M, Houston J: Prevalence of mandibular dysfunction in young adults. J Am Dent Assoc 98:25, 1979
47. Helkimo M: Epidemiological surveys of dysfunction of the masticatory system. p. 175. In Zarb GA, Carlsson GE (eds): Temporomandibular joint function and dysfunction. Copenhagen: Munksgaard, 1979
48. De Boever JA: Functional disturbances of the temporomandibular joint. p. 193. in Zarb GA, Carlsson GE (eds): Temporomandibular joint function and dysfunction. Copenhagen: Munksgaard, 1979
49. Bush FM, Butler JH, and Abbott DM: The relationship of TMJ clicking to palpable facial pain. J Craniomandib Prac 1:44, 1983
50. Greene CS, Marbach JJ: Epidemiologic studies of mandibular dysfunction: a critical review. J Prosthet Dent 48:184, 1982
51. Johnston LE (ed): New Vistas in Orthodontics. Philadelphia, Lea & Febiger, 1985
52. Perry H: Relation of occlusion to temporomandibular joint dysfunction: the orthodontic viewpoint. J Am Dent Assoc 79:137, 1969
53. Ricketts R: Occlusion—the medium of dentistry. J Prosthet Dent 21:39, 1969

54. Thompson JR: Differentiation of functional and structural dental malocclusion and its implication to treatment. Angel Orthod 42:252, 1972
55. Roberts D: The etiology of the temporomandibular joint dysfunction syndrome. Am J Orthod 66:498, 1974
56. Owen AH: Orthodontic/orthopedic treatment of craniomandibular pain dysfunction. Part 2: Posterior condylar displacement. J Craniomand Pract 2:333, 1984
57. Owen AH: Orthodontic/orthopedic treatment of craniomandibular pain dysfunction, Part 3: Posterior condylar displacement. J Craniomandib Pract 3:31, 1984
58. Funt LA, Stack BC: The F-S index of the craniomandibular pain syndrome. in Gelb H, (ed): Clinical management of head, neck and TMJ pain and dysfunction, WB Saunders, Philadelphia: 1977
59. Williamson FH: Temporomandibular dysfunction in pretreatment of adolescent patients. Am J Orthod 72:429, 1977
60. Rieder CE, et al: The prevalence of mandibular dysfunction. Part I: Sex and age distribution of related signs and symptoms, J Prosthet Dent 50:81, 1983
61. Gross A, Gale EN: A prevalence study of the clinical signs associated with mandibular dysfunction. J Am Dent Assoc 107:936, 1983
62. Ingervall B, Thilander B: Activity of temporal and masseter muscles in children with lateral forced bite. Angle Orthod 45:249, 1975
63. Moller E, Troelstrup B: Functional and morphological asymmetry in children with unilateral crossbite. J Dent Res 54(special issue A):145, 1975
64. Gibbs CJ, Lundeen HC: Jaw movements and forces during chewing and swallowing and their clinical significance. In Lundeen HC, Gibbs CJ (eds): Advances in Occlusion. Postgraduate Dental Handbook Series, vol. 14. John Wright, Bristol, 1982
65. Wright J: Integrated cranio-mandibular pain-dysfunction management. UCLA graduate orthodontic thesis
66. Darling DW, Kraus S, Glasheen-Wray MB: Relationship of head posture and the rest position of the mandible. J Prosthet Dent 52:111, 1984
67. Goldstein DF, Kraus SL, Williams WB, Glasheen-Wray MB: Influence of cervical posture on mandibular movement. J Prosthet Dent 52:421, 1984
68. Grummons D: Perspectives and persuasions regarding nonextraction orthodontic therapy. Functional Orthodontist, July/Aug 1984
69. Grummons D: After TMJ splints—then what? PCSO Bull 55:61, 1983
70. Lundeen HC, Gibbs CH (eds): Adv Occlusion 14, 1982
71. Moss ML, Rankow RM: The role of the functional matrix in mandibular growth. Angle Orthod 38:(2), 1968
72. Moffett P: The morphogenesis of the temporomandibular joint. Am J Orthod 52:401, 1966
73. Moffett BC Jr, Johnson LC, McCabe JB, Askew HC: Articular remodeling in the adult human temporomandibular joint. Am J Anat 115:(1), July, 1964
74. Grummons DC: Grumzat intermediary appliance. Funct Orthod 2(3):36, 1985
75. Jansson M: Long-term effects of orthodontic treatment. A functional, cephalometric and clinical study of Angle class II, division I malocclusion cases. Ph.D. thesus, University of Bergen, Norway, 1981
76. Ahlin JH: Extraction for treatment of malocclusion in the pedodontic patient. J Pedodont 7:(1), 1982
77. Weinberg L: Posterior bilateral condylar displacement: its diagnosis and treatment. J Prosthet Dent 36:426, 1976
78. Grummons D: Why so much jaw surgery today? Foundation for Orthodontic Research Newsletter, summer, 1986

79. Doyle MG, Stability and complications in 50 consecutively treated surgical-orthodontic patients: a retrospective longitudinal analysis from private practice. Int J Adult Ortho Orthognathic Surg 1, 1986
80. Richards LC, Brown T: Facial morphology and degenerative changes in the temporomandibular joint. J Dent Res 62:654, 1983
81. Upton L, Scott B, Hayward J: Major maxillomandibular malrelations and temporomandibular joint pain-dysfunction. J Prosthet Dent 51:686, 1984
82. Carlsson GE, Ingervall B, Kocak G: Effect of increasing vertical dimension on the masticatory system in subjects with natural teeth. J Prosthet Dent 41:284, 1979
83. Kovaleski WC, De Boever J: Influence of occlusal splints on jaw position and musculature in patients with temporomandibular joint dysfunction. J Prosthet Dent 33:321, 1975
84. Ramfjord SP, Ash MM: Occlusion. Philadelphia: WB Saunders, 1966
85. Weinberg LA: Treatment prostheses in TMJ dysfunction-pain syndrome. J Prosthet Dent 39:654, 1978
86. Weinberg LA: Vertical dimension: a research and clinical analysis. J Prosthet Dent 47:290, 1982
87. Glickman I, Weiss LA: Role of trauma from occlusion in initiation of periodontal pocket formation in experimental animals. J Periodont 26:14, 1955
88. Glickman I, Stein RS, Smulow JB: The effect of increased functional forces upon the periodontium of splinted and non-splinted teeth. J Periodont 32:290, 297 1961
89. Ramfjord SP, Blankenship J: Increased occlusal vertical dimension in adult monkeys. J Prosthet. Dent 45:74, 1981
90. Christensen J: Effect of occlusion-raising procedures on the chewing system. Dent Prac 20:233, 1970
91. Dorph G, Solow B, Carlsen O: Masticatory dysfunction after orthodontic treatment. Tandlaegebladet 79:789, 1975
92. Jansson M, Hasund A: Functional problems in orthodontic patients out of retention. Eur J Orthod 3:173, 1981
93. Larsson E, Ronnerman A: Mandibular dysfunction symptoms in orthodontically treated patients 10 years after the completion of treatment. Eur J Orthod 3:89, 1981
94. Ricketts R: Occlusion—the medium of dentistry. J Prosthet Dent 21:39, 1969
95. Andrews LF: The six keys to normal occlusion. Am J Orthod 62:296, 1972.
96. Ingervall B, Thilander B: Activity of temporal and masseter muscles in children with lateral forced bite. Angle Orthod 45:249, 1975
97. Sheikholeslam A, Moller E, Lous I: Postural and maximal activity in elevators of the mandible before and after treatment of functional disorders. Scand J Dent Res 90:37, 1982
98. McNamara DC: Occlusal adjustment for a physiologically balanced occlusion: J Prosthet Dent 38:284, 1977
99. Bancherz H: Long-term effects of activator treatment. Odontol Rev 27:64, 1976
100. Pancherz H: Treatment of class II malocclusions by jumping the bite with the herbst appliance. A cephalometric investigation
101. Pancherz H, Anehus M: Masticatory function after activator treatment. An analysis of masticatory efficiency, occlusal contact conditions and EMG activity. Acta Odontol Scand 36:309, 1978
102. Perry H: Relation of occlusion to temporomandibular joint dysfunction: the orthodontic viewpoint. J Am Dent Assoc 79:137, 1969
103. Sadowsky C, Begole E: Long-term status of TMJ function and functional occlusion after orthodontic treatment. Am J Orthod 78:201, 1980

104. Solberg WK. In Johnston LE. New Vistas in Orthodontics. Lea & Febiger, Philadelphia, 1985
105. Bucci G: Clinical evaluation of TMJ sounds in orthodontically treated subjects, M Science Thesis, University of Pittsburgh, 1979
106. Cohen WE: A study of occlusal interferences in orthodontically-treated occlusions and untreated normal occlusions. Am J Orthod 51:647, 1985
107. Posselt U. The temporomandibular joint syndrome and occlusion. J Prosthet Dent 25:432, 1971
108. Rinchuse DJ, Sassouni V: An evaluation of eccentric occlusal contacts in orthodontically treated subjects. Am J Orthod 82:251, 1982
109. RMO Diagnostic Services, Calabasas, California

9 | Growth and Development Influences on the Craniomandibular Region

Eric S. Lawrence
Gerald S. Samson

Study of the craniomandibular complex involves delicate reciprocal relationships between various anatomic zones as well as the relationship of the cervical spine to the cranium and the mandible to the cranium. The cervical spine and its influence on the craniomandibular complex has been covered in detail elsewhere in this book. The emphasis of this chapter is on the separate anatomic entities of the cranial bones, midfacial bones, and mandibular complex. Each of these areas is dependent on the others in development and function, as are the muscles of the scalp, mastication, and facial expression. The entire musculoskeletal relationship must be viewed in its entirety for a complete understanding of the interactions in determining the eventual outcome of growth in developing a particular form. All too often, these structures are studied separately without any consideration given to their functional interaction. The reader must always remember that the cranial complex, nasomaxillary complex, and mandibular complex all interact and are profoundly influenced by the relationship of the cervical and shoulder region as well as head posture and the suspension apparatus of the neck. We can then begin to appreciate the delicate balance that must occur in order to create harmony between the various anatomic zones and develop a pleasing facial form.

The concept of counterpart anatomic relationships and their interaction is the cornerstone of craniofacial growth.[1] Enlow's theories on growth and development refers to the counterpart relationship of the maxillomandibular region. In this concept, the maxilla and mandible share a feedback relationship that continues throughout the life of an individual and extends into changes that occurs during aging of the face.[2]

Full appreciation of the manifestations of a "malocclusion" requires some knowledge of the etiology of the malocclusion and the underlying skeletal and/or muscular relationships that contributed to the malocclusion.

GROWTH AND DEVELOPMENT OF THE MAXILLOMANDIBULAR RELATIONSHIP AND DEVELOPMENT OF NORMAL ARCH FORM

The maxilla embryologically forms from a center of mesenchymal condensation in the maxillary process. As the maxilla forms, bone is deposited on the lingual surface and taken away or resorbed from the nasal surface. This process of differential deposition and resorption which begins in fetal life accounts for the vertical facial growth that occurs in humans. Horizontal growth in the fetus occurs through direct deposition to all external surfaces of the maxilla in both an anterior and posterior direction. This process continues for approximately 2 years postnatally to increase the dental arch sufficiently to accommodate the primary dentition.

During the primary dentition period, a significant change in the pattern of deposition and resorption occurs. The anterior portion of the maxilla ceases to be depository, and actually begins to be resorptive. This occurs to accommodate the tremendous amount of vertical growth that must occur.[1] This leaves the posterior portion of the maxilla as the primary growth site for horizontal growth of the maxilla and its corresponding dental arches.

Vertical growth occurs to a much greater extent postnatally than does horizontal growth.[1] At birth, the position of the developing dental arches is just inferior to the orbits. Children due to small body mass, are not in need of a great amount of oxygen to fill their relatively small lungs. As growth proceeds, demand for oxygen increases; consequently, a larger nasal cavity is required to meet this demand. With this impetus, vertical growth of the maxilla increases, resulting in a development of the nasal cavity and its associated sinuses.

Growth of the face can be likened to the blooming of a flower. A face develops in a downward and forward direction from the cranial base and grows along polar coordinates (Fig. 9-1).[3] We must always remember that we are dealing with simultaneous growth in three dimensions. The mean nasal width increases 0.6 mm a year after 5 years of age.[3a] As the nasal cavity increases

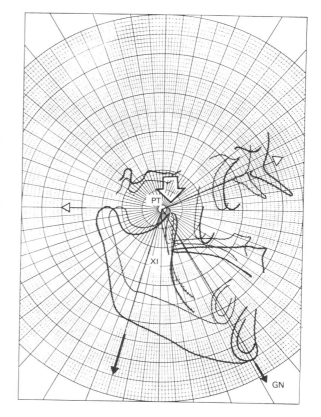

Fig. 9-1. The composite at age 8 and 18 years shows the polar phenomenon around the pterygopalatine area and the base of the body of the sphenoid at the root of the pterygoid plates. (Ricketts R: A study of changes in temporomandibular relations associated with treatment of class II malocclusion, Am J Orthod 38:919, 1952.)

in width, so does its envelope (maxilla) and so does the corresponding alveolar bone and dental arch. This process is shown clearly with the use of serial frontal cephalometric head films.

The Mandible

The growth of the mandible in a normal ideal relationship corresponds to that of the nasomaxillary complex. The mandible initially forms from mesenchymial condensation which occurs lateral to the cartilage of the first pharyngeal arch or Meckel's cartilage. This cartilage serves as a template for intramembranous bone formation prior to its disintegration. Remnants of Meckel's cartilage form the incus and malleus ossicles of the middle ear. The condylar cartilage initially forms separately from the developing mandible as a secondary cartilage. Both the mandible and the condylar cartilage begin to form embryologically at approximately 8 weeks and fuse together at approximately 4 months.[5]

Initially the entire outside surface of the mandible is depository in nature, with differential patterns of deposition and resorption beginning to occur in the

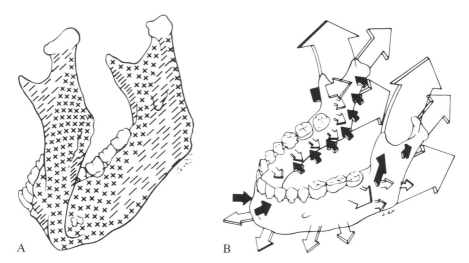

Fig. 9-2. Differential Areas of deposition and resorption. (A) pattern of deposition and resorption in the mandible. Areas of deposition (+) areas of resorption (−). (B) differences in magnitude and direction of growth that occur in the mandible. (Enlow DH: Handbook of Facial Growth, WB Saunders, Philadelphia, 1982.)

thirteenth week. These resorptive areas can be observed on the buccal (cheek) side of the coronoid process, the lingual (tongue) side of the ramus, and the posterior portion of the corpus (Fig. 9-2). The anterior portion of the ramus is also resorptive with the posterior portion being depository. This allows elongation of the mandibular corpus to accommodate the lengthening dental arch. Deposition is also observed along the anterior tip of the coronoid process.[1]

Historically, the mandible was believed to grow in a postero-superior direction, with a resultant downward and forward growth movement of the chin. This theory thus implied that a dolichofacial or vertically growing face would have a vertically growing ramus and condyle whereas a brachyfacial or horizontally growing face would have a horizontally growing ramus and condyle (Fig. 9-3). Ricketts[6] studied this growth concept using laminographs and showed a growth direction of the ramus and condyle opposite to that which was previously believed to occur. He found more horizontal development of the ramus and condyle associated with vertical facial development (dolichofacial) and more vertical development of the mandibular ramus and condyle associated with horizontal growth of the face (brachyfacial).[3] Using this information, Ricketts[7,8] formulated his theory on the arcial growth of the mandible and its projected pattern of growth. This theory was substantiated by Bjork[9] who, in an implant study, observed that often the condyles did not grow upward and backward but actually grew either straight up or upward and forward (Fig. 9-4). Further support came from Moss;[10] who suggested that the growth of the mandible followed a logarithmic spiral, Moffett,[11] who used vital staining to show that the condyle grows in a upward and forward direction;

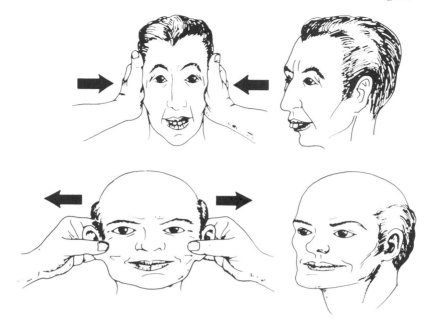

Fig. 9-3. Three major facial types are generally described. They are classified as: (**A**) dolichofacial, which is a long narrow face with a sloping forehead, prominent brow ridge, long sloping nose, and retrognathic mandible. The overall facial profile is convex. (**B**) Brachyfacial, which is a squat wide face with an upright forehead, short pug nose, and a more prognathic mandibular form. The overall facial profile is straight or concave. Mesofacial is the third facial type and is a cross between dolichofacial and brachyfacial facial types. It is considered the normal or balanced face.(Enlow DH: Handbook of Facial Growth, WB Saunders, Philadelphia, 1982.)

Fig. 9-4. Current (progressive) concept of mandibular growth and dental development as developed by Ricketts. (Ricketts R: A study of changes in temporomandibular relations associated with treatment of class II malocclusion. Am J Ortho 38:919, 1952.

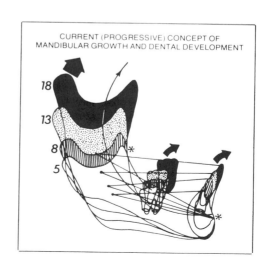

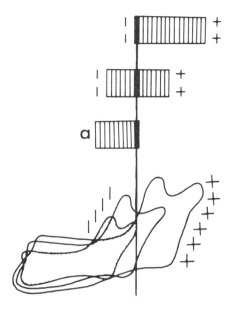

Fig. 9-5. The mandible grows in length due to extensive remodeling of the ramus. Resorption occurs along the anterior border of the ramus and is coupled with deposition along its posterior border. This increases the length of the corpus without increasing ramus width. (Enlow DH: Handbook of Facial Growth, WB Saunders, Philadelphia, 1982)

and Enlow,[1] who showed that the anterior portion of the coronoid process is depository. Ricketts[12] further supported his own theory of arcial growth by determining the actual arc of mandibular growth and formulating a method of predicting its growth. This method was tested on more than 200 patients who were followed up for a 20-year period and has withstood all further testing.

As with the maxilla, the mandible grows not only in an anteroposterior dimension, but also in a mediolateral direction. Using composites of serially taken frontal cephalograms taken from 4 to 18 years of age, Ricketts[4] showed that the growth direction of the mandible is lateral at the condylar heads and downward and outward in all other directions. When he superimposed films at the mandibular symphysis, the mandible was shown to be increased 40 mm in width at an average angle of 60°.

Growth of the mandible and the maxilla are inseparable and interdependent on each other. The mandibular corpus is the direct structural counterpart of the maxillary corpus, with the ramus relating to the pharyngeal space and the middle cranial fossa. Functionally, the ramus spans the pharyngeal space to place the mandibular dental arch in a proper relationship to the maxillary dental arch.[13] The mandibular ramus is thus the key adaptive component in the maxillomandibular relationship by relocating posteriorly to increase the corpus length or amount of space available for the dentition; by increasing in horizontal width to accommodate the expanding pharyngeal space; and by lengthening vertically to accommodate the tremendous vertical growth of the nasomaxillary complex (Fig. 9-5).

The mandible's suspension from the skull via musculature with only a tripod contact (one contact at each TMJ, with the third contact being the dental occlusion) causes the spatial position of the mandible to be subservient to that of the nasomaxillary complex. The entire mandible may be rotated in a clockwise or open direction due to an increased vertical dimension in the nasomaxillary complex (environmental conditions that may lead to this are discussed more fully later in this chapter). A similar rotation may also be caused by the angular relationship of the cranial base. If the cranial base angle (basion-sella-nasion) is open or more obtuse, the effect on mandibular position will be a downward and backward rotation of the mandible (Fig. 9-6). This type of cranial base relationship is consistent with a long narrow dolichofacial facial type. We can thus predict that in this facial type there is an inherent class II tendency that will be expressed to varying degrees depending on compensations that may or may not occur. In contrast, a short vertical dimension of the nasomaxillary complex may result in a counterclockwise rotation of the mandible and a short lower anterior facial height. Again, this relationship can also be produced with a "closing" or a more acute angulation in the cranial base angle. In this situation, the mandible assumes a more anterior position with respect to the maxilla (relative mandibular protrusion) due to its arc of closure. This condition is frequently observed in brachyfacial individuals.

A second type of mandibular rotation involves the bending of the mandible itself through remodeling. This results in a more closed ramus-corpus angle. This process is consistent with the arcial growth theory of Ricketts[8,12] and results in a more upright ramus relative to the corpus. The ramus must continue to remodel during facial growth as the horizontal enlargment of the ramus begins to slow and finally ceases while the vertical enlargment of the midface and ramus continues.[1] Most of the remodeling involving the ramus-corpus angular relationship is due to ramal changes. According to Enlow,[1] the objectives of the mandibular rotational remodeling are:

1. To render the ramus in a more upright position relative to the corpus.
2. To upright the ramus without increasing its horizontal width.
3. To provide posterior elongation of the corpus.
4. To produce a vertically longer ramus in order to compensate for vertical midfacial growth.

For mandibular rotation to be accomplished, a great amount of growth must occur in the mandibular condyle area. Fortunately, the mandibular condyle possess a secondary cartilage that can accommodate to new functional relationships by producing endochondrial bone. This unique type of cartilage forms as a separate entity from the developing mandible and later fuses into a single unit, and is thus not a derivative of Meckels' cartilage that helped form the mandible. The condylar cartilage is reactive in its growth response to maintain proper articulation between the mandible and the maxilla. As the mandible is carried down and forward, the condyle is correspondingly triggered to respond with growth in an opposite direction, thereby sustaining a proper anatomic relationship and articulation with the cranial floor[14] (Fig. 9-7). Due to the nonspecific orientation of the prechondroblasts, the condyle is free to grow in any adaptive direction to accommodate both changing vectors of ramus

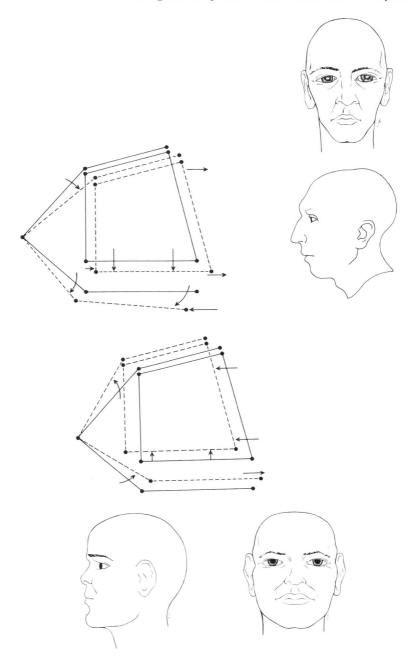

Fig. 9-6. Top: Facial type (dolichofacial) that can be expected when there is excessive vertical growth of the nasomaxillary complex. Bottom: Facial type (brachyfacial) that can be expected when there is a short midface of nasomaxillary complex. (Enlow DH: Handbook of Facial Growth. WB Saunders, Philadelphia, 1982.)

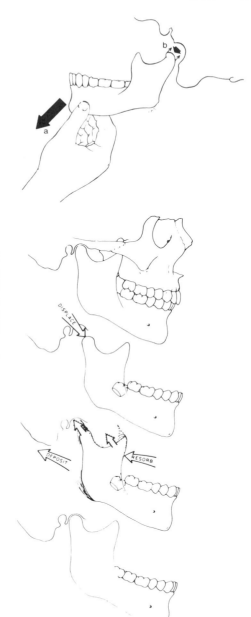

Fig. 9-7. According to the functional matrix theory, the soft tissue capsule displaces the mandible in a downward and forward direction. To maintain contact with the cranium there is a compensatory growth in a upward and backward direction. (Enlow DH: Handbook of Facial Growth, WB Saunders, Philadelphia, 1982.)

growth and individual variation based on facial type and environmental influences.

Throughout growth and development, a hierarchy of anatomic components exists in which nerves dictate muscular behavior and muscular behavior dictates bone form. Adaptive bony growth occurs in response to pressures placed on it by the soft tissue capsule, which includes the muscle, tongue, lips, cheeks, integument, mucosa, connective tissues, nerves, blood vessels, airway, pharynx, the brain as an organ mass, tonsils, adenoids, etc.[1] We can now view the nasomaxillary/mandibular relationship as a coupled complex interdependent on one another and subservient to the soft tissue capsule engulfing it. A malformation or misorientation of one component will thus necessitate compensation from another.

Graber[15] states that two-thirds of the cases of an average orthodontic practice are due to abnormal maxillomandibular relations; thus, these are frequent problems requiring orthopedic correction.

Functional Matrix

The therapeutic strategy in functional treatment is based on the mechanism and regulation of growth of craniofacial bones under the influence of functional factors. Orofacial orthopedics refers to the clinical application of the "functional matrix concept" described by Moss[16], which states that the bony facial structures are shaped and positioned as they are owing to the forces of the soft tissue capsule. Bone remodeling occurs in response to changes in the soft tissue capsule.

With regard to the functional matrix, the teeth, tongue, lips, and cheeks may be regarded as soft-tissue guide elements that control the eruption path of the teeth in accordance with a fixed genetic plan. With regard to the functional matrix as it applies to the mandible, all the musculature of the head and neck region contributes to the development of the maxillomandibular relationship. The most powerful of these muscles are the masticatory muscles. The temporalis complex exerts its force against the coronoid process of the mandible. The resultant force exerted by this muscle is directed upward and backward. The masseteric sling or complex is composed of the masseter muscle laterally and the internal pterygoid muscle medially. The fibers of both these muscles traverse in an upward and forward direction. The mandible, under the influence of these three major muscles, would appear to have a clockwise rotational tendency because there is an upward pull at the gonial angle and a upward and backward pull at the coronoid process. The muscle that stabilizes the entire system is the lateral pterygoid muscle, which functions to hold the condyle against the articular emminence (Fig. 9-8).

An example of the functional matrix theory can be seen in the postural positioning of the mandible. The mandible is suspended from the cranium by the masticatory muscle, and its position is dictated by these muscles as well as the anterior cervical musculature. In this case, the musculature may be considered the functional matrix that dictates the postural jaw position (the factors influencing the musculature are discussed later in this chapter). The musculature, by holding the mandible in a habitual position, dictates the direction in which the mandible will grow. Children with lip incompetence or a lips-apart posture generally also hold the mandible in an open or teeth-apart

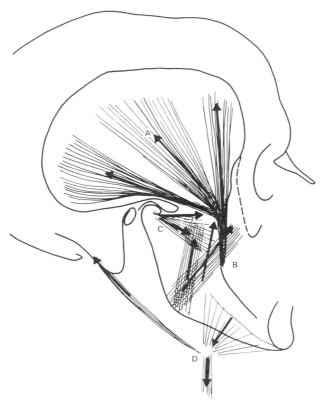

Fig. 9-8. The mechanisms of growth abnormalities in the mandible can be explained by the force couple systems involved in mandibular posture. (**A**) Mean upward and backward direction of the temporalis. (**B**) Mean upward and forward pull of the masseteric complex. (**C**) Downward and forward inclination of the pull of the external pterygoid in reciprocity to the posterior fibers of the temporalis. (**D**) Effects of the drag on the chin by the hyoid musculature. The mandible is often thought to function as a class III lever; however, it is actually a force couple system with a class I lever operating off the coronoid process and perhaps the condylar head, with the external pterygoid acting as a fulcrum. This helps explain the complex physiology of the opening and closing movements of the mandible. (Ricketts R: A study of changes in temporomandibular relations associated with treatment of Class II malocclusion. Am J Orthod 38:919, 1952.)

posture (Fig. 9-9). To sustain this position, there must be an increase in the activity of the lateral pterygoid muscles as well as in the anterior cervical musculature. This increased activity over a sustained time results in redirection of mandibular growth, almost warping the mandible in a counterclockwise or downward direction. In this situation, generally a compensatory alveolar bone growth occurs—also in the posterior dentition—resulting in an anterior openbite occlusion.

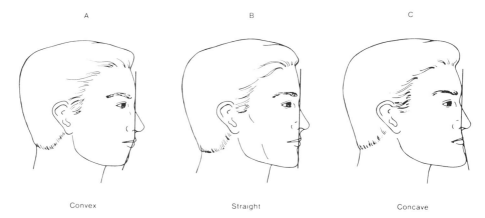

A   B   C

Convex   Straight   Concave

Fig. 9-9. Profile convexity or concavity results from a disproportion in the size of the jaws, but does not in itself indicate which jaw is at fault. A convex facial profile indicates a class II jaw relationship, which can result from either a maxilla that projects too far forward or a mandible too far back (as shown in **A**). A concave profile indicates a class III relationship, which can result from either a maxilla that is too far back or a mandible that protrudes forward, as shown in **C**. (Profitt WR: Contemporary Orthodontics. CV Mosby St. Louis, 1986.)

The field of orthopedics has taught us

1. Bone structures and mechanical stress are directly interrelated.
2. Bone remodeling induced by mechanical stress is a major biologic phenomenon.

Light continuous forces are very efficient in producing orthopedic movements. We must then consider the muscles of facial expression and perioral musculature as integral functional matrix members affecting development. The musculature we are concerned with here and which have an effect on the teeth and alveolar structures are the tongue, buccinator complex, and suprahyoids. The remaining muscles have an influence on mandibular development. Aberrant muscle function in any of these three groups may cause craniofacial and dentoalveolar deformities.

These muscular forces have long been known to have a profound influence on the dentition. Tomes[17] observed that the force in the periapical region of a tooth results in a pushing of that tooth in the direction of least resistance. The teeth appear to erupt clinically into a "channel" located between the tongue, lips, and cheeks.[18,19]

The most significant muscle group affecting the developing dentoalveolar structures from the buccal side is the buccinator complex. The buccinator is composed of three bands. The superior and inferior bands are continuous from the area of the pterygomandibular raphae across the midline to the contralateral pterygomandibular raphe. The fibers of the middle band decussate and join the fibers of the obicularis oris.[20] The three bands of the buccinator muscle envelop the entire alveolar process and act to determine the horizontal expansion of the alveolar process. Neuronal involvement signaled from stress centers in the brain may cause hyperactivity of this complex and place an inward force vector on the developing arches, resulting in a narrowing of either or both of the upper and lower dental arches. The severity of the malocclusion produced depends largely on the position of the tongue, which acts as an antagonist muscle to the buccinator complex.

FACTORS INFLUENCING THE FUNCTIONAL MATRIX

Nasal Airway Obstruction

The principle relationship between dentofacial development and nasorespiratory obstruction has long been known. In 1861, Catlin[21] wrote of the consequences of mouth breathing, describing the greater health of primitive Indians as compared with "civilized" Europeans, attributing this to the fact that the Indians slept on their backs and breathed through their noses.

Nasorespiratory obstruction may be caused by a number of factors, some of which are transitory and difficult to control, such as allergic rhinitis, and others of a more structural nature that can easily be identified and alleviated, such as enlargement of adenoidal tissue, tonsils, and inferior turbinates. There may also be narrowing of the external nares or a deviation of the nasal septum restricting proper nasal respiration.

The nasopharynx is small in the infant and develops as the child's body size enlarges and requires more oxygen.[1] The anteroposterior dimension of the nasopharynx is stable after two years of age and is measured between the posterior nasal spine of the hard palate and the anterior arch of the atlas.[22,23,24] After a stable relationship is formed in the anteroposterior direction, all subsequent growth and enlargement is primarily vertical in direction until the maxilla completes its growth.

The *adenoidal tissue* is located in the posterosuperior aspect of the nasopharynx and is composed of lymphoid tissue. It is a portion of the lymphoid tissue known as Waldeyer's ring which is also composed of the lingual tonsils and the palatine tonsils. The adenoids are generally the body's, first line of defense against invading viruses and bacteria entering through the nasal airway. Due to this position, the principle problem of the adenoids are infection and hypertrophy. Swelling of 2 to 3 cm can often be observed. This degree of swelling can interfere with the passage of air through the nasal cavity.[25] Adenoid tissue is not radiographically evident until approximately 6 months to 1 year of postnatal life.[24]

Subtelny[24] followed 15 subjects longitudinally with serial radiographs over varying periods of time to study the growth of adenoidal tissue. In no subjects was adenoidectomy performed. Subtelny[24] observed that adenoid tissue grows predominately downward and forward, progressing rapidly during the second and third year of life. During this time, it may occupy as much as one-half the nasopharngeal cavity with a peak mass occurring between the ages of 11 and 15 years. The tissue then regresses as the child passes through puberty and approaches adulthood.[26] Obstructive problems arise when the adenoid tissue develops at a faster rate than vertical growth of the maxilla.[24] The tissue in this condition may extend anteriorly to the posterior choanea. Subtelny's observations have been substantiated by Ricketts.[27] They both contend that the adenoid mass must be assessed relative to the dimensions of the nasopharynx to evaluate obstruction.

The *nasal septum* is normally located in the midline and divides the nasal cavity in half. Deviations of the septa away from the midline may be developmental in origin, but are usually the result of trauma, be it an incidental blow to the nose or even the trauma of passing through the birth canal. Josephs,[28] in his study on the effects of nasal obstruction on facial growth, noticed a greater incidence of septal deviation in allergic as opposed to nonallergic children. This corollary finding may be attributed to environmental influences (not associated with trauma) associated with the allergy which will be addressed later.

The *nasal turbinates* are a series of four structures stacked on top of one another and projecting from the lateral nasal wall. The function of the turbinates is to increase the amount of surface area of the nasal tissue that is covered with ciliated epithelium and to induce turbulence into the inspired air to facilitate warming, humidifying, and filtrating actions. The inferior turbinate is first to be exposed to the arriving onslaught of air and is thus most susceptible to infection and swelling. The turbinates, which are extremely vascular, have been observed to engorge and constrict on a 4- to 6-hour cycle. Thus, the turbinate size may vary depending on the time of day, and observations of hypertrophy should be made on more than one occasion.[29] Hypertrophy is chronic noncyclable swelling usually associated with upper airway resistance. This condition is generally resistant to conservative means of treatment and usually requires surgery or aggressive medical therapy to improve the condition.

The *lingual tonsils* are located in the posterior portion of the mouth at the lateral base of the tongue. Considerable controversy exists over their significance in respiratory obstruction; currently, they are believed to be of minimal significance to nasal airway obstruction unless they are extremely enlarged. The greater significance of tonsilar enlargment is its effect on tongue position. Due to the close proximity of the tonsils and the tongue base, tonsilar enlargment can cause a forward displacement of the tongue in the oral cavity. This removes the tongue from its normal resting position and upsets the equilibrium in the functional matrix.

Effects of Nasal Airway Obstruction on Craniofacial Growth

Many investigators and clinicians have observed a close association between nasal obstruction, facial maldevelopment, and dental malocclusion.

Ricketts[27] serially followed several patients in his practice and made the following observations on both treated and untreated patients. He observed the following characteristics common to these patients, which he describes "respiratory obstructive syndrome."

1. Primary unilateral or bilateral crossbite
2. Functional unilateral crossbite with mandibular deflection
3. Presence of enlarged adenoids or tonsils or history of it
4. Openbite
5. Lowered tongue position
6. Tongue thrust
7. Narrow upper arch
8. Chronic mouthbreathing
9. Secondary problems in the TMJ and maxilla
10. Pseudo-class I condition in bilateral crossbite with anterior mandibular deflection
11. Head tipped backward on cervical column
12. Narrow nasal cavity
13. Opening of the mandibular angle

Although Ricketts' findings are consistent with those of other clinicians, a direct cause-and-effect relationship was not established. What was needed was controlled animal experimentation. The best controlled and most notable work was that of Harvold et al[30,31,32,32a] who conducted a series of primate experiments on young growing rhesus monkeys. In one experiment, they caused the animals to be obligate mouth breathers by obstructing their nasal passage with silicone plugs. They followed these monkeys for a period of 3 years, collecting a series of photographs, dental casts, radiographs, and electromyographic recordings. Harvold et al observed that the monkeys with nasal blockage kept their mouths open continuously, whereas the control animals kept their mouths closed. Cephalometric analysis showed a significant increase in the distance from nasion to the chin in the mouth breather. The distance from nasion to the hard palate also increased, but the distance from the hard palate to the chin did not. This demonstrates that the lowering of the mandible to open an oral airway was followed by a downward migration of the entire maxilla. The lower border of the mandible became more steeply inclined in the experimental group as the gonial angle increased. Although these findings were consistent throughout the entire experimental group, the extent and severity of the malformations varied. The differential treatment response appeared to be linked to the manner in which the animal adapted to the nasal obstruction. Another study conducted by Harvold[30] placed acrylic blocks in the palatal vault of 36 rhesus monkeys to assess the change involved with abnormal tongue position. This condition is not unlike that which may be experienced with enlarged tonsils. The acrylic blocks created a continuous stimulus to the tongue, resulting in an altered tonus of the muscles involved in postural positioning of the mandible. The new stimuli caused the animals to respond initially by lowering the mandible. After only 6 months of this behavior, a statistically significant difference in the ratio between facial height and mandibular length was noted. The mandible in all the experimental animals changed dramatically due to bone resorption at the gonial angle and bone apposition at the chin. After 1 year, the experimental animals showed a greater increase in facial height, an open gonial angle, and prominent bone apposition to the chin, resulting in an increase in the mandibular symphysis. There was a significant morphologic change involving notching at the gonial angle.

Based on a series of experiments on primates, Harvold[33] postulated that oral respiration in monkeys is associated with the recruitment of certain muscles of the orofacial system usually not used for that purpose. The muscle development depends, within certain limits, on the use of the muscle. The change in bone morphology as well as tooth position depends on bone reorganization. The interaction between muscle function and bone development is expressed by Wolff's law.[34]

Harvold's findings in animals have been observed clinically in humans and supported by the views of Balyeat and Bowen,[35] Todd and Broadbent,[36] Linder-Aronson,[37] Subtenly,[38] Quinn,[39] and Ricketts.[4] The reader is reminded that total airway obstruction and total mouth breathing is rare in humans.

Tongue and Head Posture

A large factor influencing the development of the facial skeleton commonly associated with nasal airway obstruction is the posture of the tongue.

The tongue normally occupies a neutral position in the oral cavity. Ricketts,[40] in a study of 40 patients, noticed that the tongue is normally in contact with the soft palate in the posterior with its center located no lower than halfway between the crowns of the upper molars and the palatal vault. In this position, the tongue provides an outward force on the developing dentition to balance the constant inward force placed by the cheek musculature, predominately the buccinator. Under ideal conditions, an equilibrium exists in which the teeth are positioned in a "neutral space" between these opposing forces.[24,35] In another study, Eastman[41] measured the tongue position (resting) cephalometrically and found that individuals with seasonal allergies had a lower tongue posture than did normal subjects.

Owing to their location and contiguous relationship to the surface of the throat, enlarged facial tonsils may displace the tongue forward to maintain an adequate oropharyngeal space for respiration.[27,38,42] This occurs as the enlarged tonsils cause the soft palate to rest on the upper pole rather than the dorsum of the tongue, resulting in a downward and forward displacement of the dorsum. The forward posturing of the tongue may be even more marked when the nasopharynx is filled with adenoids.[27]

Previously, we discussed the relationship of the adenoids to the nasopharynx. A discrepancy in the anteroposterior dimension of the pharynx itself has significant bearing on the morphology of the soft palate. If a deep nasopharynx exists, a more obtuse cranial base angle is apparent and the soft palate is flat or straight. When a shallow nasopharynx exists, an acute cranial base angle exists with the soft palate angled sharply downward from the posterior nasal spine. This relationship was originally observed by Ricketts[43] in patients with cleft palates and was substantiated by Subtenly.[24] They both observed that in cases with an acute drop to the palate a displacement of the tongue in an anterior and inferior direction occurred, which parallels Harvold's findings in his experiments involving placing acrylic blocks in primate palates.[30]

HEAD POSTURE

The postural position of the head in relation to the cervical spine is another factor that has been ignored by most dental clinicians. Studies linking head posture to changes in craniofacial morphology have been performed by Solow and Tallgren,[44] Opdebeek et al,[45] and Posnick.[46] Clinical support for this research is derived from the observation of increased craniocervical angulation in subjects with adenoidal-induced nasal obstruction as described by Ricketts,[27] Koski`and Lahdemaki,[47] and Quinn and Pickrell.[39]

Schwartz[48,49] found that extension of the head in relation to the body, particularly during sleep, led to distal displacement of the mandible and development of a class II malocclusion. Bjork[50–52] noted that persons with flattened cranial bases and retrognathic facial profiles also carried the head in an extended position. Solow and Tallagren[53] observed that differences in craniofacial morphology between subjects with large and small craniocervical angulations were similar to those between large and small mandibular plane inclinations. Both Shelton[54] and Mew[55] described twins whose differing facial morphology was attributed to abnormal posture of the head and neck in one of the twins. In 1979, Linder-Aronson and Woodside[37] showed a relationship between abnormal head posture, enlarged adenoids, blocked nasal airway, and malocclusion. They studied lateral and PA cephalometric radiographs of 120 patients in the Burlington Growth Study. This study consists of longitudinal records taken every 2 to 3 years between the ages of 6 and 20 years. Linder-Aronson and Woodside found that in patients (22) with an increasing lower anterior facial height the mean size of the airway through the nose was narrower than in control subjects. The researchers concluded that the lower anterior facial height is dependent on the growth direction of the mandible and the neuromuscular factors influencing mandibular posture, such as mouth breathing and head posture. In their experiment, Linder-Aronson and Woodside made no reference to the facial type involved in the study, which may have influenced their results. Vig,[56] in another study of humans, found that after artificial nasal obstruction, the head quickly assumes an extended posture; Vig claimed that the process of lowering the mandible to compensate for nasal obstruction actually results in a reduction of size of the oropharynx. To compensate and thus restore the airway volume, the hyoid bone must be elevated and moved anteriorly. This repositioning is accomplished by changing the head posture (tilting backwards) or by sustained muscular contraction. Harvold et al[30,31] in primate studies also observed an extended head and neck posture with nasal respiratory obstruction. An undersized mandible may also have influence on the airway, causing the head to tilt back.[57]

Ricketts[4] hypothesized that a possible alteration in the entire postural kinetic chain of the head may result from a blockage of the nasopharynx, and further conjectured that changes in mandibular position could be associated with failure of adenoidal and tonsillar involution. In a study of 35 patients aged 3 to 12 years (18 females and 17 males) Ricketts took cephalometric head films both pre- and postadenotonsilectomy. He intended to compare the tongue heights relative to the palate, postural alterations of the soft palate, positional change of the hyoid bone, and changes in head posture. He observed both functional and postural changes. In the majority of cases, the tongue and hyoid bone elevated and the soft palate tended to raise during rest. The resting posture of the entire head tipped down a mean of 2° and, as this occurred, the palate appeared to lower and move downward over the tongue.

Even though most studies have linked postural changes of the head and neck to airway resistance, head and neck postural changes may be a primary condition, thereby influencing the functional matrix and dentoalveolar–craniofacial morphology. For further understanding of primary changes in head and neck posture occuring in postnatal years and in adult years, see Chapters 10 and 12.

Children today may be less physically active than their ancestors. The sitting position is the position most commonly assumed, be it all day at school or at home while doing homework or watching television. This position contributes to stress in the head–neck and shoulder region. The same environmental stresses that affect the adult population also affect the younger population. Children today, due to the complex society in which they live in industrialized countries, have tremendous pressure placed on them to perform and excel. This creates a very stressful psychological condition in the children, which may be manifested in aberrant tone and function of the facial and neck musculature which in turn may lead to skeletal and/or dental malformations.[58]

FUNCTIONAL FACTORS AFFECTING TMJ DEVELOPMENT

The temporomandibular articulation develops with age. At birth, the temporal articulation surface is almost flat because the articular eminence and postglenoid process have not yet developed well. Between the ages of 6 months and $2\frac{1}{2}$ years the mandibular fossa increases in depth from less than 2 mm to about 4 to 5 mm.[59] This time period coincides with the development of the primary dentition and the change in the functional requirement of the TMJ. Hinton[60] reported that orthopedic and other manipulations of the lower jaw engender distinct adaptive responses in the tissues of the temporal component. This follows Moss's functional matrix theory[61] that remodeling changes of the articular eminence and mandibular fossa are caused by altered biomechanical stress.

Naso-airway obstruction may also play a role in abnormal condylar development. The body's survival system always predominates, and in threatening life-situations, the body compensates to alleviate the problem. This phenomenon is observed with nasorespiratory obstruction. According to Ricketts,[62] to decrease resistance and increase air volume, the mandible must translate forward. This facilitates mouth opening and results in retraction of the chin. In this situation the lateral pterygoid muscle is believed to stabilize, protect, or modify the respiratory airway by providing a mechanism for protruding the mandible. In children, this survival mechanism may be very damaging to the developing condyles and articular eminence. Due to trauma of this position in function, both the condyle and eminence may be stunted in growth. A smaller eminence would affect the amount of posterior disclusion in lateral excursions, whereas damage to the condyle may cause a lack of vertical mandibular growth, causing a decreased posterior facial height and resulting in a deficient skeletal relationship.

Most of these concepts are conjectural—possible sequences of events as yet unproven. Ricketts based his contention on a study of 180 pathologic cases in which he observed a lack of normal condylar growth and width to the mandible associated with forward positioning of the condyles. In extreme cases of a small eminence, he observed that the condyles may move so far anteriorly that they may actually articulate with the greater wing of the sphenoid bone, resulting in a "sphenomandibular" articulation for function. Rubin[63] studied seven monkeys under splint therapy constructed to create prematurities. After 55 days of splint therapy, the monkeys' condyles were displaced mesioinferiorly, with flattening of the articular eminence and condylar head. Although this experiment lacked controls and histopathologic documentation of the changes, it does provide some support to Ricketts[62] hypothesis of trauma causing bony adaptation in the joint structure.

Due to their anatomic location, the condyles are vulnerable to trauma. Any fall or blow to the chin may be transferred through the mandible into the condyle and articular fossa. This type of macrotrauma may be common in children as they play and learn to walk and may lead to significant damage to the developing TMJ. Ricketts[62] claims that both macrotrauma and microtrauma have significant long-term effects, describing microtrauma as intraoral trauma resulting from problems in occlusion, loss of tooth support, or functional interferences that continually insult the joint structure through condylar displacement. Ricketts further reports that both microtrauma and macrotrauma affect the chondrogenic area of the condyle and may lead to degenerative joint disease and directly influence the growth of the condyles, subsequently producing growth deformity. In addition, actual condylar resorption may occur with mandibular trauma. The clinical significance of the dysfunction arises in its possible effects on the growth of the mandible.

Growth deformity in the TMJ complex may result in either a flat eminence or a small condyle in a large fossa. In either case, no functional eminence is present during the early phase of mandibular movements; consequently, there is a lack of separation of the posterior teeth. This may be one explanation for dental attrition in the early mixed dentition. As Ricketts states:

> Lack of eminence height or absence of functioning joint also is a factor in clinical diagnosis, for traumatic joint conditions ostensibly can occur even in children. For instance, a patient with a slight Class II malocclusion who also has a slight airway limitation in the pharynx might adapt to a forward mandibular position. No functional eminence results, particularly in the young, and the condyle may begin to be pathologically traumatized.[6]

One of the most extensive studies conducted on TMJ growth disturbance and associated dysfunction was published in 1985 by Dibbits,[64] who contended that if dysfunction causes shortening of the ramus through remodeling, it can also cause a disturbance of growth in children. Dibbits study, conducted over 15 years, involved 175 children (94 female and 71 male) 139 of whom he examined yearly for 4 consecutive years and 102 of whom he was able to recall 10 years later for follow-up examinations. He observed that TMJ dysfunction occurred during the period of time when the child was actively growing. He also found a significant group of patients with a deformed condylar projection that he termed arthrosis deformans juvenils (ADJ). Dibbits found this dysfunction group to be more retrognathic and, on the average, to have a smaller mandibular length, shorter ramus and posterior facial height, larger gonial angle, and steeper mandibular plane. These changes became evident as early as 7 years of age. In these children (ADJ), the condylar cartilage appears not to contribute to the growth of the condyle. The growth that does occur appears to be based on a backward rotation of the mandible.[65] The mandible thus develops an adaptive growth pattern to continue to fulfill the basic functional requirements due to growth of its counterparts (discussed in ref. 1). The findings of Dibbits on condylar growth direction correlate with those of Bjork[66] and Ricketts.[27]

Dentoalveolar changes as a consequence of nasorespiratory obstruction may in itself adversely affect the functioning of the TMJ. A common result of mouth breathing is a narrow maxillary arch and possible development of a posterior crossbite. To maintain the best possible occlusal contact, the body compensates for this skeletal discrepancy by flaring the upper molars bucally. In this situation, the mandibular arch may be normal or wider than normal due to the new tongue position. The main consequence of this action is that the flaring of the maxillary molars causes their mesiolingual cusps to "hang down" beyond the occlusal plane and to act as an interference in lateral mandibular movements. This type of interference is very damaging to the integrity of the joint.

The effects of muscular forces acting with airway obstruction may lead not only to dental deformity and joint disorders, but may also be an obstacle to successful treatment. Elimination of nasal airway obstruction alone may lead to successful resolution of skeletal openbites. Linder-Aronson[67] studied 60 patients 5 years after adenoidectomy and reported that both the lower facial height and angulation of the mandibular plane decreased during the postoperative period. He described this as a "normalization of the orofacial complex." Ricketts[68] in a study of 30 children posttonsiladenoidecomy reported that an average adenoid reduction of 8 mm resulted in a decreased dimension from the tongue to the cervical vertebrae, skull base and hard palate of 2 to 3 mm. The tongue was retracted upward and backward. Ricketts also observed spontaneous correction of posterior crossbite following removal of the lymphoid tissue. Quinn[42] reported a unique case of a patient with an Angle class II cusp relationship, anterior openbite, lingual axial inclination of the anterior teeth and alveolar process, a forward position of the tongue, and cervical deformity. Nine months following adenoidectomy, the molar relationship was corrected, openbite was reduced, and axial inclination of the lower incisors improved along with tongue position and cervical posture without any orthodontic intervention. Brodie[23] observed that following adenoid removal, the soft palate once again rested against the posterior surface of the tongue.

The importance of a proper nasal airway is cited in a rare occurrence reported by Bushey,[69] who reported the case of monozygotic twins, one of whom developed nasal obstruction. This twin developed excessive anterior facial height and deformity; the other twin, a nasorespirator, did not.

Clinical Recognition of Nasorespiratory Distress

It is beyond the scope of this chapter to cover adequately or provide an indepth analysis of the diagnosis of nasorespiratory obstruction. Quick screening signs exist, however, which can be observed by any clinician, who can then properly refer the patient to an otolaryngologist for definitive diagnosis and treatment.

The first step in assessing possible respiratory problems is acquisition of a good health history. This simple procedure can often pinpoint the problem or rule out various possibilities. Concern is focused on the possibility of foreign object obstruction as well as various forms of rhinitis. Allergic rhinitis is a common cause of nasal obstruction or congestion in our modern society. Airborne allergies such as those to dust and pollen receive daily attention as various over-the-counter remedies are marketed. Equal emphasis should be placed on food allergies because they may have an even more significant effect on developing children. Marks,[70] a pediatric allergist, speculates that a large part of infant and childhood nasal congestion is the result of an allergic reaction to cow's milk. He contends that the infant immune system is incapable of coping with the large foreign proteins of cow's milk; consequently, an allergic response occurs. Diet control has also been proposed by Smith[71] who states that most cases of otitis media are caused by milk allergies. He has also studied hyperkinetic children and reports that both diet and allergies are contributing factors affecting their behavior.

Next, the clinician should observe the patient sitting at rest to determine extraoral mouth breathing characteristics. The most telltale sign is lip incompetence, in which the lips are separated at rest. This often results in hypotonic lip musculature due to the lack of exercise of lip muscles against each other. Children with chronic nasal congestion develop a nasal crease that results from an "allergic salute." This salute is performed by small children who consistently rub the nose in an upward direction due to nasal itching, thereby producing this crease. Chronic rubbing may also cause chronic nasal septum deviation.

The shape of the nose itself is also diagnostic. Mouth breathers tend to have narrow external nares due to the lack of functional development. Without use, there is no need for the development of the nasal cavity. These patients thus appear to have a "shallow" midface in comparison with their other facial structures. A narrow nose is often present as part of congenital premaxillary, dental, or palatal malformations since embryologically the upper incisor teeth and part of the palate, as well as a portion of the nasal septum, arise from the premaxilla area.[71]

Children with long-standing allergies also have "allergic shiners" or darkened areas beneath their eyes. Their eyes also appear watery and tear frequently. This, together with the other facial characteristics, gives these patients a dull, sad facial appearance.

The interior of the anterior portion of the nose can easily be examined with the patient in a reclining position; the inferior portion of the nares becomes exposed. Initially, the nasal septum should bisect the nares and divide them equally. A septum not in the midline is termed deviated and can cause significant nasal obstruction. Visualization of the interior of the anterior portion of the nasal cavity can be achieved either by properly positioning the examination light or by using a penlight. A nasal speculum or a cotton swab can be used to examine the anatomy. Under normal, healthy conditions, the turbinates should appear pink and glistening. With chronic allergic rhitis, the turbinates become pale or bluish and are often edematous.

Definitive clinical examination on the patients mode of respiration can be determinined with simple nasal patency tests as described by Bushey.[72] The first test involves having the patient seal the lips for 1 to 2 minutes; the examiner can then readily assess the ability and ease of nasal breathing. A second approach is to seal the patient's lips and alternately collapse each nostril to evaluate nasal and/or pharyngeal obstruction. Humming while closing alternate nostrils acts to amplify potential obstructions. A third technique involves the use of a cold mirror to observe the relative amount of condensation of the humidified air on each side of the nose. Cotton may also be held under each nostril, and its relative movement can be observed. These tests, although crude and simple, do test the proper functioning of the nasal airway.

CLINICAL RECOGNITIONS OF DYNAMIC OROFACIAL DYSFUNCTION

Individuals of any age should have reasonable facial balance and symmetry. The clinician should assess the facial structures and posture from all possible dimensions. In the craniofacial region this involves frontal, superior, inferior, lateral, and oblique evaluations. Clinical evaluation must be correlated with any radiographs the clinician believes are indicated. In this method, both soft and bony tissues are intregrated during evaluations. The maxillary and mandibular midlines should correlate with the frontal midline of the face. An intraoral evaluation should reveal symmetrically shaped upper and lower dental arches. A broad U-shaped arch form is most desirable. Functional evaluation of the mandible must be completed carefully. This examination should include opening, closing, and mediolateral movements, as well as digital palpation and evaluation of TMJ function, as covered in Chapter 4. The TMJ should exhibit smooth and flowing movements free of joint sounds. The soft tissue of the face, including the submandibular region, should be carefully examined. Careful investigation of causes of any scars on the facial area, especially the chin, are an obvious indicator of previous trauma. Chipped or restored anterior teeth may also indicate trauma; in these instances, the child must be questioned regarding any traumatic incidents.

Regardless of age, the cuspids should meet in a class 1 relationship. This is true in primary, mixed, and permanent dentitions. The patient should not exhibit any crossbite (i.e., the buccal or outside cusps of the upper teeth should be just "outside" the lower teeth throughout the dental arch). Any openbite should be carefully noted. An openbite means teeth do not overlap vertically when the mandible is fully closed. Openbites may occur anteriorly, posteriorly, or both.

PATIENT SCREENING

After a sufficient extraoral and intraoral evaluation has been completed, the clinician must determine whether the patient should be referred to an orthodontic specialist. It is essential to discuss the desires and expectations of treatment with the patient. Establishing both the childs' and parents' chief complaint will be paramount in outlining the corrective procedure indicated for the individual (e.g., it may become obvious that the patient is not interested in corrective measures beyond a certain point). That point or that range of treatment options must be clearly assessed by the clinician.

For the clinician who is not a dentist, a determination of correct dental relationships is challenging. This is particularly true when a growing patient is assessed. These patients have a wide variety of dental situations, ranging from a complete primary or deciduous dentition in children aged 3 to 5 years to a mix of primary and permanent teeth in children aged 6 to 11 years.

In determining individual growth potential, the clinician must remember that an individual has three distinct ages: skeletal, chronologic, and dental.

The skeletal age is an assessment of the velocity and degree of general body development that may be performed by a combination of techniques involving radiographic assessment of the head and wrist, endocrine profile, and presence of secondary sex characteristics in males and females. Chronologic age is a determination of the age since birth. Dental age is assessed by determining the degree to which the roots of the teeth have developed. Thus a patient may be skeletally 12 years of age, chronologically 10 years of age, and dentally 8 years of age. We consider such patients skeletally advanced and dentally delayed in development.

When evaluating a growing patient, the clinician must be suspicious of any unusual facial appearance. Viewing the profile of a child, one would expect to see a mild amount of convexity, with the lower jaw appearing slightly recessive in comparison to the upper jaw, since the lower jaw lags behind the upper jaw in development. As a child matures, proportionally more growth occurs in the lower jaw as it "catches" up with the upper jaw growth to develop a straight profile. The clinician must be familiar with the "average" child's profile to be able to distinguish between normal from abnormal development (Fig. 9-9). An unusually small or short lower jaw will likely be accompanied by excess overjet of the dental structures. Patients with such conditions should be referred to a dental specialist. In addition, a child with a notably straight profile at an early age (less than 10 years of age) may be developing a class III discrepancy. This is reflected by "underjet" of the dentition or anterior crossbite. When suspicious or unsure, the clinician is advised to refer the patient to an orthodontist.

Intraoral examination may reveal several characteristic malformations associated with mouth breathing. Often, gingival hyperplasia or periodontal disease exists owing to the constant drying of the gingival tissues as the patient respirates orally. The dentition may have an anterior openbite. This may be of dental or skeletal origin and can be closely associated with lip incompetence.[73] A narrow maxillary dental arch may develop, with a unilateral or bilateral posterior crossbite. The crossbite may be a consequence of both upper arch narrowing and lower arch widening due to altered tongue position. A high palatal vault is associated with this condition because the dentoalveolar structures have increased in vertical height. Moving posteriorly, the relative enlargement of the palatine tonsils can be evaluated. This is easily accomplished by depressing the tongue. Large tonsils can often meet at the midline and, if infected, are red with white speckles. The larger the tonsils, the greater the potential for anterior tongue displacement.

Although the nasopharynx is three-dimensional, a two-dimensional cephalometric radiograph is helpful in assessing its dimensions. To decrease inaccuracies and to broaden the scope of analysis, it is advantageous to obtain both a frontal and a lateral cephalometric radiograph. The frontal x-ray film gives an objective view of the nasal septum as well as of the width of the nasal cavity and the maxilla. Using the Ricketts' cephalometric analysis, this can be correlated to the patient's facial type to determine if abnormal growth exists. The lateral cephalometric radiograph allows measurement of the amount of adenoidal enlargement relative to the nasopharynx. It also permits visualization of the posterior aspect of the inferior turbinate when hypertrophy of this region exists. This structure is located at the posterosuperior aspect of the hard palate. Enlargement of this structure appears as a "grapelike" structure or, as it has been termed, a "mulberry enlargement." Enlargement of the inferior turbinate, especially when coupled with adenoidal enlargement, can significantly reduce the volume of the nasopharynx. Enlargement of the palatine tonsils can also be observed as a shadow extending beyond the soft palate into the oropharynx. The position of the soft palate and tongue can also be clearly observed. Thompson[74] and McKee[75] reported that the tongue had a stable reproducible position above the maxillary molar crowns and in contact with the soft palate. In patients who are mouth breathers, the tongue can be observed inferior to this position.

The lateral cephalogram may also be used to classify the facial type to determine the effect that nasorespiratory obstruction may have on craniofacial growth. Expected effects such as a steep mandibular plane angle, small mandibular arc, short posterior facial height, long lower anterior facial height and increased maxillary height will be much more prevalent in a weak-muscled, vertically growing, dolichofacial type as opposed to a strong-muscled, horizontally growing, brachyfacial type.

MAXILLARY AND MANDIBULAR DISCREPANCIES

The dental class II discrepancy is highlighted by substantial overjet, in which the upper teeth extend significantly in front of the lower anterior teeth. When this type of malocclusion is discovered, the actual area of discrepancy may not be totally obvious (e.g., the upper teeth may be anterior to their proper position or the lower teeth may be posteriorly related to proper position, or a combination of both factors may exist). The relationship is called a class II dental discrepancy when the teeth are at fault. A complicating factor may be the relationships of the upper and lower jaw structures. If the maxilla is forward and the lower jaw is retruded, a skeletal discrepancy exists. Therefore, it is possible to have a class II discrepancy that may be a combination of the upper jaw forward, the lower jaw back, the upper teeth forward, and the lower teeth back. In class III malocclusion, the same type of disharmonies are possible. The maxilla may be posteriorly related, the mandible anteriorly related, the maxillary dentition retrusive, the mandibular dentition protrusive, or any contribution of these factors. Detailed dentofacial analysis by an orthodontist will reveal the areas and degrees of discrepancies. For the adult patient, a skeletal discrepancy may be substantial enough to warrant surgical repositioning of one or both jaws. For growing patients, discrepancies of the dentofacial structures are similar but usually less severe.

Functional appliances used in dentofacial orthopedics have been widely used in Europe with great success for many years. Their use in the United States was limited to the use of a headgear until the late 1970s when Mc-Namara[76] introduced the functional regulator to this country after observing its success in Europe. The use and misuse of these appliances, which include the Frankel, Bionator, and Herbst (and variations of them) has resulted in a wide variety of both good and bad treatment responses, all of which have been documented in the orthodontic literature. This has led to factionalism within the orthodontic profession.

An in-depth analysis of this controversy is beyond the scope of this chapter.

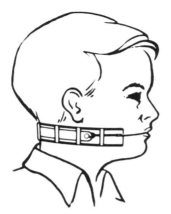

Fig. 9-10. The cervical pull headgear can be manipulated to have its main effect on either the maxilla or the mandible. (Ricketts RM: Biogressive Therapy, Rocky Mountain, 1979.)

The root of the argument is whether these appliances can be used to stimulate deficient mandibular growth toward normal. This question is one that still must be answered and toward which much of the present research is being directed.

In addition, it may be possible to redirect the proportionate facial development of the child and decrease or avoid surgical correction. This brings us to a realm of orthodontics referred to as "dentofacial orthopedics"—an area of some controversy.

Dentofacial orthopedics implies the ability, or at least the intent, to alter the developing skeletal structures. Probably the most proven method of facial orthopedics control involves the use of the headgear (Fig. 9-10). This device uses a stout wire structure attached to the teeth. Attached to the wire is a neck strap or headpiece through which orthopedic pressure is applied through the teeth to the facial bones. The headgear may be used in a variety of methods and in a variety of dentofacial discrepancies. Most commonly, the headgear is used to redirect development of the maxilla to correct a class II problem.

Another method of correction involves the use of functional appliances (Fig. 9-11). These devices usually fit entirely inside the mouth and tend not to have extraoral areas that provide resistance. Functional appliances operate on the principle that the form of the dentofacial structures is substantial as related to the functional aspects of those components (e.g., the mandible may be functioning retrusively).[77,78] Therefore, if the mandible is caused to function in a more forward position, it should grow to that position. This contention is a practical application of the functional matrix theory.

The most recent investigations in the use of these functional devices has revealed an obvious differential in the degree of correction and method of treatment response.

Although functional appliances will correct various dental discrepancies, the basis for correction is unclear.

To attempt clinical modification of dentofacial development, the patient must be diagnosed and treated during active growth of the dental structures. The more severe the discrepancy appears, the earlier the child should be re-

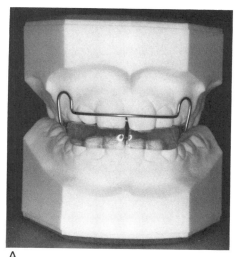

A

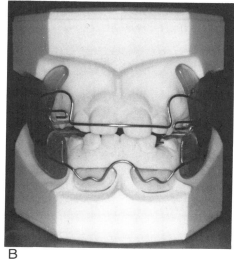

B

Fig. 9-11. The three most commonly used functional appliances used to stimulate mandibular growth. (**A**) Bionator; (**B**) Frankel Functional Regulator (FR-11), (**C**) Herbst appliance.

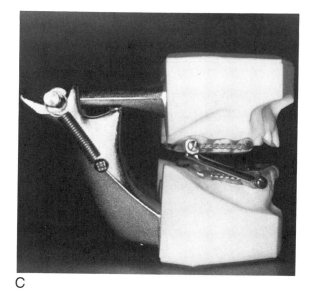

C

ferred to the orthodontist. No longer is it considered appropriate to wait until all permanent teeth have erupted before referring a patient to an orthodontist. The most optional time for correction will probably be lost if the patient is advised to wait. For a developing class II problem, the patient should be referred for consultation as early as 3 or 4 years of age. Although corrective measures may not be started at this age, the orthodontist will have the opportunity to note the severity of the discrepancy and have an accurate basis for evaluating the child's condition during further development; for the class

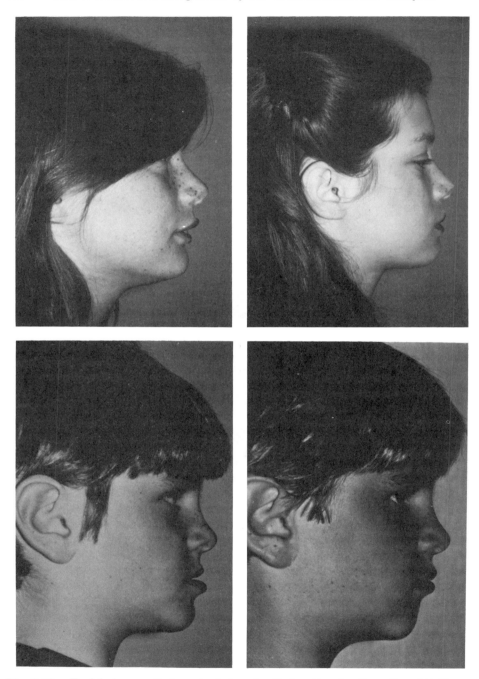

Fig. 9-12. Facial changes that can be induced with functional orthopedics. (A) Functional orthopedics was used in this patient to stimulate horizontal mandibular growth and provide a more pleasing facial profile. (B) Functional orthopedics was used in this patient to stimulate maxillary growth to correct a developing class III malocculsion. The profile produced is considered normal for a 6-year-old.

III patient, the situation is similar. The more severe the discrepancy, the earlier the patient should be referred. Corrective measures for class II malocclusions are usually instituted between the ages of 7 and 9 years. These types of corrections are referred to as "phase I" procedures, and involve establishing ideal skeletal, dental, functional, and facial proportions through dentofacial orthopedics. Most contemporary orthodontists will attempt to avoid removal of permanent teeth. When possible, the removal of permanent teeth is resorted to in only the most severe instances of dental crowding. Extractions of permanent teeth may be avoided if the patient is seen early enough to attempt a phase I correction. This does not mean that the individual will not need to be treated with complete orthodontics after all permanent teeth have erupted. When an early phase of correction is used treatment later is less time-consuming and usually does not involve extractions of permanent teeth. The result is also far more stable because the situation was not allowed to become severe before correction was started. An early phase of treatment may last between 9 and 18 months. Following this phase, a stabilizing device called a retainer is fitted for the patient, who is then monitored for balanced dentofacial development (Fig. 9-12).

The use of functional appliances for nongrowing patients is both controversial and risky. Predictable and stable results *have not* been reported in orthodontic literature.

CONCLUSION

Substantial evidence has been presented in this chapter correlating the effects of upper airway obstruction on head posture and craniofacial growth. We believe that the effects on both growth and development of the craniomandibular region cannot be denied and may strike at the etiologic factors of early craniomandibular and TMJ dysfunction. The absolute cause-and-effect relationships are not simple and will continue to be an area of much speculation and intense research. Further studies correlating head–neck postural changes and craniofacial morphology in the absence of upper respiratory obstruction warrants such investigation.

In evaluating and treating a child, a clinician's main objective is to encourage optimal balance and harmony of the craniomandibular and craniocervical structures. This includes optimal development and function during the most active growing years as well as stable function through proper balance during the adaptive changes of aging.

ACKNOWLEDGMENTS

We have been profoundly influenced by the work and teaching of Dr. Robert Ricketts and Dr. Donald H. Enlow, both of whom are giants in the field of growth and development. We both wish to extend our appreciation to these scientists for the use of many of their illustrations to help clarify this complex subject.

REFERENCES

1. Enlow DH: Handbook of Facial Growth. WB Saunders Philadelphia, 1982
2. Behrents RG: Growth in the Aging Craniofacial Skeleton. Craniofacial Growth Series Monograph 17. Center for Human Growth and Development, The University of Michigan, Ann Arbor, 1986
3. Ricketts R: A study of changes in temporomandibular relations associated with treatment of class II malocclusion. Am J Orthod 38:919, 1952
4. Ricketts RM: The interdependence of the nasal and oral capsules. In McNamara JA (ed): Naso-Respiratory Function and Craniofacial Growth, Craniofacial Growth Series, Monograph No. 9. Center for Human Growth and Development, The University of Michigan, Ann Arbor, 1979
5. Ten Cate AR: Oral Histology. CV Mosby, St. Louis, 1985
6. Ricketts R: Various conditions of the TMJ as revealed by cephalometric laminography. Am J Orthod 36:877, 1950
7. Ricketts R: Planning treatment on the basis of the facial pattern and an estimate of its growth. Angle Orthod 27:14, 37, 1957
8. Ricketts R: A principle of arcial growth of the mandible. Angle Orthod 42:368, 1972
9. Bjork A: Variations in the growth pattern of the human mandible; longitudinal radiographic study by the implant method. J Dent Res 42:400, 1963
10. Moss ML: Functional analysis of human mandibular growth. J Prosthet Dent 10:1149, 1960
11. Moffett BC, Wright DM: Orthodontic research at the University of Washington on postnatal growth history in human temporomandibular joints. Am Assoc Orthod. San Francisco, California 1968.
12. Ricketts R: Mechanisms of mandibular growth: a series of inquiries on the growth of the mandible. In McNamara JA (ed): Determinants of Mandibular Form and Growth. Craniofacial Growth Series, Monograph No. 4. Center for Growth and Development, The University of Michigan, Ann Arbor, 1975
13. Enlow DH: The Human Face. Hoeber Medical Division, Harper & Row, New York, 1968
14. Enlow DH: Rotation of the mandible during growth. In McNamara JA (ed): Determinants of Mandibular Form and Growth. Craniofacial Growth Series Monograph No. 4, Center for Human Growth and Development, The University of Michigan, Ann Arbor, 1975
15. Graber TM: Overbite—the dentist's challenge. JADA 79:1135, 1969
16. Moss M, Rankow R: The role of the functional matrix in mandibular growth. Angle Orthod 38:95, 1968
17. Tomes CS. On the development origin of the V-shaped contracted maxilla. Month Rev Dent Surg 1:2, 1872
18. Profitt WR: Equilibrium theory revisited: factors influencing position of the teeth. Angle Orthod 48:175, 1978
19. Profitt WR: The facial musculature in its relation to the dental discussion. In Carlson DS (ed): Muscle Adaptation in the Craniofacial Region Craniofacial Growth Series, Monograph No. 8. Center for Human Growth and Development, The University of Michigan, Ann Arbor, 1978

20. Frederick S: The effects of buccinator muscle on mandibular and maxillary advancements. Presented at American Association of Orthodontists Convention, Las Vegas, 1985.
21. Catlin G. Breath of Life or Malrespiration and its Effects upon the Enjoyment and Life of Man. John Wiley, New York, 1861
22. Hellman M: A preliminary study as it affects the human face. Dental Cosmos 69:250, 1927
23. Brodie A: On the growth pattern of the human head from the third month to the eighth year of life. Am J Anat 68:209, 1941
24. Subtenly J Daniel: The significance of adenoid tissue. Angle Orthod 20:59, 1954
25. Lanier B, Tremblay N: An approach to the medical management of chronic mouth-breathing. In McNamara JA (ed): NasoRespiratory Function and Craniofacial Growth. Craniofacial Growth Series. Monograph No. 9. The University of Michigan, Ann Arbor, 1979
26. Diamond O: Tonsils and adenoids: why the dilemma? Am J Orthod 5:495, 1980
27. Ricketts R: Respiratory obstruction syndrome. Am J Orthod 54:495, 1968
28. Joseph R: The effect of airway interference on the growth and development of the face, jaws and dentition. Int J Orofac Myol July, 1982
29. Ritter F: Physiology of the nose, paranasal sinuses and middle ear. In Middeton E (ed): Allergy: Principles and Practice. Vol. 1, CV Mosby, St. Louis, 1978
30. Harvold EP, Chierici G, Vargervik K: Experiments on the development of dental malocclusion. Am J Orthod 61:38, 1972
31. Harvold EP, Vargervik K, Chierici G: Primate experiments on oral sensation and dental malocclusion. Am J Orthod 63:494, 1973
32. Harvold EP: Neuromuscular and morphological adaptations in experimentally induced oral respiration. In McNamara JA (ed): Naso-Respiration Function and Craniofacial Growth, Craniofacial Growth Series, Monograph No. 9. Center for Growth and Development, The University of Michigan, Ann Arbor, 1979
32a. Harvold EP, Experiments on Mandibular Morphogenesis. In McNamara JA (ed): Determinents of Mandibular Form and Growth, Craniofacial Growth Series, Monograph No. 4, Center for Human Growth and Development, The University of Michigan, Ann Arbor, 1975.
33. Harvold EP: In search of understanding basic mechanisms of orthodontic treatment. Ann Brit Soc Study Orthod Torquay, 1981
34. Enlow DH: Wolff's Law and the factor of architectonic circumstance. Am J Orthod 54:803,1968.
35. Balyeat R, Bowen R: Facial and dental deformities due to perennial nasal allergy in childhood. Int J Orthod 20:445, 1934
36. Todd TW, Cohen MD, Broadbent B: The role of allergy in the etiology of orthodontics deformity. J Allergy 10:246, 1939
37. Linder-Aronson S, Woodside DG: The growth in the sagittal depth of the bony nasopharynx in relation to some other facial variables. In McNamara JA (ed): Naso-Respiratory Function and Craniofacial Growth, Monograph No. 9. Center for Human Growth and Development, The University of Michigan, Ann Arbor, 1979
38. Subtelny J: Effects of disease of tonsils and adenoids in dentofacial morphology. Ann Otol Rhinol Laryngol, suppl., 19:50, 1975
39. Quinn GW, Pickrell KL: Mandibular hypoplasia and airway interference. N C Dent J 61:19, 1978
40. Ricketts R: Laminography in the diagnosis of temporomandibular joint disorders. J Am Dent Assoc 79:118, 1953

41. Eastman GA: A cephalometric study of tongue posture in individuals with nasal allergies. Master's thesis, University of Michigan, 1963
42. Quinn G: Airway interferences and its effect upon the growth and development of the face, jaws, dentition and associated parts. The portal of life. North Carolina Dental Journal, Winter-Spring, 1978
43. Ricketts R: The Cranial base and soft structures in cleft palate speech and breathing. Plastic Reconstr Surg 14:47, 1954
44. Solow B, Tallgren A: Head and posture and craniofacial morphology. Am J Phys Anthropol 44:417, 1976
45. Opdebeek H, Bell WH, Eisendeld J, Misheleurich D: Comparative study between the SFS and Lds rotation as a possible morphogenetic mechanism. Am J Orthod 74:509, 1978
46. Posnick TB: Craniocervical angulation and morphologic variables in children: a cephalometric study. MSD Thesis, University of North Carolina, Chapel Hill, 1978
47. Koski K, Lahdemaki P: Adaptations of mandible in children with adenoids. Am J Orthod 68:660, 1975
48. Schwartz AM: Kopfhaltung and Kiefer. A Stomatol 24:669, 1826
49. Schwartz AM: Prophylaxe and Fruhehandlung der Bissanomalien. Fortschr Orthod 1:635, 1931
50. Bjork A: Cranial base development. Am J Orthod 41:198, 1955
51. Bjork A: The relationship of the jaws to the cranium. p. 104. In Lundstrom A (ed): Introduction to Orthodontics. McGraw-Hill, London 1960
52. Bjork A: Roentgencephalometric Growth Analysis. p. 237. In: Pruzansky S (ed): Congenital Anomalies of the Face and Associated Structures. Charles C. Thomas, Springfield, Illinois, 1961
53. Solow B, Tallgren A: Dentoalveolar morphology in relation to craniofacial posture. Angle Orthod 47:157, 1977
54. Shelton RL, Haskins RC, Bosma JF: Tongue thrust in one of monozygotic twins. J Speech Hearing Dis 24:105, 1959
55. Mew JRC: A case report of idential twins with marked facial differences that became less after treatment to one of them. Int J Orthod 15:6, 1977
56. Vig PS: Experimental manipulation of head posture. Am J Orthod 77:258, 1980
57. Mew JRC: Facial form, head posture and the protection of pharyngeal space. In McNamara JA (ed): Clinical Alteration of the Growing Face, Craniofacial Growth Series, Monograph No. 14. Center for Human Growth and Development, The University of Michigan, Ann Arbor, 1983
58. Tully WJ. Abnormal Functions of the Mouth in Relation to the Occlusion of the Teeth. In Walthers D (ed): Current Orthodontics, John Wright & Sons, Bristol, England 1966
59. Wright DM, Moffett BC: The postnatal development of the human temporomandibular joint. Am J Anat 141:235, 1974
60. Hinton R: Adaptive response of the articular eminence and mandibular fossa to altered function of the lower jaw: An overview. In Carlson DS (ed): Developmental Aspects of Temporomandibular Joint Disorders. Craniofacial Growth Series, Monograph No. 16, Center for Human Growth and Development, The University of Michigan, Ann Arbor, 1985.
61. Moss M: The functional matrix: functional cranial components. p. 85. In Kraus BS, Reidel R (eds): Vistas in Orthodontics. Lea & Febiger, Philadelphia, 1962
62. Ricketts R: Clinical implications of the temporomandibular joint. Am J Orthod 52:416, 1966

63. Rubin R: Mode of respiration and facial growth. Am J Orthod 78:504, 1980
64. Dibbets J, Vander Weele LT, Boering G: Craniofacial morphology and temporomandibular joint dysfunction in children. In Carlson DS (ed): Development Aspects of Temporomandibular Joint Disorders, Craniofacial Growth Series, Monograph No. 16. Center for Human Growth and Development, The University of Michigan, Ann Arbor, 1985.
65. Dibbets JMH: Juvenile Temporomandibular Joint Dysfunction and Craniofacial Growth: A Statistical Analysis. Stafleu and Tholen, London 1977
66. Bjork A: Prediction of mandibular growth rotation. Am J Orthod 55:585, 1969
67. Linder-Aronson S: Effects of adenoidectomy on dentition and nasopharynx. Am J Orthod 65:1, 1974
68. Ricketts R: Respiratory obstruction and their relation tongue posture. Cleft Palate Bull 8.3, April, 1958
69. Bushey RS: Alternation in certain anatomical relations accompanying the changes from oral to nasal breathing. Master's thesis, University of Illinois, 1965
70. Marks MB: Allergy in relation to orofacial dental deformities in children: a review. J Allergy 36:293, 1965
71. Smith L, Ware L: Embryology Applied Anatomy and Physiology. p. 1015. In Bluestone C (ed): Pediatric Otolaryngology. Vol. II. WB Saunders, 1972
72. Bushey R: Adenoid obstruction of the nasopharynx. In McNamara JA (ed): Naso-Respiratory Function and Craniofacial Growth, Craniofacial Growth Series, Monograph No. 9. Center for Human Growth and Development, The University of Michigan, Ann Arbor, 1979
73. Linder-Aronson S: Adenoids: their effect on mode of breathing and nasal airflow and their relationship to characteristics of the facial skeleton and the dentition. Acta Otolaryngol 265:Suppl. 3, 1970
74. Thompson JR: A cephalometric study of movements of the mandible. J Am Dent Assoc 29:925, 1942
75. McKee TL: A cephalometric radiographic study of tongue position in individuals with cleft palate deformity. Angle Orthod 26:99, 1956
76. McNamara JA: Functional determinants of Craniofacial size and shape. In Carlson DS (ed): Craniofacial Biology, Craniofacial Growth Series, Monograph No. 10, Center for Human Growth and Development, The University of Michigan, Ann Arbor, 1981
77. Frankel R, Frankel C: A functional approach to treatment of skeletal open bite. AJO 84:54, 1983
78. Frankel R: Biomechanical aspects of the form/function relationship in craniofacial morphogenesis: a clinical approach. In McNamara JA (ed): Clinical Alteration of the Growing Face, Craniofacial Growth Series Monograph No. 14. Center for Human Growth and Development, The University of Michigan. Ann Arbor, 1983

10 | Postural Applications in the Child and Adult

Neurodevelopment Aspects

Barbara Connolly

A person's postural behavior is the result of the interactions of primitive reflexes, postural reactions, body alignment and underlying muscle tone. Primitive reflexes and postural reactions, by interacting together, provide a basis for normal voluntary movement and development of motor skills. In addition, proper alignment of body parts and normal postural tone allows smooth and coordinated movement. Normal postural tone may be defined as the muscle tone that is sufficient to support posture while allowing movement in and from the posture.[1]

The process by which infants develop an upright posture can be described as an "upward spiral."[2] The primitive postures and movements of the newborn are modified and integrated into complex posture and movement strategies. In addition, spontaneous actions, primitive postures, and movement strategies of the newborn are adapted into purposeful behaviors through the integration and modification process.

Four major components of this developmental process are the infant's ability to assimilate, accommodate, associate, and differentiate.[2] Assimilation is defined as the sensory process of receiving information external to and within the infant. Accommodation is the response or motor process by which the infant adjusts the body to react to the incoming stimuli. The process of relating sensory information with the motor act being experienced and the calling up of past experiences is defined as association. Finally, differentiation may be described as the discrimination of individual elements of a specific behavior and acting on this information in performing a new behavior. All these components of the process must be functional in the person if normal development is to occur.

In the developmental continuum, new skills are believed to be modifications of past reactions. An infant who is provided with a new experience by the environment is believed to adapt to the environment with an acquired behavior. The central nervous system (CNS) then integrates the sensory feedback from the new experience and develops the required behavior. The integration of the old and new behaviors thus provides the basis for the new modification.

The development of movement also progresses from patterns of mass involuntary movement to controlled voluntary movement. These movements occur in a cephalocaudal and proximal–distal direction and in a gross–fine sequence. The following review illustrates the pattern of movement that occurs in the developing infant.

DEVELOPMENT OF AN UPRIGHT POSTURE

At birth, the newborn is influenced by neonatal reflexes that produce stereotyped and predictable movements. In prone position, the general posture is flexion. The child's face or cheek usually rests on the supporting surface, although occasional erect bobbing of the head occurs. The upper extremities are flexed and held closely to the body. The lower extremities are also flexed, with the hips held high and not resting on the surface. Some kicking postures may occur in the legs, as may other random movements. In supine position, the infant demonstrates a similar flexed symmetrical posture (Fig. 10-1). The head is turned to the side at an angle of approximately 45°. The upper extremities are flexed and adducted, although the hands are loosely fisted. In the lower extremities, flexion, abduction, and external rotation occurs. Movements that occur in this position include head rotation and random extremity movement. In prone and supine positions, the newborn's posture responds automatically to changes in head and body movement through the influence of primitive reflexes. The asymmetrical tonic neck reflex (ATNR) may occur as the infant's head is turned (Fig. 10-2). An increase in extensor tone may occur in the arm and leg on the chin side, and an increase in flexor tone may occur in the arm and leg on the occipital side of the head owing to the ATNR influence. The Moro reflex responses of arm abduction and extension followed by arm adduction and flexion should occur when the infant's head is dropped backward. Neck righting reflexes may also be seen. As the infant bobs the head erect in prone position, a involuntary turning of the head may cause the infant to "flip" over either to a side-lying or supine position owing to this primitive reflex.

When the newborn is pulled to sit, no antigravity flexor control is evident

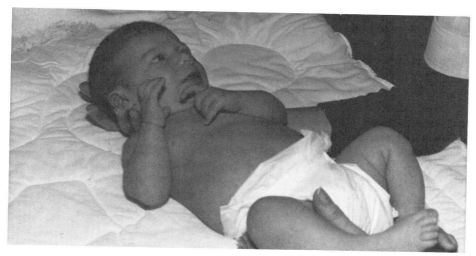

Fig. 10-1.   Flexed, symmetrical posture in supine position.

(Fig. 10-3). Once sitting is attained, the infant's head flops forward, and minimal attempts may be made to lift the head. The infant's back is completely rounded while sitting. When a newborn is held in an upright position, the posture is generally one of flexion. The neck is flexed so that the chin is near the infant's chest and the upper extremities are flexed at the elbows and adducted toward midline. When the feet touch the floor, however, the infant bears weight on the lower extremities due to the presence of primary standing, and small step-

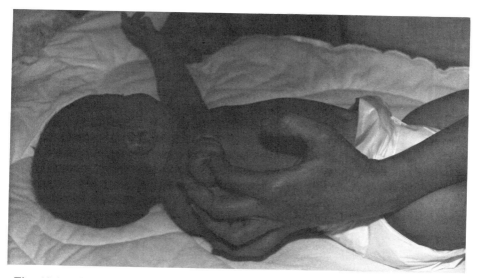

Fig. 10-2.   Asymmetrical posture noted when head is turned and infant is supine.

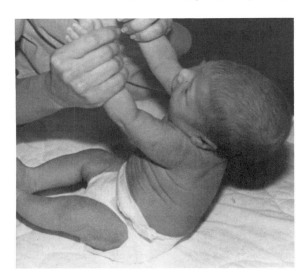

Fig. 10-3. Head lag in newborn when pulled to sit.

ping reactions may be noted if the infant is tilted forward. In this automatic walking, the infant will have little space between the feet and crossing of the legs may occur.

This early phase of development begins at birth and lasts until several months after birth. During this period, the infant engages primarily in bilateral or reciprocal flexion and extension of the limbs, with some rotation in the neck region. By the end of this phase, however, the infant has moved from a semiflexed to a fully extended posture. During this time, some of the primitive reflexes that influence the child provide protective roles, whereas others fulfill survival roles. Other primitive reflexes aid in the distribution of muscle tone in specific postural patterns, as in the case of the ATNR.

The second general phase of development is a transitional period, during which the infant develops strategies to move the body in and around in space.[2] The period begins a few months after birth when the infant begins to develop weightbearing activities such as pushing up on the elbows in prone position. The strategies used in this period develop by means of chain reactions that include vertical righting reactions (labyrinthine head righting, body on head and optical righting), rotational righting reactions (neck righting and body on body), support reactions (positive supporting) and protective reactions. Holt[3] reports that Peiper describes chain reactions as:

> The initial chain reflex . . . and . . . all the ensuing reflexes and the postures dependent upon them follow strict laws; these bring the child through reflexes of which he is not conscious into the exact position under the given conditions to maintain the equilibrium which would otherwise by lost.

The vertical righting reactions that are present during this stage help develop a vertical chain of movement that begins in the neck extensors and proceeds to the trunk and hips.

The last general phase of early motor development occurs at approximately 6 to 7 months of age when the baby is able to maintain postures independently. Midline stability reactions are adapted from the early vertical reactions, and rotational righting reactions occur. The equilibrium reactions develop to help the infant regain midline stability when alignment of midline is disturbed. This regaining of midline stability is achieved through a series of movement–countermovement postural sets that are inherent in adequate equilibrium reactions. Equilibrium reactions should entail rotation of the head and upper trunk to midline, with the lower trunk segments counterrotating. The extremities on one side should extend and adduct while the opposite extremities should extend and abduct in response to the need to protect and support the body if balance is lost.

Development may also be described as movement progressions such as prone progression, sitting progression, and erect locomotion.[4] In the prone progression as described by McGraw, the infant progresses from the flexed posture of the newborn to initial spinal extension when the head is momentarily lifted. Advanced spinal extension occurs when the extension spreads beyond the cervical area to the muscles of the lumbar area. Sustained head lifting occurs, with the baby supporting on either the forearms or palms while in prone position. During this head lifting, the crest of the ilia rests on the supporting surface and the legs are relatively quiet. In the prone on forearms and prone on hands positions, vertical righting reactions activate extensors of the neck and develop their movement against gravity. The midline extensors of the neck are primarily used until the infant begins to turn the head when the ATNR influence occurs with a change in the distribution of tone in the arms. The Landau reactions may be used during the time the infant is in prone position to expand axial extension further to the pelvis and the lower extremities. Propulsion forward first by use of the arms and then by the legs follows the period of time when the child primarily bears weight on the forearms or hands in prone position. The last stage of the prone progression involves assumption of the hands and knees position, deliberate but unorganized progression, and finally organized progression.

Sitting is a vertical antigravity posture that the child develops in the progression to standing. In the newborn, the pull to sit maneuver elicits a full head lag and, once the infant is in a sitting position, positioning of the chin on the chest occurs. Soon after the newborn period, however, alignment of the head and trunk may occur momentarily in supported sitting as the infant tries to use axial extension. At about 3 months of age, initial head lag may occur, but alignment of the head may occur near the end of the range. The initial head lag may be indicative of the tonic labyrinthine righting reaction or a lack of controlled neck flexion against gravity. Voluntary flexion occurs in the neck as the child is pulled to sitting at approximately 5 months of age. During this time, flexion in the trunk is also noted as the child is pulled to sitting. While the infant plays in a supine position, hand to feet as well as feet to mouth

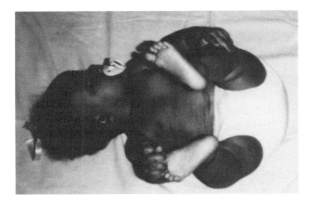

Fig. 10-4.   Feet to mouth behavior of infants.

behaviors also occur (Fig. 10-4). These activities help the infant develop antigravity flexor strength in various postural situations. By 5 to 6 months, supported sitting should occurs with the child sitting with support on the extended arms placed in front of the child. During this sitting, the baby has weight on the fisted hands with primarily head and upper trunk extension.

Full progression to sitting occurs when the child rolls from supine to prone

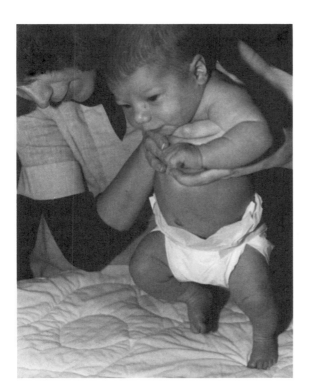

Fig. 10-5.   Automatic walking of newborns.

position and then rotates up into a side sitting position. This final stage in the sitting progression usually occurs by 9 months of age. In the independent sitting position, the infant may bring the arms up and use remnants of the pivot prone posture to get more extension in the back. Midline stability and equilibrium reactions provide background stability for the infant and allow reaching out with the hands while in this position.

The achievement of erect locomotion occurs in five distinctive phases.[4] The newborn, when placed in a standing position, is generally flexed until the feet are allowed to touch the surface, when automatic walking may occur (Fig. 10-5). During this newborn period, the infant adapts fetal axial extension through foot contact on the surface to elicit a primitive upright posture. During the inhibition or static phase of stance, the infant attempts to hold the head more in line with the body plane when supported in an upright position and may even be able to extend the neck. Reflex stepping is suppressed or inhibited during this phase, and the infant may drag the feet when moved forward instead of attempting to step. In the third or transition phase, the infant will bear weight and attempt to bounce up and down while supported. The infant may also stand in one position and stamp a foot up and down. The final two phases of erect locomotion involve deliberate stepping by the infant and independent walking.

SECONDARY CHANGES DUE TO DEVELOPMENT OF UPRIGHT POSTURE

Oral and Pharyngeal Mechanisms

With the development of an upright posture in the child, secondary changes also occur in oral and pharyngeal mechanisms. The changes in these mechanisms are determined by growth of the infant and also by the position of the infant. The assumption of an upright position is particularly important in determining the relationship of certain oral and pharyngeal relationships.

Structure

The structures of the nose, mouth, larynx, and pharynx provide pathways for the infant's interactions with the external environment of air and food. This area in the newborn infant undergoes continuous growth prenatally and continues to grow postnatally.

Anatomically, the nose of the infant differs from the adult in proportion and in much of its skeletal and mucosal structure. The nasal bones and narial cartilages are fully formed in the infant but are small. The nasal mucosa and submucosa are thick and vascular. During infancy, the nasal chambers enlarge in both vertical and transverse diameter, and by the sixth month of postnatal life the posterior choanae have doubled in size. During childhood, the greatest growth in the nasal area is in a vertical direction, with most of the growth resulting from downward displacement of the bony palate.

In the infant, the mesopharyngeal and hypopharyngeal walls are well muscled and relatively thick. The mouth, like the nose, is relatively short when compared with that of an adult. The epiglottis approximates the uvula and is at the level of the first cervical vertebrae. The larynx of the infant differs from the adult in its position, the form of its major cartilages, and its submucosa. In the newborn, the hyoid and larynx are approximated, the thyroid and cricoid cartilages are vertically small, and the laryngeal submucosa are thick and firm.

During the first year of life, major changes occur in the peripheral structures of the oral and pharyngeal mechanisms due to the growth of the child and possibly in response to the achievement of upright posture.[5] The pharynx elongates in relation to the cervical vertebrae due to the vertical growth of the bodies of the cervical vertebrae and a general descent of the skeletal landmarks of the pharynx. The upper pharynx enlarges and is associated with a downward and forward displacement of the pharyngeal palate.[5] The oral cavity enlarges around the tongue due to the growth of the maxilla and mandible and to eruption of teeth. The tongue itself is displaced downward by the descent of the hyoid. The result of this movement is the availability of space for more motion of the tongue. This change also allows release of the general and sustained apposition of the tongue to the oral palate.

Function

The oral and pharyngeal mechanisms have three functions: positional, respiratory, and feeding. Positional function of the pharyngeal airway is crucial to the survival of the newborn infant. If the newborn infant is placed supine and is breathing through the nose, the pharynx is patent from the posterior nasal choanae to the laryngeal aditus. The laryngeal vestibule is open to the cords. The airway for the infant is directly achieved by the hyoid, tongue, and mandibular musculature and indirectly by the musculature that achieves positioning of the head and neck. In the term infant, the pharyngeal area has greater positional mobility because the TMJ has no temporal fossa and is extremely mobile in the horizontal plane. Therefore, the primary mechanism for stabilization in this area is skeletal muscle. The mandible is stabilized by the masseter, temporalis, and the medial and lateral pterygoid muscles. The hyoid is stabilized through the activity of submental muscles, and stylohoid, posterior digastric, and pretracheal muscles.

This relationship of craniocervical posture and airway adequacy is illustrated by a study of children without neuromotor disorders but with malocclusion problems that was done by Solow et al in 1984. Head posture correlated to malocclusion problems such as small linear mandibular dimensions, mandibular retrognathism, and a large inclination of the mandible in relation to the anterior cranial base.[6] In these children, the radiographically determined measure of the free airway between the maxilla and the adenoid tissue showed correlations that indicated a strong relationship between airway adequacy and craniocervical angulation. Perhaps a growth-coordinating mechanism exists that is responsible for the determination of the necessary balance between flexors and extensors in the child, resulting in adequate craniocervical posture in the child.

Pharyngeal airway function occurs not only by the patency of the pharynx and laryngeal vestibule but also by stable closure at the pharyngoesophageal area and at the junction of the pharynx and the mouth (Fig. 10-6). The closure at the junction of the pharynx and the mouth along with the downward and forward displacement of the palate results in nasal portal respiration. This closure also prevents unwanted penetration of oral contents into the pharyngeal airway during feeding.

The postural arrangements of the upright human evolve from the structural and spatial arrangement of the cranium with the cervical vertebrae, and from the relationship of the mandible with the cranium and the hyoid, tongue, and, larynx, with the hyoid and cranium as determined through the anatomic as well as functional development in the young child.[5] Any alterations in the development of the child in the oral and pharyngeal area can affect the functioning of the oral cavity in the adult (e.g., although there are no clear-cut explanations of how growth and development are modified by variations in airflow in humans, children who are mouthbreathers tend to have variations in the normal craniocervical posture).[7] Solow and Tallgren[8] as well as Thompson and Vig[9] found correlations between cranial extension–flexion and the vertical development of the facial skeleton and dentoaveolar structure in studies of children and adults.

In the infant, the pharynx and the intrinsic larynx function as an upper respiratory chamber and enlarge in tidal inspiration and constrict in expiration. If any respiratory distress occurs, the infant's tongue and hyoid come into play and move forward with inspiration and return with expiration. As the child matures, however, the pharynx and tongue decrease in their movements during unphonated respirations.

Nose breathing is present in the newborn probably due to less nasal respiratory resistance in the infant as compared with adults. Oral tidal respiration occurs within the first 3 to 5 months of postnatal life. The oral positioning of the tidal inspiration and expiration is a developmental achievement that occurs due to the positioning of the area of the pharyngeal palate, the superior constrictor, and the pharyngeal portions of the tongue. It is accomplished as a part of the overall maturation of the oral structures.

Feeding is a major and critical function of the pharyngeal and oral area. The order of developmental achievements in feeding include pharyngeal swallow, oral sucking, labial prehension and closure, and mature sucking. At birth, the pharynx is mature for swallowing activities, although few sucking movements may initially be apparent. In the swallowing action, the palate is drawn upward and backward as the pharynx wall is drawn forward to appose the palate. The body of the tongue moves posteriorly and upward to appose the soft palate and adjacent hard palate. As the lower portion of the pharynx, hyoid,

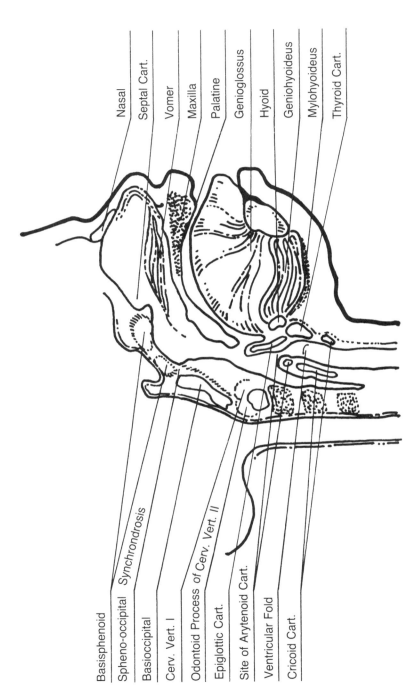

Basisphenoid

Spheno-occipital Synchrondrosis

Basioccipital

Cerv. Vert. I

Odontoid Process of Cerv. Vert. II

Epiglottic Cart.

Site of Arytenoid Cart.

Ventricular Fold

Cricoid Cart.

Nasal

Septal Cart.

Vomer

Maxilla

Palatine

Genioglossus

Hyoid

Geniohyoideus

Mylohyoideus

Thyroid Cart.

Fig. 10-6. Paramedian section of the pharangeal, oral, and nasal area.

and larynx are drawn upward, the bolus is moved to the esophagus and is transported from the oral cavity.[5] In the newborn infant, this pharyngeal swallow should be well coordinated with little or no distress apparent in the infant.

RESPIRATORY CHANGES

Changes in the respiratory patterns of children as they progress from the prone or supine to the upright position occur due to maturational changes as well as postural changes. Anatomic differences in the respiratory system of children as compared with that of adults include smaller airway size and smaller lumen size. In addition, because of the lack of smooth muscle development, which occurs by 3 to 4 years of age, infants and young children have weakness of the bronchioles. This weakness may contribute to airway collapse and air trapping. Studies have also shown that peripheral airway conductance, or the ease with which air flows through an airway, increases substantially at about 5 years of age.[10] Infants' chests are rounded, not oval, and have ribs that are more horizontal than those of adults. Sternal retraction may be noted in infants because the sternal cartilage is poorly developed and less supportive. Due to these differences between infants and adults, belly breathing is demonstrated by young infants. By 2 years of age, however, children should begin lifting the upper chest during inhalation owing to the contraction of the diaphragm, followed by lateral costal expansion which causes the upper chest to rise.[11] Continued belly breathing in children may indicate that the muscles of the upper chest and neck are not able to fix the rib cage against the pressure created by diaphragm movement.

Positions other than the upright posture have marked effects on the functioning of various respiratory apparatus due to the influence of gravity. In the upright position, gravity acts in an expiratory direction on the rib cage and in an inspiratory direction on the abdomen. In the supine position, however, gravity has an expiratory effect on both the rib cage and abdomen. In the supine position, as compared with the upright position, there is less gravitational effect on changes in lung volume because the height of the abdomen is less. In supine, position, the diaphragm is displaced into the rib cage and, as a consequence of this movement, the resting expiratory level of the pump changes from its upright value of approximately 35 percent of the vital capacity to a value of approximately 20 percent.[12] Therefore, less positive muscle pressure is needed for inspiration and expiration in the supine than in the upright position.

The most efficient muscular pattern for inspiration is through the use of the diaphragm, with the assistance of the external intercostals. If breathing becomes difficult owing to a disease process or a musculoskeletal problem, however, the accessory muscles of inspiration may be brought into play to augment ventilation.[11] When this occurs, the person is apt to use mouth breathing, which may lead to malpositioning of the jaw and other oral structures.

POSTURAL ASSESSMENT IN CHILDREN

One should begin postural assessment of children by obtaining a developmental history of the child. The times when the child first lifted the head in prone position, first sat independently, first crept on hands and knees, and first walked are important factors in determining if the child has developmental delays. If delays exist, the child may inhibit problems (although perhaps subtle, with postural alignment. Adult postural alignment should be evident in children by 10 to 11 years of age; if this alignment is not apparent, more in-depth questioning of the developmental history of the child should be undertaken.

The assessment of posture in very young children begins with evaluation of the head position. Although problems with development of normal movement are believed to occur most often in children with neuromotor disorders, similar compensations may occur in other children. Abnormal neck hyperextension may be evident in children when head/neck flexion components do not develop. Hyperextension of the neck is normal in children between 1 to 3 months of age but should be counterbalanced with the development of neck flexors by 3 months. This abnormal degree of neck hyperextension can lead to a blocking of normal mobility of the scapula because the child elevates the shoulders to help stabilize the head. In addition, when the child is sitting with neck hyperextension, the lack of "chin tuck," or contraction of the neck musculature, leads to opening of the mouth with a forward jutting of the jaw.[13] Hyperextension of the neck may also lead to craniofacial morphologic changes such as mandibular retrognathism.[6]

The child who has a forward head may have problems similar to the child who has neck hyperextension. Again, the primary problem is one of lack of chin tuck, with a resultant elongation of the neck extensors. Such a child initially experiences problems with a forward thrusting of the jaw but may develop chronic problems such as mandibular retrognathism.

Head and neck asymmetry problems may be observed in the child in prone, supine, sitting, or standing positions. For the child with this problem, bilateral symmetrical head and neck flexor action has not developed and the child is unable to hold the head in midline.[13] For these children, the ATNR may be present, although it should have been integrated by 4 to 6 months of age except under times of extreme stress. If the head remains constantly turned to one side, the spine may also rotate, setting the stage for the development of scoliosis. The continued presence of the ATNR may also cause deviation of the mandible.[14]

Problems with movement of the shoulders occur often if the child is experiencing abnormal positioning of the head and neck. Patterns of abnormal movement may include exaggerated shoulder elevation and increased scapular adduction.[13] In the child with abnormal shoulder elevation, the arms do not move forward because of poor development of the shoulder flexors. Tightness of the muscles between the scapula and humerus is present. The upper extremities are kept in an internally rotated position. With the abnormal shoulder elevation, increased scapular adduction may also be used to reinforce axial extension and stability. For a child with these problems, increased work to maintain adequate ventilation may be evident since the shoulder girdle lacks full range of motion (ROM).[11]

Postural alignment problems occur at the hips when excessive anterior or posterior pelvis tilting exists. An increased anterior pelvic tilt is apparent in the normal 4-month-old child but is soon balanced by the development of the abdominals and hip extensors. For a child of any age who continues to experience an increased anterior pelvic tilt, the lower extremities are abducted, flexed, and externally rotated when the child is in prone, supine, sitting, and standing positions. An increased lumbar lordosis exists, and the abdomen tends to protrude. Poor hip mobility is a common finding. A child with an increased posterior tilt to the pelvis has the basic problem of too much extension in the lower trunk and hips. The extensor muscles are too tight and are not elongated. A co-contraction of the abdominals and hips extensors does not develop. This lack of co-contraction is particularly apparent while the child attempts sitting. As compensation in sitting, the child either sits on the base of the spine rather than on the buttocks or sits in a reverse tailor position.

Postural assessment of the child in standing may reveal any problems with posture that have been described in the preceding paragraphs. Even in the young child of 18 months, the head should be over the sacrum, although there may be a slight forward positioning. In the 18-month-old child, the hips may be slightly flexed, producing an increased lumbar lordosis as compared with adult postures.[15] The young child characteristically has a protruding abdomen due to the position of the pelvis. A wide base of support typically exists. The scapula may be prominent in the young child as the child attempts to use adduction of the scapula to increase axial extension. In the normally developing child, however, relaxation of the shoulder adductors should occur at times as normal extension develops.

In the child of approximately 7 to 8 years of age, more of the adult posturing should be apparent. More lordosis will be evident than that in adults, however, and the head may continue to be slightly forward. Poor posture includes a forward head, kyphosis, depressed chest, lordosis, prominence of the scapulae, or hyperextended knees.[15]

By age 10 to 11 years, the child should have a posture that resembles adult posture. The ideal body alignment when the child is facing forward should be as follows:[16]

Head erect—not turned or tilted to side
Level shoulders
Hips level with equal weight on both legs
Patella facing straight forward

The posterior view of the child should reveal the following:[16]

Head erect
Straight cervical, thoracic, and lumbar spines

Level shoulders
Neutral positioning of the scapulae with the medial borders parallel
Hips level with equal weight on both legs
Legs and heelcords straight

The normal posture of the child as viewed from the side should include:[16]

Head erect with the chin above the notch between the clavicle with a slight forward curve in the neck
Shoulders in line with the ears
Upper back erect
Abdominal wall flat
Slight lordosis in the low back
Pelvis in a neutral position (not anteriorly or posteriorly tilted)
Knees slightly flexed
Feet pointed straight ahead or slightly toeing out

POSTURAL SCREENING

Several screening tools are commercially available for postural assessment; however, screening can be done using self-developed formats.[17] Each child should be assessed with the shirt removed and the pants loosened. Ideally, the child should be standing during the assessment. Each child's evaluation should include assessment of the symmetry of iliac crests, shoulder elevation, shoulder girdle position, waist creases, and arm-to-body spaces (Figs. 10-7 and 10-8). Leg lengths should also be assessed. Alignment of the head over the gluteal cleft is an important assessment for problems of a forward head, hyperextension of the neck, and curvature of the spine. Forward bending should be observed in each child for the existence of thoracic or lumbar prominences that might indicate scoliosis. The assessment of the ATNR in the quadruped reflex-inhibiting posture should also be performed, since children with scoliosis have a positive ATNR in this position.[18]

Children who have neuromotor problems or overall developmental delays may experience many postural deficits. A child with hypertonicity has delayed integration of primitive reflexes such as the tonic labyrinthine or ATNR, which may cause asymmetrical posturing of the head, trunk, and extremities. In addition, the decreased thoracic mobility evident in children with severe spasticity may limit inspiration and expiration, causing the child to use accessory respiratory musculature, which leads to more problems with posturing of the head into a forward position. The continuation of primitive oral feeding patterns in some children with hypertonicity (hyperactive gag reflex, tongue thrusting, tonic bite reflex, and sucking reflex) may lead to malalignment of the oral structures as well.

In children with hypotonicity or low muscle tone, delayed integration of primitive reflexes may be evident. As in the case of the child with spasticity

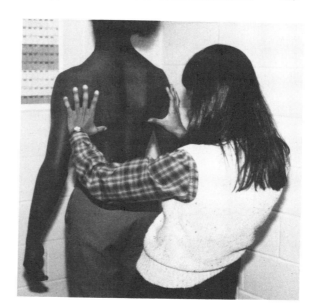

Fig. 10-7. Postural alignment screening for level scapula.

and delayed integration of reflexes, the child with hypotonicity may have problems with overall postural alignment and particularly with asymmetries or limitations of movements. Shallow breathing may occur owing to the poor expansion of the rib cage caused by weakness of the diaphragm and use of the respiratory muscles during inspiration and expiration. Feeding problems in

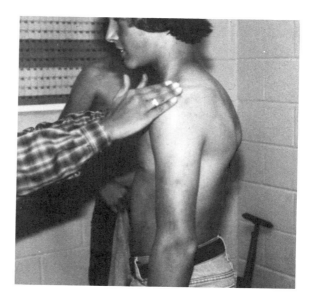

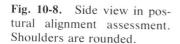

Fig. 10-8. Side view in postural alignment assessment. Shoulders are rounded.

children with poor muscle tone in the oral area include hypoactive gag reflex, open mouth, protruding tongue, and incoordination with swallowing.

Scoliosis, one of the leading causes of postural problems in children, may be caused a variety of mechanisms. Structural scoliosis is a combination of lateral deviation or bending, rotation, and anatomic changes of the spinal vertebrae. Scoliosis is usually progressive, but becomes more stable at the termination of the child's growth. The more severe curves, however, may progress after maturity through degenerative joint changes.[19] Categories commonly used to describe the etiology of scoliosis are as follows:[19]

1. Osteopathic—scoliosis as the result of an abnormality in the body parts of the spine caused by disease, trauma, or congenital malformation.
2. Myopathic—scoliosis caused by a disease in the muscles themselves.
3. Neuropathic—scoliosis caused by a muscle imbalance secondary to a neurological lesion such as polio or cerebral palsy.
4. Idiopathic—scoliosis resulting from no demonstrable cause.

Children who have undergone radiation should be watched closely for the development of scoliosis or kyphosis due to possible destruction of growth centers due to the radiation. In addition, children who have had open heart surgery, thoracoplasty, pneumonectomy, or rib resections may be at risk for development of spinal deformities.[19]

Children with scoliosis may eventually have chest deformities that compromise lung function by restricting the space in which the lung functions. Respiratory dysfunction owing to the scoliosis may lead to compensations in the patterns of breathing and thus to abnormal craniocervical posturing. Children with scoliosis need to be closely observed for asymmetries that may occur due to the scoliosis or the compensatory patterns of movement and of breathing that can adversely affect position of the head and neck. Any deviations noted by the therapist from the normal postural alignment previously described should be recorded.

POSTURAL TREATMENT

The blocks to movement that were described earlier in this chapter commonly occur in children with neuromotor or developmental problems owing to genetic or environmental factors. These postural problems noted at the head, shoulders, and pelvis may also occur in the normally developing child, and the treatment of the postural deficit is similar to that of the child with neuromotor dysfunctions. The neurodevelopmental treatment (NDT) approach aims at facilitating normal movement and normal postural reactions in the child while inhibiting abnormal movement and primitive reflex patterns. In addition, the NDT approach emphasizes normalization of muscle tone as much as possible through stimulation activities. For the child with neck hyperextension or a forward head, the NDT approach elongates the neck extensors while activating the neck flexors.[13] Tucking of the chin during developmental activities is stressed. The "forward jaw" or retrognathic jaw position that occurs in these head postures is modified by obtaining better active head control, especially through the chin tucking.

During feeding, the child's head should be slightly flexed and brought forward. Sucking activities are enhanced and the intraoral negative pressure is increased if the child's head is forward slightly. Stroking of the cheeks by the therapist's fingers additionally enhances slight forward positioning of the child's head. Swallowing is extremely difficult if the head is tilted backward owing to the relationship of the pharyngealesophageal area when the head is hyperextended. Tilting the head backward can cause food to be aspirated into the lungs. Chin tucking during both sucking and swallowing ensures an open pathway for the ingestion of both fluids and solids.[20] During feeding, the trunk should be approximately vertical to minimize the effort of stabilizing musculature, to facilitate breathing, and to provide adequate stability. No hyperextension of the trunk or lateral deviation of the spine should be allowed in the sitting posture.

In the child with head and neck asymmetry, the aim of treatment is to increase head, neck, and spine mobility through attainment of midline orientation of the head. All developmental activities are done with the child's head in midline. Initially, the therapist should assist the child in maintaining the midline posture, either through manual control or adaptive equipment. The child, however, is expected to assume control of the position independently as soon as possible.

In feeding, the head should be held in midline to prevent forward thrusting of the jaw and tongue due to primitive reflexes such as the ATNR. Jaw control by the therapist using increased tactile and proprioceptive input may be necessary to maintain the head in a midline position during feeding if the child is unable to hold the midline position independently.[20] With jaw control, the child will tend to use the upper lip and keep the tongue inside the mouth, thus facilitating a better sucking and swallowing pattern.

If the child experiences abnormal shoulder elevation, scapular adduction, or scapular abduction, activities should be aimed at lowering the shoulder level and obtaining neutral positioning of the scapulae. Activities such as elongating the neck extensors followed by active flexing of the shoulders lead to lowering of the shoulder girdle. Active reaching by the child while the therapist stabilizes the scapula either manually or by adaptive equipment may assist the child in normalizing scapular mobility.

In feeding, the shoulders and arms should be brought slightly forward and downward to prevent hyperextension of the head and trunk. The forward positioning of the scapulae also allows the arms to move freely as needed during self-feeding.

If the child has blocking of movement at the hips, either by excessive anterior pelvic tilting or posterior pelvic tilting, the NDT approach emphasizes treatment of the underlying muscle weakness or tightness that has produced the malposition. In the child with too much anterior tilting, the problem of poor abdominal development is treated. The abdominal musculature is stimulated to increase strength and control. In the child with too much posterior pelvic tilting, the basic problem is that the extensor muscles of the back are too tight and are not elongated. Activities for elongating the back musculature, such as total flexion postures, are used to attain a neutral pelvis.

In feeding, the position of the pelvis may be the key to overall positioning of the child. The pelvis should be in a neutral position so that the child has a stable trunk with no hyperextension, hyperflexion, or lateral deviation. In the sitting position, the hips and knees should ideally be flexed to 90°, thus preventing the abnormal extension pattern caused by excessive posterior tilting. The ankles should be flexed to 90° and the feet should be supported on a flat surface. Once the feet are stabilized, the child should have better stability at the hips as well.

Specific activities that are suggested for improvement of oral control in children with problems with tongue control, jaw control, and sucking and swallowing difficulties are described in detail in various texts.[21,22] Assessment of the child's reflex development, postural tone, and postural alignment should be done prior to attempting any of the suggested activities. In treatment of the oral mechanism, the entire child must be considered owing to the interrelationships of total body position and tone with oral functioning.

Other approaches to postural treatment of children address the problems of malalignment from an alignment, muscle length, and muscle strength view point rather than the reflex-movement-pattern viewpoint of NDT. The intent of the activities suggested by these approaches are markedly similar, however, to the intent of NDT. In faulty head and shoulder positions, the cervical spine extensors are stretched if they are short. These activities are important in treating the child with a forward head position that has not occurred as a result of a neurological problem. The cervical spine flexors are strengthened if they are weak. The thoracic spine extensors are strengthened if rounding of the shoulders exists.[15] If a lordotic posture exists, stretching of the low back muscles is indicated if these are tight and strengthening of the abdominal musculature is performed by pelvic tilt exercises or by trunk curls.[15] If an excessive posterior tilt to the pelvis exists, activities for tilting of the pelvis forward are recommended. Prone hyperextension is avoided since it may increase posterior pelvic tilting.

In scoliotic deformities, postural exercises are aimed at elongating the spine by decreasing the lumbar and cervical lordosis that occurs.[23] Activities for stretching tight lateral trunk musculature and for strengthening the opposite weak lateral trunk musculature are recommended. Activities to decrease any asymmetry are to be included in the therapeutic program. If the scoliosis is functional and not structural (e.g., no bony abnormalities), faulty habits that tend to increase the lateral curve should be corrected.

Orthotic devices may be used in controlling postural deficits in some children. In children with neurological impairments, a cervical spine orthosis may be used if the child has (1) poor anteroposterior head control, (2) tonal or postural torticollis, or (3) exessive cervical mobility.[24] Orthotic treatment for the thoracic spine is usually given for stability. The thorax may not be stabilized in some children with neurological problems; if the stabilizer seems to increase the intensity of primitive reflexs by an orthotic device.[24] For the lumbosacral spine, a lumbosacral corset may be used in children with either an increased anterior or posterior tilt. Use of the corset may cause diaphragmatic alienation and impedence to the downward excursion of the diaphragm during inhalation, however.[24]

Breathing exercises may be recommended for children who have postural deficits, particularly when chest deformities compromise lung function. Scoliosis appears to cause the most thoracic deformity and respiratory dysfunction in children. In scoliosis, the pulmonary function can range from normal in mildly involved children to severely reduced in children with severe rotational scoliosis. Physical therapy for children with scoliosis should include exercises to improve deep breathing and to increase thoracic mobility.[25] These activities are important for children with scoliosis because of the decreased vital capacity caused by the mechanical disadvantage of the muscles of inspiration. Moreover, if the scoliosis is severe, the child's breathing may be rapid and the total volume of air moved may be small. The work of breathing may be abnormally high owing to the abnormal resistance to mobilization of the chest wall.

SUMMARY

This review of the neurodevelopmental aspects of posture should alert physical therapists working with children with postural problems to the dental problems that may result if cooperative interventions with other health professionals such as dentists, otolaryngologists, or allergists are not undertaken. The child with postural malalignment problems may not respond as positively to physical therapy treatment if problems with craniofacial morphology or upper airway resistance problems such as allergies, tonsils, and adenoids are not addressed. The physical therapist may need to refer children with these additional problems to other appropriate practitioners if success is to be realized in the physical therapy program.

Dentists should be alerted to the possibility of postural alignment problems other than in the craniocervical area if the child has craniofacial morphology. If the child has problems with a forward or asymmetrical posturing of the head, the dentist should consider referring the child to physical therapy for a complete postural assessment. Moreover, if lateral curvature of the spine is suspected, as evidenced by unequal hip prominences or arm-to-body space, head and neck not centered over the sacrum, uneven shoulder elevation, uneven waist creases, or obvious spinal deformity, the child should be referred to physical therapy for further screening.

Adult Posturing

Shirley A. Sahrmann

Posture, defined as the relative arrangement of the different parts of the body,[26] has been a subject of interest to the scientist, clinician, artist, soldier, and to any individual concerned with appearance. The scientist's interest ranges from the biomechanics of balancing segments against the forces of gravity and the neuromuscular reflexes controlling balance, to the psychosocial behavior associated with specific postures. Clinicians, such as orthopedists, neurologists, and physical therapists derive their diagnosis in part from observations of posture and movement. The artist, whether the medium is painting, sculpture, theatre, or dance is able to convey many personal attributes of a subject merely by a well-chosen and presented posture. Most persons form a strong impression of a new acquaintance based on appearance, an important component of which is carriage or bearing. Strength, power, competence, and general well-being are somehow conveyed by an erect well-aligned appearance, which is the basis of military posture.

Posture as a subject of study reached its peak in the late 1800s and early 1900s.[27] During that era, scientists were concerned with the mechanics of maintaining and regulating the upright position. Some clinicians made extravagant claims that many ailments of the body, particularly those of the intestinal and respiratory systems, could be directly attributed to faulty posture.[28–31] These claims were based on individuals with extreme conditions and lacked scientific proof that slight irregularities in posture could affect the abdominal organs. Shepard[30] believed that the value of good posture was purely cosmetic. Kraus and Raab[32] and Kendall et al[33] were strong proponents of the concept that many musculoskeletal pain syndromes such as back, shoulder, and neck pain result from lack of strength of postural muscles and consistent postural faults.

The historical emphasis on good posture that was part of many school physical education programs is no longer prevalent.[27] The casualness of today's life style and emphasis on comfort is almost inconsistent with the formality and discipline usually characteristic of good posture. The lack of scientific data supporting the necessity and value of good skeletal alignment and proper postural muscle exercise have certainly contributed to the current situation. So too, health priorities for the past several generations have been on major medical diseases and only recently have musculoskeletal disorders such as back, neck, and shoulder pain syndromes that appear to have a basis in faulty posture become the focus of attention. The impetus for this attention is the growing cost associated with lost time on the job and medical care of regional pain syndromes.

In 1947, the American Academy of Orthopaedic Surgeons appointed a posture committee whose report included the following definitions. Good posture is defined as that state of muscular and skeletal balance that protects the supporting structures of the body against injury or progressive deformity irrespective of the attitude (erect, lying, squatting, stooping) in which these structures are working or resting. Under such conditions, the muscles will function most efficiently and the optimum positions are afforded to the thoracic and abdominal organs. Poor posture is a faulty relationship of the various parts of the body that produces increased strain on the supporting structures and in which there is less efficient balance of the body over its base of support.

GRAVITY PLUMB-LINE ASSESSMENT OF POSTURE

Plumb-line measurements were used by Braune and Fischer[34] to determine the center of gravity of the human body. These early anatomists also derived the centers of gravity of individual body segments. The center of gravity is the point of intersection of the sagittal, coronal, and horizontal gravity lines. Their studies, of frozen cadavers aligned the lateral gravity line with the joint centers (Fig. 10-9). Because this position could be assumed by a living person, Braune and Fischer termed the posture *Normalstellung*. Later workers unfortunately interpreted this to mean ideal posture. Braune and Fischer never suggested that this alignment was intended to be a standard or guideline. Fick,[35] another early biomechanist, did not believe that there was a *Normalhaltung*, or normal posture.

Later investigators, Hellebrandt[36] among them, used a more dynamic method to determine the center of gravity. The method was to determine the three cardinal orientation planes by using data derived from a balance board and the equation for partial weights. The method was originally devised by Reynolds and Lovett,[37] Hellebrandt's studies showed that the height of the center of gravity was approximately 55 percent of the total height, with little variability regardless of the person's build or height. The average location of the gravity line was 5.08 cm (approximately 2 inches) anterior to the lateral malleolus when the "best" posture was assumed by the subjects and not coincident with the malleolus. The dispersion around the mean was great. In the comfortable natural stance, the mean distance of the gravity line from the malleolus was 14 percent greater. In 85 percent of the subjects, the mean projection fell slightly in front of the geometric center of the base of support, toes disregarded; in 15 percent it fell slightly behind the geometric center but always

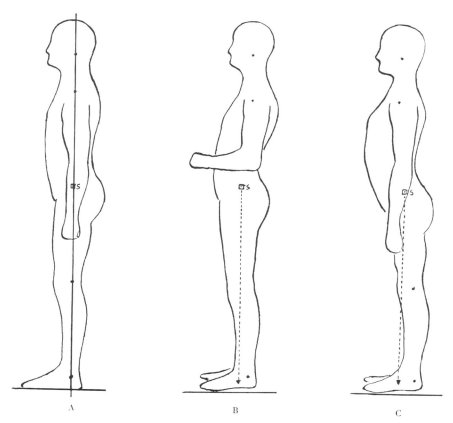

Fig. 10-9.   Three standing positions (Redrawn from Braune and Fischer). (A) Perpendicular standing, constructed from investigations on frozen cadavers. For the convenience of computations it was adopted as a basic position and was (misleadingly) called normal stance. (B) Comfortable posture. (C) Military position. Projection of centers of joints. S = Projection of center of gravity of body as a whole. (Brunnstrom S: Center of Gravity Line in Relation to Ankle Joint in Erect Standing. Phys Ther Rev 34:109, 1954, with permission from the American Physical Therapy Association)

in front of the axis of the ankle joint. This indicated that a perpendicular dropped from the average center of gravity falls remarkably close to the geometric center of the base. The relationship between the projection of the center of gravity remains within 7 percent of the geometric center of the support base regardless of the heel height of shoes or the size of a load carried on the back.[38]

In most subjects, the gravity line was unequally distributed between the feet, falling to the left in 80 percent during natural stance. When a best posture was assumed, the gravity line fell to the right, which was believed to be an overcompensation. In an attempt to explain the stance asymmetry, Hellebrandt postulated that it might be compensatory for a right-sided morphologic preponderance. Her studies of limb preference, strength, and limb size found a

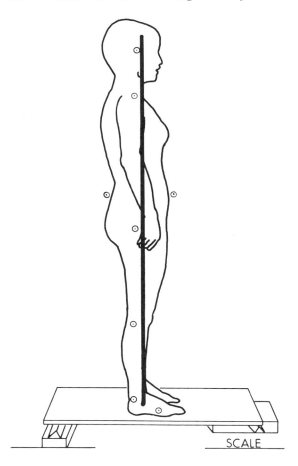

Fig. 10-10. Measuring bony segments from markers to center of gravity.

small but statistically insignificant greater size of the right limbs of right-handed individuals.[39] Postural sway is an inherent part of the upright posture, and it is not surprising that the average position of the constantly shifting trajectory is not exactly over the center of the base of support and is actually more likely to reflect an overcompensation rather than an undercompensation. Postural sway oscillations are of larger amplitude in the anteroposterior direction than in the lateral direction. This sway must be regulated by an automatic mechanism.

Basler[40] also found that the tension in the calf muscles needed to equilibrate gravitational forces at the ankle was less than one-seventh of the maximum voluntary contraction of the calf muscles. Postural sway, particularly in the anteroposterior direction, presents difficulty in obtaining quantitative measures of postural alignment when viewed from the side. A recent study[41] showed that quantitative measures of vertical alignment could be reliable when the actual gravity line was used for vertical reference (Fig. 10-10). The method used in the study was placement of markers on eight bony landmarks (TMJ, acromion, posterior superior iliac spine, anterior superior iliac spine, greater trochanter, fibular head, lateral malleolus, fifth metatarsal) of subjects who were standing on a balance board so that the projection of the gravity line could be determined at the time a photograph was taken. This method, which takes into account the sway, alleviates the problem presented by a vertical line of reference.

The Vertical Line of Reference

A common method for analyzing posture is to assess the relationship of body segments and joints to the vertical reference line. This line is not the actual gravity line as previously described, which must necessarily be obtained by the method described. Rather this line is a compromise between the actual gravity line and the plumb line of Braune and Fisher that coincided with the exact centers of the joints. The Braune and Fischer posture can only be assumed temporarily under artificial conditions because the position is unstable. The line of reference advocated by the Kendalls for posture analysis (Fig. 10-11) is located just anterior to the lateral malleolus (1 inch in front of the ankle center) rather than the 2 to $2\frac{1}{2}$ inches that is typical of the actual gravity line. The advantage of the Kendall location is its ease of consistent location; it also places the reference line closer to the major joint segments. The Kendalls' line of reference is used in back, front, and side views. The line in the side view represents a plane that hypothetically divides the body into front and back sections of equal weight. Along the course of the line are certain points of reference. The base point is the fixed reference point because it is the only stationary or fixed part of the standing posture. The points of reference are slightly in front of the ankle joint, slightly anterior to a midline through the knee, through the greater trochanter of the femur, approximately midway through the trunk, through the shoulder joint, and through the lobe of the ear. The lower limb reference points are not the centers of the joints because the "on-center" position (Braune and Fischer's gravity line) is not a stable one. Rather the "off-center" positions contribute to the stability of the body in a standing position by contributing to the extension moment of all three lower limb joints. The passive elements or the joint structure itself provides stability when an extension moment occurs. Kendall points out that dorsiflexion at the ankle with the knee straight is normally 10 to 15°. Thus, when a person stands barefoot, with feet nearly parallel, the lower leg does not sway forward on the foot (ankle dorsiflexion) more than about 10°. In standing, the femur and lower leg relationship should not exceed 10° of postural deviation backward. The hip joint also has about 10° of hyperextension and, in standing, the joint motion of the pelvis on the femur is restricted to about 10° of postural deviation forward. Because the gravity line passes slightly anterior to the knee joint axis and slightly posterior to the hip joint, these joints are passively forced into extension. Restraint of these forces is provided by muscle tendons and ligaments.

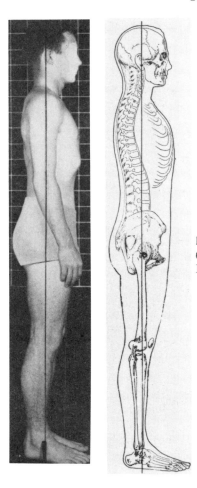

Fig. 10-11. Ideal plumb alignments: side view. (Kendall FP, McCreary EK: Muscles: Testing and Function. Williams & Wilkins, Baltimore, 1983.)

Thus, any stretching of these structures should be done carefully or the joints will exceed their normal range and the forces acting upon them will create stress on inappropriate surfaces.

The placement of the line of reference 1 inch in front of the ankle, as suggested by Kendall,[33] would be approximately half the distance to the projection of the actual gravity line and thus would be closer to the joint centers. A recent study by Woodhull et al.[42] calculated the positions of the partial centers of gravity above the knee and hip as a measure of how the body is balanced above these joints. Their measurements confirmed that slight gravitational torques exist, tending to extend these joints (1.4 cm in front of the knee and 1.0 cm behind the femoral trochanter). Data were also taken from dancers, who had significantly higher variances in alignment of the ear, shoulder, hip, knee, and ankle. The differences of the dancers individually and as

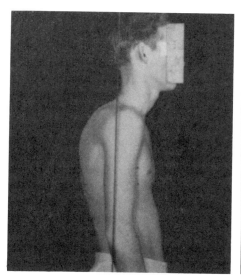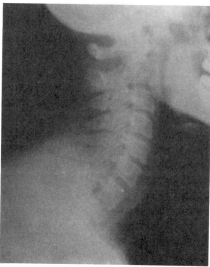

Fig. 10-12.   (A) Forward head. Subject shows an extremely faulty alignment of neck and thoracic spine. Degree of deformity is suggestive of an epiphysis. Patient was treated for pain in the posterior neck and occipital region. (B) In forward head position, cervical spine is in hyperextension. Narrowing of interspaces is most marked between C4 and C5, and between C5 and C6 where C5 and C6 nerve roots emerge. (Kendall FP, McCreary EK: Muscles: Testing and Function. Williams & Wilkins, Baltimore, 1983)

a population were believed to be an indication of the force of habits in modifying posture.

Because increases in the gravitational torques would increase the stresses on supporting tissues as well as on the joint itself, it is reasonable to conclude that good alignment is advantageous. The line of reference does provide a useful method for assessing alignment. As with any standard, an absolute fixed value is not to be expected; rather, a range of values is reasonable. Few persons, if any, can be expected to meet the standard. Although intrinsic variations do exist, minimizing the deviations from the reference line is to the advantage of the individual. Practice in postural assessment enables the clinician to distinguish between structure and postural faults (e.g., actual bowing of the tibia and fibula need to be distinguished from postural bow legs). Structural deviations often become exaggerated and predispose individuals to additional alignment changes. As with measurements of any biological system, few scores precisely meet the standard; clearly, however, the larger the deviation from the standard the more likely the development of pathology. Certainly, the person with a very forward head is more predisposed to cervical degenerative changes than is the person with good alignment (Fig. 10-12).

THE PREVALENCE OF FAULTY POSTURE

Kendall et al. stated that they never examined anyone with perfect posture.[33] More recently, Alderman found postural faults in 93 percent of the 83 high school students used in the study.[43] The most common faults were: forward head, 62 percent; round shoulders, 36 percent; lateral asymmetry of shoulders, 31 percent; lordosis, 29 percent; pelvic tilt, 23 percent, and kyphosis, 21 percent. More than one deviation was found in 62 percent of the students. The increased flexed posture of the aged is obvious even to the casual observer. The forward head and thoracic kyphosis are particularly obvious faults.

Forward Head Posture

One form of forward head posture (FHP) is characterized by an exaggeration of the normal cervical curve, resulting in a lordosis (Fig. 10-13). The muscle imbalances associated with this type of cervical posture are shortness of the neck extensors and elongation of the neck flexors. Assessment of head and neck alignment should also be done with the subject seated because a very different picture may be apparent. If person sits in a position with the hips slid forward in a chair and the thoracic spine flexed, the cervical spine may be flexed usually at the joints between the fifth, sixth, and seventh vertebrae (C5, 6, 7) but extended in the upper segments; thus, the entire cervical spine is not lordotic. A variation of faulty neck alignment exists if the person's occupation requires looking down or working over a desk. In this situation, the neck extensors will probably be elongated and the flexors may be short. Thus, the clinician must assess the person's work posture and the time spent in that position. The person's sleeping posture can also contribute to the poor posture. There is a strong tendency to maintain the posture that is the most familiar. Therefore, a person with a forward head will often use a large pillow which further promotes the FHP. The standing posture assessment can cause a misleading impression if the person spends most of the time sitting rather than standing or walking.

Careful observation of movement is another important assessment component. In addition to assessing ROM the clinician should assess the segments producing the motion, particularly in flexion. Persons with shortened neck extensors most often produce most of the movement of C5, 6, and 7, with minimial change in the rest of the cervical spine. This occurs because most often the lower cervical segments are in flexion while the upper segments are maintained in extension by the tightness of the neck extensors and are thus less flexible than the lower segments.

Forward shoulders and thoracic kyphosis are also major contributors to the FHP. Correction of the faulty position of the upper trunk is necessary for correction of the forward head.

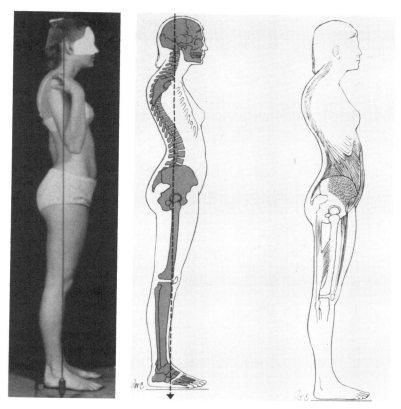

Fig. 10-13. Kyphosis—Lordosis posture. (Kendall FP, McCreary EK: Muscles: Testing and Function. Williams & Wilkins, Baltimore, 1983.)

REQUIREMENTS FOR MAINTAINING GOOD POSTURE

Posture can be considered the base from which movement takes place. The condition of muscles can be inferred from the posture or skeletal alignment. Knowledge of muscle conditions provides guidelines about the quality of movement of specific segments (e.g., observation of forward shoulders with medial rotation of the humerus suggests that shoulder flexion elevation will be performed with excessive elevation of the humerus in the glenoid fossa and excessive abduction of the scapula.) The intrinsic relationship between skeletal alignment, muscle length and strength, and movement means that all components are important for good posture. Optimal alignment is assessed by noting deviations from the vertical line of reference. Optimal muscle function is assessed by detecting alterations from the standards in length, strength, and endurance. Optimal movement is assessed by observations of variations in the precision of joint segment participation during isolated motions and in the interplay of multisegments during total body movement. Although individuals with musculoskeletal pain syndromes have a specific regional problem, most often this is only one of several faulty segments. Because the body must maintain a balance of its segments and the center of gravity within the base of support, compensations must be made if one segment is in faulty alignment (e.g., if the head is forward, the thorax must be shifted slightly backward to maintain the center of gravity within the base of support. Very often, the symptomatic segment is not the etiology of the imbalance but only one of the manifestations, just as fever is only one of the symptoms of a systemic infection. Faulty position of the shoulders and thoracic spine can only result in faulty position of the head and neck. Good alignment of the head and neck is theoretically possible but not likely when alignment of the pelvis is faulty. Thus, the most effective correction and prevention can only be achieved by a program that addresses all components. The kinetic chain properties of the body require a program of corrective exercise for the whole body.

Faulty segmental alignment can either be associated with shortness of muscles pulling the segment into poor alignment or with excessive length of the antagonist muscles, or both conditions may be present (e.g., forward shoulders can result from tightness of the pectoralis minor muscle pulling the scapula into protraction or from excessive length of the lower and middle trapezius, or from both alterations in muscle length). Sedentary persons with forward shoulders usually have excessive length of the middle and lower trapezius muscle rather than shortness of the pectoral muscles. By contrast, in the laborer or the racquet sport athlete, the pectorals are usually tight, and the trapezi are stretched. This is consistent with the findings that tight muscles occur because they are used in shortened positions and are not stretched by the segments to which they attach returning to their ideal position. Treatment of conditions of the head and neck should include simultaneous correction of muscle imbalances of the shoulders and upper trunk. The position and movement patterns of these structures are major determinants in neck and head alignment.

Flexibility is the key to preventing both acute and chronic musculoskeletal problems. Because aging and repetitive activity associated with work or fitness activities reduces flexibility, most often a stretching program is necessary. Indeed, stretching could be considered as important to musculoskeletal health as brushing is to dental health. Intrinsic factors, such as inherent flexibility, in some individuals do not predipose them to tightness; thus, their daily activities suffice for maintaining ideal ROM; however, this is not true for most persons. The opposite condition also exists: Some individuals stretch excessively and thus compromise the stability of their joints. This is particularly true in dancers and gymnasts. Unfortunately, although many books appropriately emphasize the importance of stretching, they provide neither guidelines for the ideal range nor enough detail for stretching the correct muscles. Thus, the dancer often has excessively stretched hamstrings and shortened back muscles, and the runner has shortened hamstrings and an excessively stretched back. Both of these types of imbalances are produced by forward bending or other types of "hamstring" stretches.

The segments and muscles groups that should be examined for length changes are: (1) head and neck—flexors and extensors, (2) shoulder—flexors, extensors, and rotators, (3) trunk—flexors and extensors, (4) hip—flexors, extensors, abductors, and rotators, (5) ankle—plantarflexors. Changes in muscle length are commonly associated with changes in strength.[44] Therefore, examination for length also includes strength tests. The middle and lower trapezius and external oblique abdominal muscles often test weak when they have become elongated. This relationship is called "stretch weakness" by Kendall and McCreary.[45]

Stretched muscles can become strained and thus painful. In addition, the synergists of the lengthen muscles often become shortened and give rise to trigger points (e.g., the upper trapezius, rhomboids, and levator scapulae are common sites of trigger points. Although temporary relief can be obtained by symptomatic treatment, long-term improvement requires exercises to shorten the lengthened muscles and to stretch the shortened muscles to restore proper balance.

For postural relationships, the most important factor that contributes to balance is not absolute strength but the relative strength of synergists and antagonists. Many persons are weak and yet have good posture because the musculature about specific segments has comparable degrees of tautness, with the joints in good alignment. Other persons may be quite strong, but the strength of the flexors may exceed that of the extensors and thus cause a faulty joint position. Maintaining balance both in the passive length and in the contractile strength of opposing muscle groups is the key.

In addition to balance, there should be adequate strength and endurance to enable the person to participate in work and recreational activities safely. Segments are not usually held in alignment by persistent muscle contraction; thus, endurance is not a major factor in good posture. Nonetheless, prevention of musculoskeletal problems is best accomplished by maintenance of adequate resources in strength and endurance, which can minimize injury resulting from the fatigue, stress, and strain of activity. The relatively sedentary life style of most persons usually requires an active program of exercise to achieve these resources. Increasing importance is being given to the role of endurance training in the prevention of many chronic illnesses of the blood vascular system, such as heart disease, high blood pressure, and diabetes. Prevention of osteoporosis is in part a function of exercise. Such training is not possible when an injury exists. A well-designed program of exercise including posture and flexibility exercises in addition to endurance training is a must for anyone interested in health maintenance and illness prevention.

POSTURE CORRECTION IN THE ABSENCE OF PAIN

The key concepts are that good posture and alignment minimize stress and strain and maximize efficiency in the use of the muscles, joints, and the entire body. High-intensity and high-repetition activities can accelerate the degree of stress and strain. Any clinician or even inquiring friend knows that few persons are without periodic musculoskeletal pain. Attention is given to this pain only when concern is raised about a potentially serious underlying condition or interference with work. Because shoulder muscles are constantly in use even in the most sedentary of persons, painful conditions are quite common. So, too, because of the attachment of the shoulder girdle muscles to the cervical vertebrae and to the cranium, neckache and headache are associated symptoms. Faulty length of shoulder girdle muscles contributes to the stresses on the cervical spine because it is the spine that must withstand the forces generated by contraction of the shoulder muscles that attach to it. The value of a well-designed program of exercises for the neck and shoulder girdle cannot be overestimated when the potential of pain and cervical disease is so high in conditions of faulty alignment and muscle imbalance.

The cumulative effects of the changes associated with periodic muscular or joint pain may take years to produce permanent tissue damage. Osteoarthritis is believed to be the result of subtle and chronic biomechanical abnormalities.[46,47] The extent of the various musculoskeletal pain syndromes depend on the degree and the constancy of the faults. Faulty postures are used as indicators of pathology or dysfunction of the nervous, muscular, and skeletal systems. The obvious postures of the hemiplegic and the patient with Parkinson's disease are important diagnostic signs to the neurologist, as are the faulty alignment of the muscular dystrophy patient and the person with scoliosis or arthritis. These conditions are ones in which the systemic pathology produced the alignment change. Only rarely is appropriate recognition given to faulty alignment as a source or a perpetrator of pathology rather than as a result of pathology. This is best explained by the priorities for our health-related research efforts. Because most of these conditions do not influence length of life and various types of medications can be used for symptomatic short-term relief, no major effort has been made to study such problems. This situation is beginning to change, however, because of the increasing cost to employers of required care for employees with pain syndromes not caused by disease.

Hadler has pointed out the prevalence of "regional musculoskeletal disorders," which are conditions that occur in a person without systemic disease.[48] Such persons represent the major portion of the patients who visit family physicians, primary care internists, industrial physicians, rheumatologists, orthopedists, osteopaths, and physical therapists. These disorders are of increasing interest because they impair function in the workplace and because of the growing cost associated with lost work time and medical care. The lack of a specific disease associated with these disorders only compounds the difficulty for both the clinician and the patient as well as the third-party payer.

Regional musculoskeletal disorders can be considered to arise from the cumulative effects of repetitive activity and associated muscle imbalances. Various pathological conditions have their basis in the cumulative effects of small, seemingly innocuous agents. The well-known relationship between pulmonary and heart disease and cigarette smoking is one example. Evidence also seems to be accumulating that a similar relationship exists between cancer and dietary substances. The chronic, repeated faulty stresses on bone either in the form of compression or tension that result from poor posture and the associated muscle imbalances is another example. As in the patient with scoliosis or polio who has exaggerated abnormal biomechanics, these stresses can eventually be a source of eventual tissue pathology, as in osteoarthritis. The paralysis of the polio patient provides an exaggerated example of how abnormal biomechanics can have their origin in muscle imbalances rather than in an inherent bony defect or some type of generalized disease process such as rheumatoid arthritis. Usually, the imbalances are subtle and not as obvious as in the polio patient.

Poor posture is certainly prevalent in our society. Our life style has encouraged a relaxed attitude that is carried over into posture. This does not imply that disease or malfunction of organs are present; or even place the individual at risk for such pathologies. What poor posture does suggest is the potential for developing a regional musculoskeletal pain syndrome. Such a syndrome may arise early in life as an accompaniment to rigorous physical activity either as part of work or recreation or later in life as the result of years of cumulative stress. The current emphasis on prevention and maintaining a healthy life style has aroused the interest of many persons in exercise. A balanced exercise program that is almost always directly related to the quality of the individual's posture is an important factor in maintaining musculoskeletal health and in prevention of several systemic diseases. Certainly, persons who complain of upper neck and/or cervical pain should be referred to the medical and dental practitioners who can best assess the factors contributing to the problem and institute corrective treatment.

REFERENCES

Neurodevelopmented Aspects

1. Bobath B: Abnormal Postural Reflex Activity Caused by Brain Lesion. Wm. Heinemann, London, 1975
2. Gilfoyle EM, Grady AP, Moore JC: Children Adapt. Charles B. Slack, Thorofare, NJ, 1981
3. Holt K: Movement and Child Development. p. 2. Clinics in Developmental Medicine, Vol. 55. JB Lippincott, Philadelphia, 1975
4. McGraw MB: The Neuromuscular Maturation of the Human Infant. Hafner Publishing, New York, 1969
5. Bosma JF: Structure and function of the infant oral and pharyngeal mechanisms. p. 33. In Wilson JM (ed): Oral Motor Function and Dysfunction in Children. University of North Carolina, Chapel Hill, NC, 1978
6. Solow B, Siersbaek-Neilsen S, Greve E: Airway adequacy, head posture, and craniofacial morphology. Am J Orthod 86:214, 1984
7. Vig PS: Respiratory mode and morphological types: some thoughts and preliminary conclusions. In McNamara J (ed): Nasorespiratory Function and Craniofacial Growth. Monograph No. 9. Craniofacial Growth Series. Center for Human Growth and Development, The University of Michigan, Ann Arbor, MI, 1979
8. Solow B, Tallgren A: Dentoalveolar morphology in relation to craniocervical posture. Angle Orthod 47:157, 1977

9. Thompson B, Vig P: Associations between craniofacial morphology, intermaxillary space variables and head posture. IADR 57:1253, 1979

10. Doershuk CF, Fischer BJ, Matthew LW: Pulmonary physiology of the young child. In Scapelii EM (ed): Pulmonary Physiology of the Fetus, Newborn, and Child. Lea & Febiger, Philadelphia, 1975

11. Tecklin JS: Physical therapy for children with chronic lung disease. Phys Ther 61:1774, 1981

12. Minifie FD, Hixon TJ, Williams F: Normal Aspects of Speech, Hearing and Language. Prentice Hall, Englewood Cliffs, NJ, 1973

13. Bly L: The components of normal movement during the first year of life. p. 85. In Slaton D (ed): Development of movement in infancy. University of North Carolina, Chapel Hill, 1981

14. Simmons NN: Disorders in oral, speech and language function. p. 531. In Umphred D (ed): Neurological Rehabilitation. CV Mosby, St. Louis, 1985

15. Kendall FP, McCreary EK: Muscles: Testing and Function. 3rd Ed. Williams & Wilkins, Baltimore, 1983

16. Kendall HO, Kendall FP: Developing and maintaining good posture. Phys Ther 48:319, 1968

17. Lezberg SF: Early screening for spinal deformity. Clin Manage Phys Ther 3:24, 1983

18. Connolly BH, Michael BT: Early detection of scoliosis: neurological approach to using the asymmetrical tonic neck reflex. Phys Ther 64:304, 1984

19. Hoppenfeld S: Scoliosis: A Manual of Concept and Treatment. JB Lippincott, Philadelphia, 1967

20. Morris SE: Oral motor problems and guidelines for treatment. In Wilson J (ed): Oral Motor Function and Dysfunction in Children. University of North Carolina, Chapel Hill, 1978

21. Smith MAH, Connolly BH, McFadden S, et al: Feeding Management of the Child With a Handicap: A Guide for Professionals. University of Tennessee for the Health Sciences, Memphis, 1982

22. Wilson JM (ed): Oral Motor Function and Dysfunction in Children. University of North Carolina, Chapel Hill, 1978

23. Caillet R: Exercises for Scoliosis. p. 430. In Basmajian JV (ed): Therapeutic Exercise. 3rd Ed. Williams & Wilkins, Baltimore, 1978

24. Huber SR: Therapeutic application of orthotics. p 616. In Umphred D (ed): Neurological Rehabilitation. CV Mosby, St. Louis, 1985

25. DeCesare J: Physical therapy for the child with respiratory dysfunction. p. 334 In Irwin S, Tecklin JS (ed): Cardiopulmonary Physical Therapy. CV Mosby St. Louis, 1985

Adult Posturing

26. Webster's Seventh New Collegiate Dictionary. G & C Merriam, Springfield, MA, 1963

27. Clarke HH: (Ed) Physical Fitness Research Digest. Series 9, No. 1. President's Council on Physical Fitness and Sports, Washington DC, 1979

28. Goldthwaite JE: Body Mechanics. 5th Ed. JB Lippincott, Philadelphia, 1952

29. Karpovich PV: Physiology of Physical Activity, 5th Ed. Charles C Thomas, Springfield, IL, 1959

30. Shepard RJ: Alive Man: The Physiology of Physical Activity. Charles C Thomas, Springfield, IL, 1972

31. Kelly ED: Adapted and Corrective Physical Education. 4th Ed. Ronald Press, New York, 1965

32. Kraus H, Raab, W: Hypokinetic Disease, Charles C Thomas, Springfield, IL, 1961

33. Kendall HO, Kendall FP, Boynton DA: Posture and Pain. Williams & Wilkins, Baltimore, 1952. Reprinted by RE Krieger, Melbourne, FL, 1971

34. Braune W, Fischer O: Uber den Schwerpunkt des menschlichen Korpers mit Rucksicht auf die Ausrustung des deutschen Infanteristen. Abhdlg D Kg Sach Wissenschaften 26:561, 1889

35. Fick R: Hundbuch der Anatomie und Mechanik der Gelenke, Bardeleben's Handbuch der Anatomie des Menschen. Vol 2. Jena Gustav Fischer, 1911

36. Hellebrandt FA, Tepper RH, Braun GI, Elliott MC: The location of the cardinal anatomical orientation planes passing through the center of weight in young adult women. Am J Physiol 121:465, 1938

37. Reynolds E, Lovett RW: A method of determining the position of the center of gravity in its relation to certain body landmarks in the erect position. Am J Physiol 24:286, 1909

38. Hellebrandt FA: The influence of the army pack on postural stability and stance mechanics. Am J Physiol 140:645, 1944

39. Hellebrandt FA, Nelson BG, Larsen EM: The eccentricity of standing and its cause. Am J Physiol 140:205, 1943

40. Basler A: Die Schwelinie des menschlichen Korpers und ihre Verschiebungen. Pfluegers Arch Physiol 221:768, 1929

41. Hall C, Sahrmann SA, Norton BJ: Reliability of a technique for measuring postural alignment. Phys Ther 66:755, 1986

42. Woodhull AM, Maltrud K, Mello BL: Alignment of the human body in standing. Eur J Appl Physiol 54:109, 1985

43. Alderman MK: An investigation of the need for posture education among high school girls and a suggested plan of instruction to meet these needs. Master's Thesis, University of Texas, 1966

44. Gossman M, Sahrmann SA, Rose SJ: Review of length associated changes in muscle: experimental evidence and clinical implications. Phys Ther 62:1799, 1982

45. Kendall FP, McCreary EK: Muscles: Testing and Function. 3rd Ed. Williams & Wilkins, Baltimore, 1983

46. Bollet AJ: An essay on the biology of osteoarthritis. Arthritis Rheum 12:152, 1969

47. Howell DS, Moskowitz RW: Symposium on osteoarthritis. Arthritis Rheum, suppl., 20:S96–S103, 1977

48. Hadler NM: Medical Management of the Regional Musculoskeletal Diseases. Grune & Stratton, Orlando, FL, 1984

11

Physical Therapy Concepts in Evaluation and Treatment of the Upper Quarter

Therapeutic Modalities

Jeffrey S. Mannheimer

Pain is the prime impetus that causes a patient to seek medical help. Prior to such consultation, many patients use over-the-counter medication or apply various types of heat and cold. Throughout history and even in current medical practice, the same management technique for the treatment of many types of pain, including that of craniomandibular origin, frequently consists solely of symptomatic intervention. We constantly see craniomandibular patients whose previous therapy has been consistent application of various symptomatic modalities without regard to the cause of pain or use of specific therapeutic interventions geared to its etiology. Furthermore, such modalities are frequently provided without regard to proper sequencing, dosage, or application and may be administered by unlicensed individuals; the charge for such treatment is often costly and unjustified.[1]

It is the specific intent of this section to present the proper use of adjunctive physical therapy modalities within the framework of a comprehensive approach geared to the management of patients with craniomandibular and cervical spine pain/dysfunction.

Comprehensive management consists of a thorough upper quarter and craniomandibular evaluation to analyze posture, neuromuscular function, and biomechanics. This is followed by patient education and instruction, manual individualized restorative techniques to reduce or correct compression, impingement and entrapment forces, adjunctive physical therapy procedures, nonmedicinal pain management techniques, and preventative maintenance.

The proper use of one or more adjunctive physical therapy modalities can significantly enhance achievement of the treatment goals. Pain reduction is only one benefit obtained by the use of thermal agents, massage, vibration, and electrical stimulation. The specific physiological effects of these modalities may also assist in the performance of manual and/or mechanical therapeutic interventions geared to functional restoration, postural corrections, and a decrease in inflammation and edema. Proper sequencing of each modality to obtain maximal benefit may require applications prior to, during, or after specific manual therapeutic techniques.

The specific modalities that offer distinct therapeutic benefits and that are easily applicable to the craniomandibular and cervical region are moist heat packs, cold packs, vapocoolant sprays, ultrasound, high- and low-voltage electrical stimulation, iontophoresis, phonophoresis, transcutaneous electrical nerve stimulation (TENS), noninvasive electroacupuncture and electromyographic biofeedback. Prior to a discussion of each modality, the general indication for their adjunctive use is discussed.

INDICATIONS FOR ADJUNCTIVE USE OF THERAPEUTIC MODALITIES

Pain Relief

All of the aforementioned modalities can be used to reduce discomfort. Pain is primarily produced as a result of direct or indirect macro- or microtrauma to a specific tissue or group of tissues, such as a joint capsule, muscle, ligament, connective tissue, etc. Other etiological factors such as infection, systemic disease, endocrine imbalance, fatigue, and emotional tension may also be causative agents. Trauma may be spontaneous, causing direct tissue damage or gradual as a result of abnormal posture. Our concern is particularly the tissue structures that comprise the TMJ and its relationship to the head and neck.

Direct soft tissue or joint trauma produces a generalized acute physiological response of guarding (muscle spasm) and inflammation. The inflammatory response consists specifically of impeded circulation and lymphatic clearing with a concomitant reduction in oxygen and nutrient supply plus metabolite retention. Prolonged pain and guarding can lead to shortening and restricted motion of soft tissue structures such as connective tissue, muscle, and joint capsule. This restricted mobility contributes to the development of trigger points, joint hypomobility, and possible nerve entrapment, further compounding the pain process.

Pain reduction may occur simply from the counterirritation properties of one or more of the previously mentioned modalities and/or by a direct reduction of inflammation, edema, metabolite retention, and muscle guarding, and the resultant restoration of normal function.

Trigger Point Desensitization

The literature pertaining to the etiology, pain mechanisms, and treatment techniques relative to trigger points is quite extensive. The best total single reference source is the excellent text by Travell and Simons.[2] A trigger point is considered to be a small hypersensitive region in muscle, ligament, fascia, or joint capsule that can be a source of referred pain. Pain is described as a localized deep dull ache with a surrounding hyperalgesia.[2,3] An active trigger point when pressed, massaged, pinched, needled, stretched, or subjected to intense heat or cold will produce the symptomatic triad of a localized deep ache, hyperalgesia, and referred pain.[2,3] Pain referral may occur within dermatomal and myotomal distributions in a segmental or extrasegmental fashion that can even cross the midline of the body, as illustrated by the sternocleidomastoid (SCM) pain pattern.[2,3] Travell has documented the common referral patterns related to the major masticatory and cervical musculature.[4]

A knowledge of trigger point referral patterns can help to determine the muscular source of origin. Trigger points, however, are primarily a secondary manifestation of trauma and are not usually the primary causative factor, but frequently promote persistent pain complaints.[3] Well-known patterns of referral from the masseter, temporalis, and pterygoids to the ear, teeth, mandible, temporal, and infraorbital region, as well as related cervical trigger points, can compound the entire pain pattern.

Trigger point pain referral patterns cannot be totally eliminated solely by the desensitization techniques presented here. The key to total elimination is restoration and maintenance of proper posture, body mechanics, and resting position of the entire craniomandibular and cervical spine region. Individual applications of single modalities to trigger points will produce only short-term periodic relief unless the rehabilitation program is comprehensive.

Tissue Preparation

Thermal modalities that elevate tissue temperature when properly used prior to soft tissue stretching, joint mobilization, traction, and therapeutic exercise provide therapeutic effects that can greatly enhance the performance of these techniques and procedures. Thermal agents commonly used by physical therapists consist of those that produce superficial heat (infrared, paraffin, whirlpool, and moist heat packs) as well as deep penetrating heat (shortwave or microwave diathermy and ultrasound).

Moist heat packs, infrared lamps, and ultrasound are the only such modalities that we recommend for application to the craniomandibular/cervical region. Infrared and moist heat packs do not penetrate more than 1 cm below the skin surface and therefore only produce temperature elevation of superficial tissue.[5] Moist heat, however, may be advantageous for use prior to the application of ultrasound and can assist in the reduction of muscle spasms. Moist heat applied simultaneously with electrical stimulation can also enhance circulation.

Deep heating agents such as shortwave and microwave diathermy are contraindicated in the presence of metal and therefore cannot be used when fillings or oral appliances containing metal exist.[6–8] Ultrasound, however, can provide sufficient tissue penetration and is easily directed to a small area such as the TMJ or the suboccipital fossa without being contraindicated.[9]

The generalized therapeutic benefits of heat are reduction of muscle spasms, reduction of pain due to chronic dysfunction, and increase in the extensibility of periarticular soft tissue. A combination of these effects when obtained prior to or during techniques used to increase joint range of motion (ROM) are excellent indications for the adjunctive use of moist heat and ultrasound.

Enhancing Proprioceptive Input

If muscle guarding, capsular adhesions, and concomitant joint hypomobility exist, active movement is severely hindered. The central nervous system (CNS) is thus deprived of proprioceptive input. Nociceptive input therefore predominates, owing to tissue irritation from edema, retained metabolites, impaired circulation, and decreased lymphatic clearing. Any attempt at active or passive movement causes an immediate increased excitation of pain fibers.

Normally, a balance exists between proprioceptive (mediated by large-diameter, fast-conducting afferent fibers) and nociceptive input (mediated by smaller diameter, slowly conducting afferent fibers) at the dorsal horn of the spinal cord. According to the tenets of the gate control theory, inhibition to the transmission of nociceptive impulses occurs when sufficient proprioceptive input exists at segmentally related spinal cord segments.[10] The degree of afferent stimulation necessary to produce nerve depolarization is normally high for small fibers and low for large fibers. Depolarization thresholds, however, reverse themselves when sensory deprivation exists. In an acute closed lock of the TMJ (anteriorly dislocated disc without reduction), normal mandibular movement is strongly impeded. This greatly decreases or eliminates the continuous flow of normal proprioceptive input and promotes constant nociceptive input as a result of soft tissue restriction, reflex muscle guarding, and metabolite retention. An imbalance of large vs. small fiber afferent input thus occurs, favoring the small nociceptive fibers and producing a decrease in their depolarization threshold and a concomitant increase in nociceptive input when active mandibular movement is attempted.

Adjunctive use of thermal and electrical modalities can decrease the inflammatory response, thereby improving circulation and promoting a decrease in nociceptive activity. Furthermore, the use of manual joint/and soft tissue mobilization as well as hold–relax stretching techniques during and/or immediately following thermal or electrical modalities allows increased active movement and proprioceptive input.

The nucleus caudalis of the trigeminal nerve has a substantia gelatinosa region that is similar in structure and function to as well as continuous with that of the dorsal horn of the spinal cord.[11–14] Thus, increased proprioceptive activity from the TMJ follows the same neurophysiological principles as that of any other spinal or peripheral synovial joint. In addition, the proximal fibers of cranial nerves V, VII, IX, and X are associated with the trigeminal sensory nucleus and have sympathetic connections with the upper cervical spine through the nucleus caudalis. A significant percentage of the fibers from the trigeminal sensory nucleus cross the midline, and a lesser degree remain ipsilateral. This extensive anatomic relationship and neural pathway interaction can account for the myriad effects associated with the patient who sustains a whiplash injury or develops a forward head posture (FHP).

Promote Healing

If inflammation and pain can be decreased, circulation increased, and irritation and compression forces eliminated, normal function and healing can occur. Restoration of proper active movement must, however, be maintained and facilitated by the promotion of normal head and neck posture as must provision of normal movement and positioning of the condyle with the disc in the TMJs.[15–17] Failing to add instruction in proper body mechanics, postural corrective exercises, and activities of daily living (ADL) adaptations at home, work, or play can easily impede the healing process and cause dysfunction and pain to recur to the cervical spine and its concomitant influence on the craniomandibular region. Ongoing stress and strain of joint and soft tissue structures of the craniomandibular and cervical spine must be eliminated, as is discussed later in this chapter.

SPECIFIC EFFECTS OF INDIVIDUAL THERAPEUTIC MODALITIES

Previous publications discuss in detail the biophysical and neurophysiological mechanisms of each adjunctive modality discussed in this section (these publications are listed in the references). My intent is to use these available data as they relate to the modalities that offer benefits specific to the craniomandibular, TMJ, and cervical spine areas.

Superficial Heating Agents

Superficial heating agents applicable to use at the craniomandibular and cervical region consist of moist heat packs and infrared lamps. Moist heat packs represent the least expensive, reusable source of superficial heat that can be applied to the cervical spine or TMJ region. These are available with a cervical contour for easy conformation to the involved area. When properly heated in a thermostatically controlled water tank (140 to 160°F), direct applications of a moist heat pack produces skin and subcutaneous tissue heating only to a depth of 0.5 to 1 cm.[5]

Moist heat packs transfer heat to the body by conduction. The local effects of moist heat produce an elevation in skin temperature and subcutaneous tissues that reaches a maximum in 6 to 8 minutes. Heating of the underlying muscle tissue, if it occurs, requires at least application for 15 to 30 minutes. Muscle that is covered by a significant amount of adipose tissue will, however, experience only a 1°C increase in temperature after such an application.[5]

Studies conducted with dry heat applications, such as by fluidotherapy (circulation of warm air and fine cellulose particles in a container) to the hand or foot have demonstrated an elevation of up to 9°C.[5] Fluidotherapy, however, is not applicable to the head or neck. Joints of the hand or foot as well as the TMJ have only a small degree of soft-tissue covering; therefore, a greater elevation in temperature may occur from superficial heating at these areas.

The increase in tissue temperature from moist heat produces cutaneous vasodilation, with a resultant increase in local circulation. The circulatory enhancement can assist in the removal of inflammatory by products such as prostaglandins, bradykinins, and histamine. This in turn serves to reduce nociceptive activity by a reduction in substances that irritate or excite interstitial chemoreceptors.

Because elevation of muscle temperature by superficial heating agents is minimal, a reduction in muscle spasm through decreased α motoneuron activity is unlikely. Michlovitz, however, proposes that an increase in skin temperature alone may provide an indirect method of decreasing α motoneuron activity by causing a decrease in γ efferent firing. This results in muscle spindle relaxation and a concomitant decrease in afferent firing from it.[5]

The use of an infrared lamp in lieu of a moist heat pack is only recommended when a patient cannot tolerate the weight, pressure, or touch of a moist heat pack against the face or neck. Infrared emits radiant energy that penetrates no more than 2 to 3 mm below the skin surface. The maximal degree of circulatory enhancement requires at least a 20-minute application. Therapeutically, infrared is not as desirable as the moist heat pack, and its effects are significantly less.

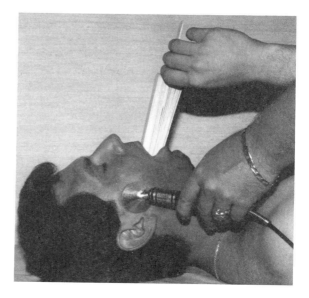

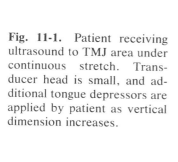

Fig. 11-1. Patient receiving ultrasound to TMJ area under continuous stretch. Transducer head is small, and additional tongue depressors are applied by patient as vertical dimension increases.

Deep-Heating Agents

In my clinical experience, ultrasound is the method of choice when deep heating is required at the TMJ or cervical spine. Ideally, an ultrasound unit with a small-diameter applicator head is more easily able to conform to the TMJ and suboccipital regions.

Ultrasound, when properly applied, can elevate tissue temperature to a depth of 5 cm or more below the skin surface.[9] Ultrasonic energy is absorbed specifically in tissues that have a high collagen content. Skin and SC fat therefore absorb little, if any, ultrasound, while ultrasound to muscle and joint capsule with high collagen levels absorb a great deal.[9] Therefore, ultrasound represents an excellent means of selectively heating deep periarticular structures.

Shortwave and microwave diathermy do not penetrate as deep as ultrasound. Ultrasound can also be safely administered if prosthetic joints or metallic implants of silver and gold, normally used in this treatment field, are present, whereas shortwave or microwave diathermy cannot.[9,18–22,22a]

At normal body temperature, collagen has the property of elasticity and high viscosity.[9,23] When its temperature is elevated to 40 to 45°C, however, collagen molecular bonding is altered, viscosity is decreased, and the respective periarticular structures are more susceptible to stretch. Optimal benefit thus requires that the TMJ be placed on stretch by use of tongue depressors while ultrasound is being applied (Fig. 11-1). Studies performed on large joints such as the hip have required intensities of 1.0 to 2.5 W/cm² for 5 minutes at each aspect of the joint to raise the temperature to the 40 to 45°C range. These intensity and duration parameters can be decreased for application to the TMJ since the degree of soft tissue between the joint and skin is considerably less than that of the hip; therefore an intensity of 1.0 to 1.5 W/cm² is sufficient.[9,19,24–26]

A temperature elevation to 40 to 45°C is required for collagen extensibility to occur. Collagen extensibility will enhance the effectiveness of intraoral mobilization techniques. The etiology, evaluation of capsular tightness, and application of the mobilization techniques are described in Chapter 6. Because bone is relatively superficial in the TMJ area, the treatment can start with an intensity of 1.0 to 1.5 W/cm² for 3 to 5 minutes; if the patient reports a deep dull achy sensation, indicative of periosteal temperature elevation, the intensity should be decreased by 10 percent, but the sensation of warmth should persist. In addition, ultrasound can also be applied at fracture sites, where it may accelerate healing.[9,27]

Alternative measures can be used if the patient cannot tolerate direct application of the transducer on the TMJ. A water-filled balloon or examination glove filled with warm water can be placed over the TMJ. Transmission gel should be applied between the TMJ and water sac as well as between the water sac and transducer.[28] Sonation over the water sac will allow transmission with little attenuation through the water sac to the TMJ. It is also recommended that the transmission gel be preheated prior to application to the skin. We use a thermostatically controlled gel heater so that a cold transmission medium is not applied after moist heat.

Ultrasound alters motor and sensory nerve conduction velocity, but because studies have not been performed with specific regard to the trigeminal or occipital nerves, no direct reference to the TMJ or upper cervical spine regions can be made. Decreased latencies have been noted, with a concomitant decrease in conduction velocity through varying dosages of ultrasound on major peripheral nerves of the upper extremity.[29–32]

An increase in pain threshold can occur after the use of ultrasound. Michlovitz attributes this to its counterirritant effect or alteration of the excitability of free nerve endings (nociceptors).[9]

Few studies have been performed comparing the pain-relieving effects of ultrasound alone with those of other modalities.[9] Many means of counterirritation and modalities that can be applied, preferably by the patient at home, will surely offer more benefit than ongoing application of single modality treatments such as ultrasound in the clinic. We continue to see patients, however, who have been previously treated elsewhere solely by application of moist heat and ultrasound three times weekly for a significant period of time. This type of therapy is merely augmenting the income of the individual clinician or facility, robbing the patient and misrepresenting the practice of physical therapy.[1]

Ultrasound can also be used to drive antiinflammatory and analgesic agents through the skin. This technique is known as phonophoresis.[33,34] The rationale for this technique is that the increase in tissue permeability produced by the ultrasound beam allows deep and local application of chemical agents to be focused selectively at distinct areas such as the TMJ. Cortisol, dexamethasone, and salicylates are commonly used antiinflammatory agents. Lidocaine is a frequently used analgesic agent.[33,34] Phonophoresis is similar to iontophoresis, which is discussed later in the chapter.

Contraindications to Superficial and Deep-Heating Agents

Contraindications and precautions to the application of various therapeutic agents may relate to systemic conditions or specific body organs or regions. For the purposes of this text, the discussion is limited to the head, face, and cervical spine. Application of both superficial and deep-heating agents should not be performed over the eyes or in areas that have impaired temperature sensation or circulatory deficits. In addition, heat should not be applied in hemophilia or immediately after trauma when increased bleeding may occur or at an area of malignancy.[5,9] Because of the close proximity of the eye to the TMJ, extra care must be taken to ensure that application of ultrasound stays outside the inferior and lateral borders of the orbit of the eye. Due to a poor blood supply to the lens and little attenuation by the aqueous and vitreous humor, heat dissipation may not be adequate and increased temperature may result in production of cataracts.[9,35]

Ultrasound is also contraindicated over growing epiphyses and should therefore not be used in children, especially with intensities greater than 3.0 W/cm^2 when applied for 3 minutes with a stationary transducer head.[9,36,37] Even though we recommend constantly moving the transducer head, a small region such as the TMJ or suboccipital fossa minimizes the amount of movement that can occur.

Ultrasound should not be used in the presence of Raynaud's phenomenon, which may be apparent on the face, particularly at the ear, nose, and lips. Care must also be exercised after TMJ surgery when decreased sensation in the trigeminal distribution frequently exists. Tables 11-1 and 11-2 summarize the use of therapeutic heat and ultrasound, respectively.

Cryotherapeutic Agents

Cold can be applied to the TMJ and cervical region by ice packs as well as vapocoolant sprays. Ice has the specific benefits of reducing edema, inflammation, and muscle spasm when applied in the acute stage immediately after trauma.[38–41] Vasoconstriction is perhaps the best-known effect of cold applications, followed closely by counterirritation properties that produce analgesia. Short application periods of cold that do not exceed 15 minutes produce arterial and venule vasoconstriction. The decrease in skin temperature and activation of thermoreceptors gives rise to a reflex excitation of sympathetic adrenergic fibers causing vasoconstriction. Furthermore, hypothalamic stimulation also results in reflex cutaneous vasoconstriction.

Blood flow also decreases by exposure to cold through an increase in viscosity. A decrease in circulation when produced after an acute injury can

Table 11-1. Therapeutic Heat

Superficial: infrared, dry/moist packs	(1 cm)
Deep: SWD, MWD, U.S.	(3–5+ cm)

Therapeutic benefits, general
   ↓ Muscle spasm when not in acute stage
   ↓ Pain secondary to chronic soft tissue dysfunction
   ↑ ROM due to ↑ extensibility of periarticular soft tissue
Specific
   ↑ Muscle temperature to 42°C results in a ↓ firing rate of type II muscle spindle afferents
   ↑ Temperature of joint capsule and muscle at bone/muscle interface
   ↑ Collagen extensibility
Precautions/contraindications
   Sensory deficit (pain and temperature)
   Children
   Malignancy
   Eye
   Circulatory impairment

SWD, shortwave diathermy; MWD, microwave diathermy; US, ultrasound; ↑, increase; ↓, decrease; ROM, range of motion.

concomitantly inhibit the production of edema. Cold also acts to reduce muscle spasm. The research literature is not conclusive in its discussion of the effect of cold on muscle tension.[39] A decrease in pain by cold applications can reflexively reduce muscle spasm by breaking up the pain-spasm-pain cycle. Joint stiffness can increase, however, with decreasing temperature.[38,39] Cold reduces spasticity temporarily, after which stretching and exercise can be performed.[39–42] Many of the cryokinetic techniques (except the use of vapocoolant sprays) of cold and stretch plus exercise will not be tolerated on the face by the TMJ, however, due to the density of sensory innervation. A complete review of all the neurophysiological studies on the subject of cryokinetics is provided by Knight.[39]

Peripheral nerve conduction velocity can be decreased by applications of

Table 11-2. Ultrasound

Heat and stretch
   Collagen primarily exhibits elastic properties and minimal viscous flow at normal body temperature
   When heated, viscosity and collagen molecular bonding ↓ , which facilitates stretch
   Greater residual ↑ in tissue length and less potential damage from preheat or simultaneous heat and stretch
   US preferred for well-defined area; little attenuation through skin/subcutaneous fat; joint capsular structures and muscle have high collagen content and thus absorb ↑ amount of US; selective heating at bone/muscle interface
Technique
   Temperature 40 to 45°C
   1.0–1.5 W/cm^2 for 3–5 min + continuous stretch
Enhancement
   Water sac/gel
   Preheat gel
   Movement of sound head
   First 1–2 min 1.0–1.5 W/cm^2 → dull deep ache ↓ 10% and maintain mild sensation of warmth

US, ultrasound; →, results in.

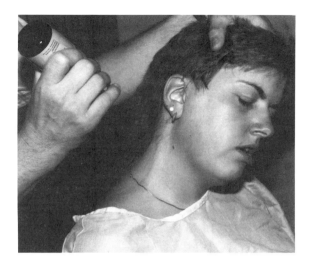

Fig. 11-2. Fluorimethane spray and stretch to the scalenes.

cold for 5 minutes or longer.[42] It has been demonstrated that with each 1°C decrease in intramuscular temperature, a decrease of 1.2 m/sec in motor conduction velocity occurs as well as a 2 m/sec decrease in sensory nerve conduction velocity. Furthermore, small-diameter afferents (nociceptive fibers) show greater sensitivity to cold than do larger diameter fibers. Cold can also decrease axoplasmic transport within the nerve. A linear decrease in sensory nerve conduction velocity occurs with decreasing cold applications until 27°C is reached after which a conduction block may occur.[39,42]

Fluorimethane and ethylchloride are the two commonly used vapocoolant sprays. Ethylchloride is basically a topical anesthetic and provides a quick means of local pain relief. It, however, is volatile and inflammable, and easily freezes the skin.[38–41,43] Fluorimethane, is neither volatile nor flammable. It is not as cold as ethylchloride, and therefore will not easily produce freezing in the area sprayed.

Fluorimethane has the specific advantage of being able to be sprayed over an area or muscle that is under a sustained stretch (Figs. 11-2 and 11-3). The cold spray produces stimulation of cutaneous and SC afferent nerve fibers that reflexively decreases γ motor unit activity, thus facilitating the passive stretch.[2] Freezing the skin overlying a muscle that is to be stretched serves to inhibit such an action. When stretch and spray is used to treat active trigger points, Travell recommends spraying from the trigger point throughout the pain referral patterns in successive sweeps while monitoring stretch of the involved muscle.[2]

Ethylchloride, however, can provide a quick and easy means of analgesia by the process of counterirritation and elevation of the pain threshold. Specifically, when ethylchloride is applied just prior to acupressure or deep pressure massage of trigger points, elevation of the pain threshold can enhance the tolerance to and effectiveness of this technique. Table 11-3 summarizes the use of stretch and spray techniques.

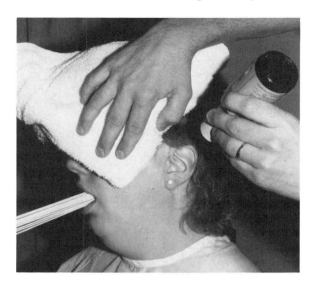

Fig. 11-3.   Fluorimethane spray and stretch to the masseter/temporalis.

Contraindications to Use of Cryotherapy

The application of cryotherapeutic agents should not be performed on patients with trigeminal neuralgia or postherpetic neuralgia of the trigeminal nerve. These sensory deprivation pain syndromes give rise to hypersensitivity and an increased response to even gentle touch that would be quickly facilitated by the application of cold. Such an adverse response would increase more rapidly to cold than to heat. In addition, any patient with pain and temperature hypersensitivity or sensory loss, such an those with Raynaud's syndrome, cold urticaria, cryoglobulinemia, and paroxysmal cold hemoglobinuria, should not

Table 11-3. Stretch and Spray

Florimethane	
↓ Muscle spasm	
Subacute/chronic stage	
Subcutaneous afferent stimulation	↑ Pain threshold
Reflex ↓ γ motoneuron firing to facilitate	Counterirritant
passive stretch	↓ Pain and facilitate motion
Contraindications	
Raynaud's syndrome	
Cold hypersensitivity	
Open wounds	
Compromised local circulation	
Technique	
30° angle	
45 cm from skin	
2–3 (sweeps)	
10 cm/sec speed	
Trigger point desensitization	
↓ Soft tissue restriction	

be exposed to cold.[38-40] Neither should patients with hypertension, circulatory impairment, or cold intolerance be exposed to cold modalities.

The skin can tolerate freezing only for 4 to 7 minutes without any sensory experience of injury other than a slight peeling of the superficial epithelial layer.[44] One should observe the patient and be aware of any complaints of burning, tingling, numbness, or blanching of the skin. Frostnip may occur from ice applications on the face, hands, or cheeks, and the first warning will be the aforementioned signs and symptoms. Frostnip occurs before frostbite and can easily be reversed by warming the involved area.[44] Because cryo-therapeutic applications are only given for short periods of time on the face, further damage such as frostbite need not be discussed.

Acupressure/acupuncture

Acupressure, like acupuncture, has a long history of clinical documentation. Many publications relate to the value of these techniques in the reduction or alleviation of headaches, TMJ, and dental and cervical spine pain of varied etiologies.[45-49] The specific effects of acupressure or acupunctural technique is to provide pain relief through the counterirritation principal, gate control theory or liberation of the body's own natural opiates called endorphins.[50-52]

The Japanese technique of acupressure is known as Shiatsu, which actually means finger pressure.[52] Traditional Shiatsu and Chinese acupressure can be taught to patients for home use.[45,49,52,53] The effectiveness of ice plus acupressure seems to be much greater than either technique applied alone.[54]

A new inexpensive ($15.95 for two probes and a tube of conducting gel to minimize skin irritation) and reusable device called the Cryo-Stim (Pelton-Shepard Industries, 1326 W. Fremont St., Stockton, CA 95203) probe allows simultaneous application of acupressure massage and cold. Ice massage has previously been performed with an ice cube, a popsicle or a frozen paper cup of water. When kept in the freezer for 4 hours the tip of the Cryo-Stim probe equilibrates to the same temperature as its environment and remains effective for 10 to 15 minutes. This eliminates the need for ice and does not produce wetness.

All previously mentioned therapeutic interventions for pain relief basically consist of applications at the site of pain or injury. Acupressure techniques as well as use of the Cryo-stim probe may be applied locally, however, or can be based on traditional meridian relationships and thus applied at sites remote from the area of pain. The advantage of this is enormous if hypersensitivity exists at the pain site.

Acupuncture is a technique using SC needle insertion and manual twirling and must be administed by an acupuncturist or physician; therefore, it cannot be applied at home by the patient. The addition of electrical stimulation through lead wires from an electrical generator to the acupuncture needles may increase effectiveness. This technique is called invasive electroacupuncture.[51]

Surface stimulation of selected points through electrical probes, without skin penetration, is known as noninvasive electroacupuncture and is a form of TENS. Like acupuncture, only a small area is stimulated with successive applications at various sites.[51,55,56]

Noninvasive electroacupuncture units have adjustable frequency (pulse rate) and amplitude controls. The extremely small-diameter probe allows use of a microampere current (greater current density under the small electrode) as opposed to milliamperes with the common portable TENS units. A pulse rate of 2 or 4 Hz delivered for 30 to 60 seconds is tolerated best. Optimal results occur with amplitude raised to the highest level of comfortable tolerance. Because this somewhat noxious form of electrical stimulation is not tolerated initially at the painful site, it is recommended that stimulation begin at segmentally related distal sites.[51] If upper quarter pain syndromes exist, initial stimulation sites are the dorsal web space, midline of the wrist just proximal to the second volar crease and overlying the flexor carpi ulnaris tendon. This provides stimulation of all the major peripheral nerves of the upper extremity at their distal superficial aspects. Stimulation then progresses proximally over tender or low-resistance sites, at superficial aspects of segmentally related peripheral nerves, as well as on motor, trigger, and acupuncture points within the pain distribution pattern. I have made an extensive comparison of the anatomical and physiological relationship of acupuncture, motor, and trigger points to the peripheral nervous system; the comparison is available elsewhere.[55]

I do not necessarily follow suggested acupuncture point or meridian relationship formulas as others have recommended.[57] I evaluate each patient's pain distribution and segmental origin separately. It is also beneficial to stimulate low-resistance areas surrounding the region of pain. If the therapist starts at distal sites, the patient develops an initial tolerance to the noxious sensation at a nonpainful but frequently segmentally related site, which may also decrease discomfort in the area of pain. Thus, when stimulation is applied at the painful sites, greater tolerance is obtained, stronger intensity can be used, and better results are obtained.

Occasionally, stimulation will begin at the contralateral extremity if upper extremity referral exists. Bilateral stimulation usually augments the pain-relieving effect. Pain relief can be quite rapid with this technique, sometimes occurring after only three sites have been stimulated.[51]

The mechanisms relating to pain relief from noninvasive electroacupuncture techniques are attributed to an endorphin liberation as well as hyperstimulation analgesia.[56] At present, I am unaware of any published studies dealing specifically with this analgesic technique that examined endorphin elevation scientifically. Manufacturers of these devices as well as others that use a low-frequency, low-intensity stimulation, refer to the literature relating to invasive electroacupuncture to explain effectiveness.[51]

My experience with this technique, however, has been quite successful. Melzack believes that hyperstimulation analgesia interrupts reverberatory neural circuits and that breaking up such a cyclic mechanism with concomitant increased active exercise can offer prolonged relief.[56] Active exercise combined with proper posture and body mechanics also serves to increase proprioceptive input.

The specific effect of all the aforementioned acupunctural methods is pain relief.[58,59] Other effects have been attributed to acupuncture, however, such as ACTH liberation, which may serve to reduce inflammation and aid in the healing process; however, more scientific experimentation is necessary.[58-63]

Contraindications to Use of Acupressure

Few contraindications exist to the use of acupressure massage techniques other than the necessity to avoid application at regions of sensory deficit, hypersensitivity, circulatory impairment, or malignancy.

Electrotherapy

Electrical stimulation can be a valuable adjunctive technique for pain relief as well as reduction of edema, muscle spasm, inflammation, and metabolite retention. Various stimulation parameters and treatment modes can be programmed to provide high-frequency (50 to 150 Hz) stimulation for fast pain relief or rhythmic low rate (0.5 to 4 Hz) muscle contraction at the involved region for edema reduction, and reflex vasodilation. As with previously discussed modalities, circulatory enhancement serves to produce an influx of oxygen and nutrients, with flushing out of retained metabolites. This process also serves to reduce inflammation and (secondarily) pain.

The most common type of electrical stimulators consist of low-voltage AC–DC generators, high-voltage galvanic generators, TENS units, and noninvasive electroacupuncture and iontophoretic devices. A wide variety of models, both line and battery powered, are available from numerous manufacturers. The differences relative to waveforms, polarity, stimulation parameter ranges and modes, electrodes, and recommended usage cover a large area and are beyond the scope of this chapter. The reader can consult the references for more detailed information. Each general category of units, however, can be used in the treatment of craniomandibular–TMJ–cervical spine disorders; thus, a brief introduction and delineation is warranted.

Low- and high-voltage devices as well as interferential current generators are each capable of producing all of the aforementioned therapeutic effects. No published clinical studies compare the benefits and efficacy of one form of electrotherapy with another in similar patient populations; thus, the reader must decide through trial and error, word of mouth from peers, or claims of the manufacturers.

High-voltage units may, however, provide deeper tissue penetration due to the ability of the patient to tolerate higher amplitude (intensity) levels with these devices without significant chemical or thermal effects.[64] Variability through interrupted, surge, and reciprocal modes is available on both low- and

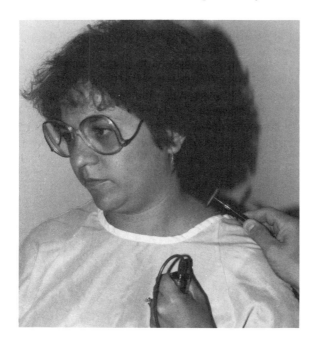

Fig. 11-4. Trigger point desensitization being performed by noninvasive electroacupuncture stimulation. Patient holds ground electrode in hand.

high-voltage units. These units can deliver current through surface electrodes of various sizes as well as hand-held probes.

Noninvasive electroacupuncture devices use a hand-held probe that functions as a point locator as well as a stimulator. The specific effect of this type of stimulation, usually delivered at a low rate (1 to 4 Hz) is to produce a relatively rapid onset of pain relief, which may occur with stimulation distal to the painful region. This is highly beneficial when stimulation at the area of pain, such as the face, cannot be tolerated.[51,55,65–70]

Hand-held probes of various sizes can also be effectively used to desensitize or break up persistent trigger points by the technique of hyperstimulation analgesia (Fig. 11-4).[56]

The transfer of ions through the skin by an electromotive force is known as iontophoresis. This technique uses a low-amperage direct current to drive ions through the skin by placement under electrodes of the same polarity. Originally a time-consuming technique due to electrode preparation, iontophoresis has been simplified by the advent of new portable battery-operated stimulators with electrodes specifically designed for injectable applications of the desired chemical agent.[71–73]

Iontophoresis, like phonophoresis, may be more advantageous than injection of a chemical agent because no tissue damage can occur through the bolus of injected fluid. In the management of TMJ dysfunction, antiinflammatory agents such as cortisol, dexamethasone, and salicylates, as well as local analgesics such as lidocaine, can be applied to the inflamed joint.[71]

Electrotherapy can also offer an effective alternative to medication for

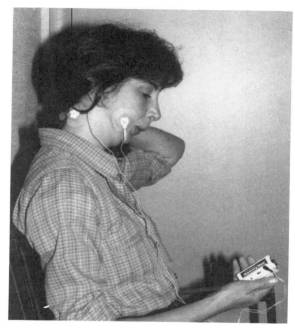

Fig. 11-5. Patient using conventional transcutaneous electrical nerve stimulation to allow tolerance to treatment. One electrode is placed in suboccipital fossa on right; the other is placed at mental foramen.

home management of pain due to myofascial pain.[74] Small, portable, battery-operated TENS units are available by doctor's prescription for rental or purchase for either acute or chronic pain syndromes.[1,66] TENS is also an effective means of postsurgical pain control when its use can significantly reduce the amount of narcotic medications and resultant side effects.

When combined with proper instruction in body mechanics and postural corrective exercises, the periodic use of TENS at home can aid in the desensitization of trigger points, relieve muscle guarding and thus promote the return of painfree ROM.[65,66]

TENS can be used adjunctively in the clinic for pain control sufficient to allow performance of specific therapeutic procedures.[66] In the comprehensive management of patients with craniomandibular–TMJ–cervical spine disorders, TENS may allow joint mobilization of the TMJ when hypersensitivity to touch or discomfort hinders performance of this manual technique (Fig. 11-5). A previous publication of mine described TENS as allowing gentle joint mobilization of the cervical spine (lateral oscillations and posterior/anterior glides) to be performed by decreasing a significant degree of discomfort.[66]

In such instances, TENS may decrease pain through gate control by selectively activating large-diameter proprioceptive afferents to inhibit or balance small-diameter nociceptive input at the dorsal horn. The additional mechanoreceptor (large-diameter fiber) activation through gentle manual oscillatory techniques may serve to increase proprioceptive input further and enhance the inhibition of nociceptive transmission. The conventional stimulation mode is recommended for the two aforementioned procedures.

TENS also has a distinct role in producing masseter and temporalis re-

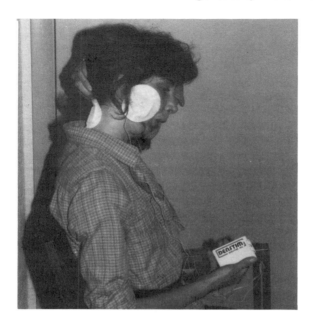

Fig. 11-6. Patient receiving very-low-rate masseter/temporalis muscle stimulation for postsurgical reduction of edema. Three electrodes are used, consisting of a positive ground electrode midline suboccipital and negative electrodes overlying each TMJ area.

laxation (reduction of guarding), as well as a reduction in postsurgical edema and pain.[66-69] A low-rate (0.5 to 1 Hz) mode producing slow, rhythmic muscle contractions is recommended for these applications (Fig. 11-6).

The simultaneous administration of moist heat and high- or low-voltage electrical stimulation can also be used effectively to decrease muscle guarding and chronic discomfort. Figure 11-7 illustrates application of this technique. The patient is in the supine position with separate electrode channels at the

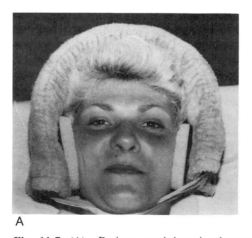
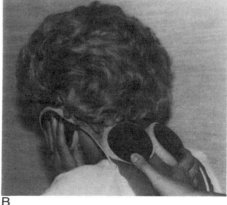

A   B

Fig. 11-7. (A) Patient receiving simultaneous administration of moist heat and high-voltage galvanic stimulation. **(B)** One channel of two electrodes is applied bilaterally at the suboccipital region; the other is placed over TMJ masseter area.

suboccipital region and TMJ/masseter area. A moist heat pack is applied over each electrode channel, serving to augment relaxation of muscle guarding, in crease tissue temperature; and easily hold the electrodes in place.

Recommended treatment time is 15 to 20 minutes, with stimulation parameters set at a pulse rate of 80 to 120 Hz and amplitude set at a comfortable level of electrical paresthesia (tingling). The unit is set in the reciprocal mode to allow 2- or 5-second alternate periods of stimulation at each site. Stimulation thus continues to switch every 2 or 5 seconds from one channel to the other during the entire treatment period.

Alternative applications can be performed using single-channel arrangements at the aforementioned areas or at the upper trapezius region. Unilateral arrangements may consist of one electrode at the suboccipital fossa and the other of the same channel at the ipsilateral TMJ/masseter region or bilaterally at the TMJ/masseter area with one channel. A wide variety of electrode placement techniques can be performed, many of which I have illustrated and discussed in previous publications.[1,66]

No appreciable difference in effectiveness has been observed clinically with changes in polarity or substitution of the high-voltage galvanic unit with a low-voltage unit.

Stimulation protocols can also include use of surging currents or pulsetrains, which can provide increased patient comfort or a mild contraction–relaxation form of stimulation for a reduction in muscle guarding. Small-diameter circular electrodes are preferred for conformity to the suboccipital and TMJ area.

Contraindications to Use of Electrotherapy

The manufacture and use of many electrotherapeutic devices is governed by the Food and Drug Administration (FDA). Portable stimulators for home use are considered class-2 medical devices and are thus strongly regulated. Manufacturers of TENS units must list the commonly known contraindications and precautions.[1,70] Electrical stimulation should not be performed on persons with a demand-type cardiac pacemaker or over the area of the carotid sinus, laryngeal, or pharyngeal musculature. Electrical stimulation may interfere with the action of the pacemaker or affect blood pressure and respiration with stimulation across the chest or anterior cervical spine, respectively. In addition, specific to the craniovertebral region, stimulation over the eyes should be avoided, as it should on the head or neck of patients with a history of transient ischemia attacks, cerebrovascular accidents, or epilepsy.[1,70] All the aforementioned contraindications apply equally to use of any of the elctrotherapeutic devices or techniques. Table 11-4 summarizes the use of electrotherapy.

Phonophoresis and Iontophoresis

In my clinical experience and practice, phonophoresis and iontophoresis are rarely used because effective pain control and a decrease in inflammation is usually obtained with other modalities discussed in this chapter. If needed,

Table 11-4. Electrotherapy

Low-voltage generators (LV), clinic and self-administration
High-voltage galvanic (HVG), clinic and self-administration
Transcutaneous electrical nerve stimulation (TENS), self-administration
Noninvasive electroacupuncture (EAP), clinic
Iontophoresis (IP), clinic and self-administration

	Stimulation parameters			
Techique	Amplitude	Frequency	Pulse Width	Electrodes
LV	0–100V	1–100 Hz	Fixed	Variable size
HVG	0–500V	1–80 Hz (twin peak)	Fixed or 5–100 u/sec	Ground required, variable size
TENS	0–80 mA	1–150 Hz	40–250 u/sec	Variable size
EAP	0–1,000 uA	1–128 Hz	Fixed	Hand-held probe
IP	0–5 mA	Continuous DC	Fixed	Variable size, medicinal application

Applications
↓ Edema
↓ Pain (acute, chronic and postoperative
↓ Muscle spasm
↓ Metabolites
↓ Inflammation
↑ Circulation
↑ Muscularly oriented occlusion
  Densensitize trigger points

however, they should be applied immediately after a 10-minute application of moist heat to the TMJ. Kahn recommends iontophoresis with Xylocaine (5 percent ointment) or hydrocortisone (1 percent ointment) under the positive electrode placed over the TMJ.[34,71] The negative (indifferent) electrode is placed on the shoulder or upper thoracic region. Recommended treatment parameters are 0–5 mA for 20 to 30 minutes. Due to possible irritation from the direct current, it may at times be beneficial to increase the milliamperage gradually to the maximal level which, if tolerated, is 4 to 5 mA. After iontophoresis, gentle mobilization and therapeutic exercise may be performed. A portable battery-operated unit called the Phoresor has simplified the performance of iontophoresis and also allows home use by the patient (Motion Control, Salt Lake City, UT). Bertolucci and Harris demonstrated effective use of this device with antiinflammatory agents in the management of musculoskeletal conditions.[72,73]

Delivery of similar antiinflammatory and analgesic agents can be provided by phonophoresis. Kahn states that deeper penetration may occur with delivery by ultrasound in comparison to electrical stimulation, but the therapeutic effect may not be as immediate. Kahn recommends an intensity of 1.0 W/cm² for 3 minutes and also suggests administering phonophoresis immediately after iontophoresis for an even better effect.[71]

Phonophoresis or iontophoresis may be effectively used over persistent trigger points as an additional means of desensitization. This will also be tolerated better than the technique of deep pressure massage for 2 to 3 minutes

Table 11-5. Phonophoresis and Iontophoresis

Selectivity drive in		
Antiinflammatory agents: corticosteroids, dexamethasone, salicylate		
Local analgesics: procaine/lidocaine hydrochloride		

Phonophoresis/Iontophoresis	vs	Injection
Tissue permeability by radiation pressure of US beam with phonophoresis		Tissue damage from bolus of H_2O
↑ Diffusion rate		

Technique: skin surface (medication + coupling agent)

Phonophoresis —	Sonation TMJ —	10% hydrocortisone ointment 1.5 W/cm^2 5 min
Iontophoresis —	TMJ/forehead —	2% lidocaine (+) 4 mA, 20 min

followed by ice for 6 to 10 minutes or hyperstimulation analgesia with electrotherapy devices. Table 11-5 summarizes the use of phono and iontophoresis.

Biofeedback

Biofeedback, unlike all the previously discussed adjunctive modalities, does not stimulate or deliver a thermal or chemical agent to the involved area. Biofeedback does the reverse; namely, it amplifies minute muscle action potentials or skin temperature to provide immediate feedback to the patient, through visual and/or auditory means, of data indicative of muscle contraction (spasm or guarding), relaxation, or hand warming. This information can be invaluable in teaching a patient voluntary self-regulation and awareness of abnormal physiological or biomechanical states that may perpetuate myofascial pain syndromes and concomitant dysfunction.

Electromyographic (EMG) feedback is the most commonly used type of biofeedback. Other forms are temperature, electroencephalographic (EEG), and galvanic skin response (GSR) biofeedback. EMG biofeedback can be a valuable aid in reducing bruxism, suboccipital or cervical spine muscle guarding, tinnitus, and postural retraining.[75-81] Appropriate referral for psychological evaluation may be necessary because stress and emotional tension can be significant factors in promoting bruxism and related muscle spasm. Behavioral intervention thus may be needed in keeping with the tenets of a comprehensive rehabilitation program.

Biofeedback devices can be either small, portable, and battery operated for home training or large sophisticated clinical models. General body relaxation training must precede specific biofeedback training. Instruction in diaphragmatic breathing, autogenic exercises, and visual imagery techniques are essential adjuncts to a successful biofeedback and stress reduction program.

SEQUENCING AND CLINICAL APPLICATION OF
THERAPEUTIC MODALITIES

The successful application of adjunctive therapeutic modalities depends on their proper sequencing within a comprehensive management program. In addition, two or more modalities used simultaneously can augment the response of each other. Finally, the treatment application and therapeutic dosage must be in line with the established biophysical and neurophysiological action of the modality or agents.

An excellent example of proper sequencing can be illustrated in the presence of an acute closed lock. TENS or another form of electrical stimulation can be used to obtain muscle relaxation. This can be augmented by simultaneous application of moist heat or, if electrical stimulation cannot be tolerated, moist heat can be administered separatley for 10 minutes to the involved TMJ as well as the cervical spine for relaxation of the musculature and initial elevation of tissue temperature. Ten minutes is sufficient, since maximal elevation of local temperature occurs within 6 to 8 minutes.[5,82] Immediately following administration of moist heat, ultrasound with sustained stretch can be performed over the TMJ while the patient periodically increases stretch by application of additional tongue depressors. The number of tongue depressors initially used should be equal to the comfortable limit of vertical opening that the patient can obtain after use of moist heat, with such opening not to excede 20 to 25 mm of vertical opening as long as the disc is anteriorly dislocated. The patient should add additional tongue depressors as relaxation occurs and vertical opening increases. If a constant stretch is not tolerated, tongue depressors may be totally or partially removed every 30 seconds during the 3- to 5-minute ultrasound application. Using ultrasound while placing the TMJ on stretch aids in decreasing muscle spasms and maintaining capsular extensibility. Such a stretch should not exceed 20 to 25 mm until satisfactory attempts at relocating the disk have been made.

When this heat and stretch technique is completed, gentle intraoral distractional mobilization to the TMJ should be performed, with appropriate instruction in a home exercise program as discussed in Chapter 6.

PAIN CONTROL AT HOME

Nonmedicinal means of pain control that patients can use independently consist of ice, vibration, acupressure, and TENS. Melzack and associates showed that a 7-minute application of ice massage solely to the dorsal web space on the side of pain decreased discomfort by at least 50 percent in patients with acute dental pain.[54] Vibratory stimulation and TENS has been extensively researched and is also at least 50 percent effective in relieving a wide variety of acute and chronic pain syndromes of head and neck origin.[83–86]

Stimulation parameters of a high rate (100 Hz) and application at the dorsal web space as well as at or close to the site of pain provided the best results.

TENS is also a valuable adjunctive technique in the management of acute cervical pain, but must not represent the sole therapeutic paradigm.[51,86]

TENS is perhaps most effective for use by the patient at home in the management of acute pain. In addition to use in definitive manual treatment of outpatients, TENS can be used to allow a quicker restoration of function by relieving muscle guarding and allowing proprioceptive input. Patients are also more willing to engage in a home exercise program when TENS is added for home use.[1,66]

A knowledge of the stimulation modes is necessary along with electrode placement sites to obtain optimal benefit with TENS. Table 11-6 presents a brief explanation of the adjustment guidelines relative to each mode. Electrical stimulation is usually not well tolerated on the head or face, yet at least one electrode may have to be placed at the site of facial pain if other arrangements are not beneficial. The initial application of TENS in this area should begin with electrode placement at the suboccipital fossa, where stimulation of the occipital nerves as well as the spinal tract of the trigeminal can be accomplished without facial stimulation.[1,66] Regardless of the specific pain syndrome involving the face, head, craniomandibular, or suboccipital region, a single channel of two electrodes placed in each depression between the cranial attachment of the SCM and upper trapezius should be the first choice.[1,66] The rationale for this electrode arrangement is related to the fact that the spinal tract of the trigeminal nerve has synaptic connections with the cervical spine at the C2 through C4 level.[11–14] Therefore, suboccipital stimulation may be able to produce pain relief at any facial or cranial region since both the trigeminal and occipital nerves can be simultaneously stimulated.

Electrode placement at the dorsal web space of the hand ipsilateral to the side of pain can be an effective remote stimulation site.[1,66,67] Segmental innervation of the dorsal web space is C5 through T1 and thus is not anatomically related to the spinal tract of trigeminal, although only one segment removed. Examination of Penfield's somatomotor and somatosensory cortices reveals an interesting relationship, however. Cortical cells that receive input from thumb and index finger stimuli lie adjacent to those of the head and face. The cortical inhibitory surround theory or "busy cortex" provides a possible explanation for the effectiveness of this remote unrelated site.[11,55,66] Significant excitation of a specific cortical region may result in inhibition and decreased sensitivity of an adjacent or surrounding cortical area. Thus, dorsal web space stimulation may produce an elevation of the excitation threshold of cortical cells representative of the face and head.

Electrode placement techniques incorporating both the suboccipital fossa and dorsal web space can also be evaluated prior to stimulation of the head or face.[66] When stimulation at sites other than the face or head fails to produce satisfactory relief, one electrode can be placed at the area of pain and the other at the ipsilateral suboccipital fossa and/or dorsal web space. A small circular electrode is recommended for facial application.[66] Clinical experience has shown that a single channel of one suboccipital electrode and the other at a superficial nerve site on the face is very effective (Fig. 11-5). In management

Table 11-6. The Stimulation Modes

	Step I	Step II	Step III	Step IV
			Adjustment Guidelines	
Mode	Pulse Rate	Pulse Width	Amplitude	Readjustment
Conventional	Preset within 50–100 Hz	Preset within 40–75 μs	Slowly activate one channel at a time and increase until a smooth comfortable electrical paresthesia is obtained.	Electrical paresthesia should be perceived throughout the distribution of the pain. Increasing the pulse width can result in a spread of paresthesia, comfort can be increased and accommodation minimized by modulation or burst features.
Strong low rate (acupuncture-like)	Preset 1–4 Hz	Preset 150–200 μs	Slowly activate one channel at a time and increase to highest tolerable level producing rhythmic muscle contractions.	Comfort can be increased by use of modulation.
Pulse-train (burst)	Preset within 70–100 Hz	Preset within 40–75 μs (low intensity) 150–200 μs (high intensity)	Slowly activate one channel at a time and increase to desired level. Paresthesia with rhythmic pulsing (low intensity) Paresthesia with rhythmic muscle contractions (high intensity) should occur.	Increasing pulse width can result in a spread of paresthesia if not perceived throughout distributions of pain.
Brief intense (should not be used on the face, head or neck)	Preset within 100–150 Hz	Preset within 150–200 μs	Slowly activate one channel at a time to highest tolerable level of paresthesia: Nonrhythmic muscle fasciculations or tetany should occur.	Increase amplitude and/or pulse width if sensation decreases. Activation of modulation can increase comfort and tolerance.

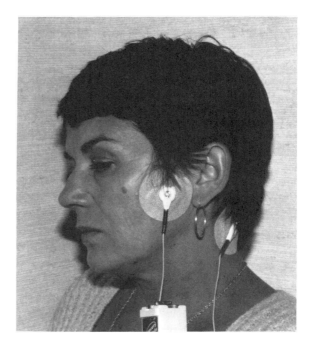

Fig. 11-8. Patient with Eagle's syndrome using transcutaneous electrical nerve stimulation for pain control at home. One electrode is placed over TMJ; the other is placed at ipsilateral suboccipital fossa (conventional mode).

of craniomandibular pain, one electrode on the TMJ or motor point of the masseter coupled with one at the ipsilateral suboccipital fossa is highly effective with the conventional stimulation mode. (Fig. 11-8). Acupuncture points exist at all these regions, but it is actually the superficial aspect of a peripheral nerve or one of its branches that provides the distinct anatomical connection to the CNS.[87,88] Many other electrode placement sites and channel arrangements can be performed with TENS. The reader is referred to the reference 66 for an in-depth examination and literature review.

Acupressure using a finger or the Cryo-stim probe is a simple technique that we often teach patients to use throughout the day for pain relief.[45,49,52–53] The best results usually occur when acupressure is initiated at the onset of craniomandibular pain. In line with the previously established protocol for electrical stimulation techniques, stimulation at distal sites is recommended initially. A typical protocol for pain relief through acupressure consists of strong manual massage with the thumb for 10 to 30 seconds in the following sequence:

1.   Massage the dorsal web space bilaterally one side at a time. Accurate placement of the thumb or probe produces the sensation of a deep ache locally as well as in the abductor digiti quinti ipsilaterally. This is attributed to stimulation of the ulnar nerve, which also innervates the first dorsal interosseous at the web space. (Superficial radial, musculocutaneous, and ulnar nerve).

2.   Make a fist and strongly pinch the small skin fold that juts out lateral

to the fifth metacarpal phalangeal joint. Use of the nails of the opposite thumb and index finger is recommended (ulnar nerve).

3.   Cup the occiput in each hand and place the thumbs in the suboccipital fossa bilaterally. Place the head in a position of axial extension and massage strongly at the suboccipital fossa (occipital nerve and spinal tract of trigeminal). The Cryo-stim probe can also be used at this region.

4.   Place each thumb in the depression lateral to the eyebrow at the superolateral aspect of the orbit of the eye. Massage strongly while maintaining the head in a supported position in axial extension (zygomaticotemporal nerve).

Acupressure should be performed to the maximal intensity that can be tolerated for 30 seconds. Seven minutes per site is recommended when using the Cryo-stim probe with mild to moderate pressure. At times, it may be necessary to repeat stimulation of each site a second or third time if benefit is not apparent after the initial application.

BIOFEEDBACK

The adjunctive use of biofeedback and relaxation training for the reduction of muscular tension has a long, well-documented history, especially in the management of headache and craniomandibular disorders.[81] In long-standing chronic myofascial pain syndromes, EMG biofeedback training may be especially helpful to teach resistive patients how to relax muscle guarding at the involved area by gaining increased awareness of the sensation of muscle contraction rather than relaxation.

Scott and Lundeen showed that healthy subjects could develop preauricular pain that was similar in quality to that of many TMJ patients by merely performing vigorous mandibular thrusting for 5 minutes.[74] This is extremely beneficial to convey to the patient who performs nocturnal bruxism. If 5 minutes of vigorous masticatory activity can cause significant discomfort, what will occur from hours of the same activity on a continual basis?

EMG biofeedback training can be used to teach general relaxation of the frontalis muscle initially. Prior to such a session, however, I recommend that the patient first be taught relaxed diaphragmatic breathing in a comfortable supine position with proper support to the cervical spine. Biofeedback electrodes can then be placed on the masseter muscles for site specific training. Scott and Gregg performed a review of the value of behavioral relaxation therapy and showed that this approach is a helpful clinical intervention.[81]

Clinical sequencing of EMG biofeedback-relaxation training may require its use on alternate days if physical therapy is also being performed. We have used relaxation training, however, as the initial therapeutic intervention for patients with acute pain such as a cervical strain or an acute anterior disc dislocation that does not reduce; definitive physical therapy techniques can then be initiated. The reduction in muscle tension may allow manual therapeutic techniques to be administered more easily. Increased awareness of the problems associated with the forward head posture can also be gained by EMG biofeedback training.

SUMMARY

This section has focused on the proper use of adjunctive therapeutic modalities as one part of the comprehensive management of patients with craniomandibular problems. The rationale, technique, treatment parameters, and sequencing for the use of each method has been provided and comprehensive treatment paradigms have been discussed. The important philosophy to remember is that each patient needs to be treated individually and evaluated thoroughly, and a therapeutic program must be initiated that combines patient education (posture, body mechanics), restoration of normal functions (manual therapy), and preventative maintenance. The methods, techniques, and modalities discussed in this section can be used to enhance the effectiveness of all aspects of the rehabilitation program.

Orthopedic
Physical Therapy

Marty Kaput

The entire body acts as an integrated whole. Although one can separate the body into its various component parts, structurally and physiologically these individual components act together. Generally, the closer in proximity these components lie, the closer together they function. The craniomandibular system is strongly influenced by the components of the upper quarter. The upper quarter describes the relationship of the cervical spine to the thoracic spine and the shoulder girdle. These areas are anatomically integrated and physiologically coordinated. Any dysfunction in one area can potentially cause a dysfunction in a related area. This disturbs the normal balance between the craniomandibular system and the upper quarter.

The upper quarter can influence the craniomandibular system in numerous ways:

1. Head and neck posture have effects on mandibular position and movement, as described in chapter 12.
2. The upper quarter is a significant area that refers pain into the classical TMJ areas. Travell has documented that trigger points in the sternocleidomastoid and upper trapezius muscles can refer pain into the facial region.[89]
3. Trott and Goss in their study of 34 patients with myofascial pain dysfunction syndrome of the masticatory system found corresponding pain and dysfunction in the cervical spine in 56 percent of their patients.[90] Cervical spine dysfunction resulting in headaches has been extensively reported in the literature.[91-93]
4. The President's Conference also recommends evaluating for musculoskeletal problems when evaluating a "TMJ" patient.[94]

Because the upper quarter is so closely associated with the craniomandibular system, evaluation and treatment in this area is often necessary to deal fully with the TMJ patient. These patients often have involvement of the myo-

Table 11-7. Evaluation
1. History
2. Structural evaluation
3. Active range of motion
4. Palpation
5. Passive range of motion
6. Provocation tests
7. Neurologic tests

fascial system in the head, jaw, neck, and shoulder areas. Establishing a better head–neck relationship will help achieve myofascial harmony. Establishing this relationship will assist the dentist in approaching an ideal craniomandibular relationship that will allow the patient to function optimally and, ideally, pain-free.

This section of the chapter has two purposes: *first* to present to the physical therapist upper quarter evaluation and treatment concepts, and, *second* to improve the dentist's awareness of the role of physical therapy in the management of patients with craniomandibular dysfunction and myofascial pain dysfunction (MPD).

EVALUATION

The physical therapy evaluation is one of the most important parts of any physical therapy regimen. This evaluation is not performed to diagnose a disease; rather, it is a clarifying examination to determine the nature and extent of the existing dysfunction. An initial evaluation is always performed, but the process does not end with this evaluation. The process must be ongoing for best management of a patient's problem. The evaluation is the foundation on which the physical therapy treatment is based.

Each therapist may have a different regimen of evaluation. The regimen should be fairly rigid so that all components of the evaluation are covered. This does not mean that the therapist will not deviate when necessary from the usual routine, but a consistent, thorough evaluation is a primary safeguard for detecting signs and symptoms of more serious pathology. The evaluation is divided into seven areas (Table 11-7). Each area supplies pertinent information regarding the patient's dysfunction. The therapist should avoid making premature judgments as to the cause of the patient's dysfunction before all data are collected. A form is useful to assist the therapist in recording the information in a logical and concise manner (Fig. 11-9).

HISTORY

The history helps the therapist to determine which systems should be examined. This portion of the evaluation allows the patients to discuss their problems with the therapist. Because most patients have complaints of pain, specific

```
┌─────────────────────────────────────────────────────────────────┐
│                     UPPER QUARTER EVALUATION                      │
│  Chief Complaint: _____  │
│  _____   │
│  _____   │
│  _____   │
│  _____   │
│  History: _____  │
│  _____   │
│  _____   │
│  _____   │
│                                                                   │
│  Structural Exam:                            Palpation:           │
│        ○        _____            _____    │
│       ▽|▽       _____            _____    │
│        |        _____            _____    │
│        |        _____            _____    │
│        |        _____            _____    │
│        ▽                                                          │
│  AROM:                         PROM:         Shoulder:            │
│               Cervical Spine:  _____     _____    │
│  Restricted |                  _____     _____    │
│  Blocked ||                    _____     _____    │
│  Pain/Restr X                  _____     _____    │
│  Hypermobile ∿                 _____     _____    │
│                                                                   │
│  Provocation Tests:                                               │
│  1) Cervical Compression __  Distraction __                       │
│  2) TOS 1st R__  L__  2nd R__  L __  3rd R__  L __                 │
│  3) Vertebral Artery R__  L__                                     │
│  4) Shoulder Locking R__  L_                                      │
│                                                                   │
│  Neurological:                                                    │
│                        Dermatone: _____               │
│                        Myotone: _____               │
│                        Reflexes: _____               │
└─────────────────────────────────────────────────────────────────┘
```

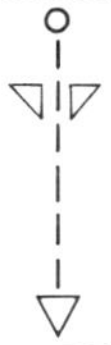

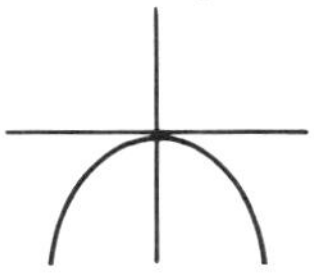

Fig. 11-9.   Upper quarter evaluation form.

questions regarding the pain will help the examiner direct the patient's thoughts (Table 11-8).

The first part of the history helps the therapist to determine the area, depth, nature, behavior and chronology of the patient's symptoms and also helps the therapist rule out signs and symptoms of more serious pathology. When pain is of a deep, boring nature, unchanged with different positions or with treat-

Table 11-8. History Questions

---

1. Do you have pain in the head, neck, or shoulder area? Upper back?
2. Do you have any pain that extends into your arms?
3. Do you have any weakness or tingling in your arms?
4. Do you have any difficulty or pain with movement of your neck?
5. Do you have any difficulty, pain, or weakness with movement of your arms?
6. Are your daily activities disturbed by the pain in your head and neck areas?
7. Is the pain constant or intermittent?
8. Is the pain of a burning nature or is it dull, sharp, or aching?
9. Where did the pain initially start?
10. Was this associated with any accident or injury?
11. Where did the pain progress to?
12. What makes your pain better?
13. What makes your pain worse?
14. What position do you sleep in?
15. Can you get comfortable at night?
16. Does the pain wake you from sleeping?
17. How do you feel in the morning?
18. Is there any pattern to your pain during the morning, afternoon, and evening?
19. How has the pain changed since the initial onset?
20. Have you undergone any previous treatment?
21. What was your response to such treatment?
22. Do you have any other medical problems?
23. Have you had any past surgery?
24. What medications are you taking?
25. Is there anything else you would like to tell me about your problem?

---

ment, more serious pathology can be suspected. Most pains of musculoskeletal origin will change with different postures and activities. Some position or movement should provoke the involved tissue and increase the pain, whereas other movements and rest positions should decrease the pain. The physical therapist should inquire specifically about the patient's work and rest postures.

The behavior of the pain can also be used to document progress. That the patient can maintain a work or rest posture longer is a sign of improvement. The extent of the pain can be used in the same manner. Generally, a more localized pain indicates an improvement in the dysfunction.[95,96]

Reports of numbness, tingling, or weakness are signals of possible neurological involvement and must be evaluated. The therapist should try to determine if the numbness is objective or subjective and if the weakness is isolated to a specific myotome or is more generalized secondary to pain or disuse.

The response of the patient to previous treatments can also be helpful in determining which treatment approaches the therapist may wish to use to begin treatment. Patients may report that previously they used heat or cold and that this significantly changed their pain. Patients also report that they had physical therapy previously from a chiropractor or dentist, and that it did not help significantly. Further questioning may reveal that this treatment was an individual modality, such as ultrasound or electrical stimulation given alone, not in conjunction with a full physical therapy regimen. A therapist who then decides to use these modalities in conjunction with a full treatment program must explain the rationale for their use to patients so that they understand that this program is different from what they previously received.

The therapist must also be aware of other medical problems that may hinder or complicate treatment. This is discussed more fully later in this chapter.

Last, the therapist should give the patient time to express any other concerns that were not specifically covered in the previous questions. Although most of the questions in the history deal with the patient's perception of the pain, the therapist cannot allow this to determine the cause of the pain. Pain itself can be misleading. Pain is often felt at a site far removed from the dysfunction (e.g., pain felt over the medial pterygoid muscle may arise from the medial pterygoid but also may be referred from the posterior cervical musculature.[89,92] The history, although important, is only one part of a total evaluation.

STRUCTURAL EXAMINATION

When evaluating a patient with upper quarter dysfunction, the therapist focuses evaluation on the upper quarter; however, because all parts of the body are interrelated and interdependent, the therapist also performs a screening examination of the lower quarter. Evaluation of these areas can be important in identifying precipitating and perpetuating factors in the patient's original complaints of pain and dysfunction.

The structural examination allows the therapist to evaluate the patient's standing posture. Posture refers to the alignment and relationship of the component parts of the body to each other. Generally, the more efficiently the body is aligned, the more efficiently it will function. Poor alignment creates an environment for mechanical stresses and strains to the various anatomical structures that can eventually lead to pain and dysfunction.

Posture is evaluated in two planes, the frontal and saggital planes. A plumb line is helpful in assessing this posture. In the saggital plane, the plumb line should pass through the tragus of the ear, the shoulder joint, slightly posterior to the axis of the hip joint, slightly anterior to the axis of the knee joint, and slightly anterior to the lateral malleolus (Fig. 11-10).[97] In the frontal plane, the plumb line should be equidistant from the medial aspects of the heels, legs and thighs, and the scapula. This line should coincide with the midline of the trunk and head (Fig. 11-11).[97] One common change that occurs in patients with upper quarter dysfunction is the forward head posture, which involves backward bending of the upper cervical spine, a decrease in the normal midcervical lordosis, and an increase in the upper thoracic kyphosis and lumbar lordosis.[98] The shoulder girdle is usually elevated and protracted, with internal rotation at the glenohumeral joints. Side tilting of the head may also be apparent and may be secondary to muscle involvement or more subtle joint restrictions.

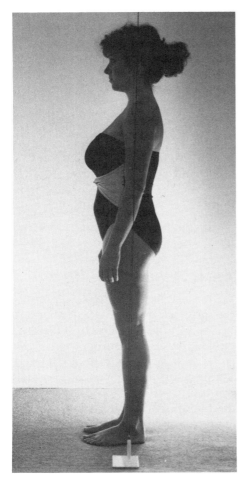 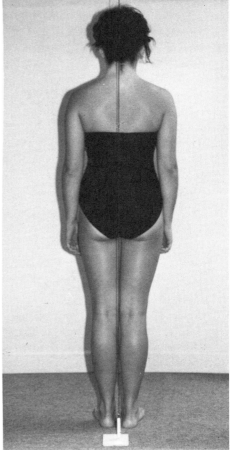

Fig. 11-10. Posture viewed from sagittal plane.

Fig. 11-11. Posture viewed from frontal plane.

ACTIVE ROM

The active mobility of the patient alerts the therapist to the willingness of the patient to move, the overall ROM, and the quality of the movement. The examiner tests cervical spine side bending, rotation, forward bending, backward bending, and nodding, with the patient in a standing or a sitting position. At the end of each ROM, if limited, the examiner should note if pain or stiffness limits motions. Slight overpressure can also be administered to note the feeling of the resisting tissues. Movements that are full, pain-free, and pain-free even with overpressure can usually be cleared of symptomatic musculoskeletal pathology. Limitations in movements may incriminate the facet joints, their capsules, ligaments, and muscles.

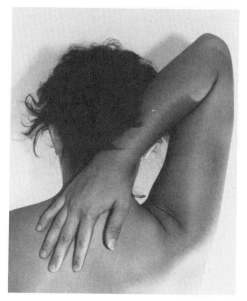
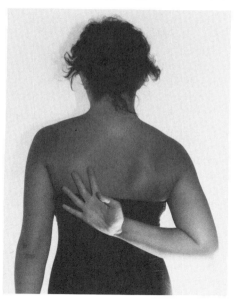

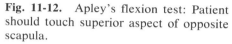

Fig. 11-12. Apley's flexion test: Patient should touch superior aspect of opposite scapula.

Fig. 11-13. Apley's extension test: Patient should touch inferior angle of opposite scapula.

With active movements of the cervical spine, the astute observer can also note some mobility in the upper thoracic region. Active mobility here is fairly limited because of the attachments of the ribs and the presence of soft tissue. Forward bending and rotation are the easiest movements to examine in the upper thoracic region. Limitations in cervical movement, especially in forward bending and rotation, can be secondary to restrictions primarily found in the upper thoracic region.

If shoulder girdle pathology is suspected, especially if the patient describes any pain in the shoulder girdle area or difficlty with movement in this area, the shoulder girdle must be ruled out as a primary cause of dysfunction. This will help to differentiate whether the pain is simply referred from the cervical spine or is local, or both. Two simple clearing tests are Apley's flexion and extension tests.[99] The flexion test (Fig. 11-12) evaluates a combined movement of shoulder flexion, adduction, and external rotation. The extension test (Fig. 11-13) combines extension, adduction, and internal rotation movements.

PALPATION

Palpation is invaluable to the therapist. The therapist palpates the skin, subcutaneous tissue, muscles, ligaments, joint lines, and superficial aspects of the peripheral nerves, seeking an area of "difference." This difference is the change from the expected normal. The skin is palpated for subjective tenderness and objective changes in temperature, moisture, and texture. Specific areas of tenderness are noted; however, this is not necessarily a reliable indicator of the primary source of the pathology. An increase in temperature is an indication of inflammation. Cool areas or dry shiny skin is more indicative of chronic conditions.[98] The subcutaneous tissue is then palpated for abnormal amounts of fat, tissue fluid, tension, localized swelling, and nodules. Fatty nodules may be present. Although frequently tender, they are not usually a primary source of dysfunction. An increase in tissue tension is often felt in the upper thoracic region when a dowager's hump exists. Localized areas of swelling are also noted. Next, the examiner palpates the specific muscle groups. Muscles are palpated for a change in muscle tone and for muscle spasm and trigger points. If the patient reports pain from palpation of the muscle, the examiner will further determine if the pain is felt locally or is referred into another area. The ligament nuchae and supraspinous ligaments are the only ligaments directly palpable in the cervical and thoracic spine. Chronic problems may produce a thickened ligament. The joint lines are also palpated. The cervical facet joints are palpated for changes in their positions and for edema. Superficial aspects of the nerves can be palpated for tenderness as well as for reproduction of the patient's symptoms (e.g., palpation in the interscaleni triangle may reproduce the patient's arm complaints).

In the upper quarter region, numerous areas can be palpated (Table 11-

Table 11-9. Palpation Sites

1.	First and second costosternal joints
2.	Sternoclavicular joints
3.	Inferior border of the clavicle
[a]4.	Sternocleidomastoid muscle—insertion and muscle belly
[a]5.	Scaleni muscles
[a]6.	Interscaleni triangle
7.	Position of the hyoid bone
8.	Superior border of the clavicle
9.	Pectoralis major/minor
10.	Coracoid process
11.	Subscapularis tendon and bursa
12.	Bicipital groove
13.	Supraspinatous tendon
14.	Infraspinatous tendon
15.	Transverse process of atlas
[a]16.	Lateral margins of the facet joints
[a]17.	Suboccipital muscle
[a]18.	Greater occipital nerve
[a]19.	Upper trapezius muscle
[a]20.	Levator scapula muscle
20.	Supraspinatous muscle belly
21.	Infraspinatous muscle belly
[a]23.	Rhomboid major and minor muscles
24.	Terres major and minor muscles
25.	Latissimus dorsi muscle at its attachment on the scapula

[a] Palpation sites for dentists.

9). The therapist must take a systematic approach so that all areas will be covered. One easy regimen is to start anteriorly and to move posteriorly.

PASSIVE ROM

Another use of palpation is detecting passive ROM. Passive mobility tests the accessory motions of the facet joints of the cervical and thoracic spine and the shoulder complex. Accessory motions are arthrokinematic movements that are necessary for full osteokinematic movement[98] A patient may be limited in the osteokinematic movement of rotation to the right of the cervical spine. This may occur for several reasons. Possible explanations are that the facet joint of the midcervical spine on the right cannot glide down and backward or that the facet joint on the left may be restricted in the up and forward gliding movement. These gliding movements are the accessory arthrokinematic movements. Obviously other factors, including pain and muscle restrictions, may be limiting the motion. Passive mobility testing helps to locate the level or levels involved and also helps to rule out facet restrictions as the cause of the dysfunction. The mobility at each level is graded as normal, hypermobile, or hypomobile. Some authorities use a more specific 0–6 grading scale with 0 describing a fused joint and 6 describing a hypermobile joint[100]

Passive mobility of the subcranial, midcervical and, upper thoracic spine can be assessed through numerous techniques. The interested reader can refer to the bibliography for a list of texts that review these techniques.[98,101–103] Three representative techniques are illustrated in Figures 11-14 through 11-16. Some skepticism exists in the medical community as to the reliability of passive mobility testing. One study by physical therapists demonstrated the intrarater reliability of passive mobility testing in the lumbar spine.[100] In an osteopathic study of the thoracic spine, five examiners agreed 79 percent of the time when distinguishing between thoracic segments with an increase in deep tissue tension as compared with normal tension.[104]

If the shoulder is involved, passive mobility of the shoulder joint complex must also be evaluated. Passive mobility of the shoulder involves moving the joint through its osteokinematic ranges of flexion, extension, abduction, adduction, horizontal abduction, horizontal adduction, internal rotation, and external rotation. The arthrokinematic glides must also be assessed together with the accessory motions at the acromioclavicular, sternoclavicular, and scapular thoracic joints.

PROVOCATION TESTS

Some of the evaluation procedures already described are used to provoke or reproduce the patient's pain. Active and passive testing as well as palpation may provoke pain, but these tests are also considered positive if there is any change in mobility or a difference from the expected normal reaction to palpation. These next tests are specifically designed to incriminate certain struc-

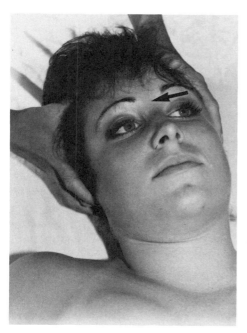

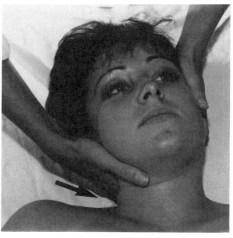

Fig. 11-15. Therapist evaluates side-bending of midcervical spine.

Fig. 11-14. Therapist palpates transverse process of C1 with index finger of right hand. As head is brought into sidebending right, C1 moves to right and becomes more prominent under therapist's palpating index finger.

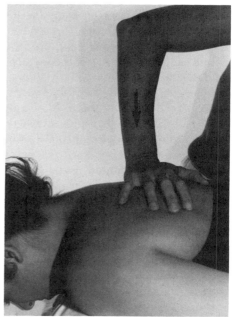

Fig. 11-16. Therapist spring-tests for passive mobility of thoracic spine.

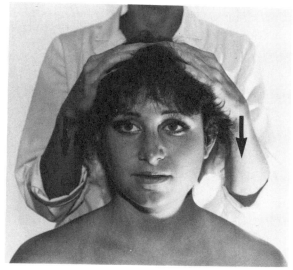

Fig. 11-17. Cervical compression testing: Therapist imparts downward compressive force through cervical spine.

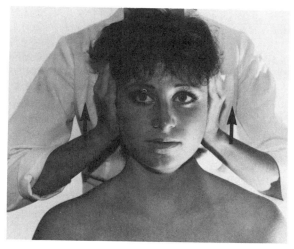

Fig. 11-18. Cervical distraction testing: Therapist imparts upward force, distracting cervical spine.

tures by recreating or intensifying the patient's symptoms. These tests include cervical spine compression, distraction, thoracic outlet testing, vertebral artery testing, and shoulder locking.

Cervical compression and distraction tests are illustrated in Figures 11-17 and 11-18. An increase in symptoms with compression testing may indicate foraminal encroachment or facet impingement. A decrease in pain with distraction testing may indicate nerve root compression or facet or disc pathology. This test can also help the therapist determine whether cervical traction would be a valuable treatment modality.

The thoracic outlet is an area closely related to the cervical spine. At this superior aperture of the thorax, compression of the subclavian vessels and brachial plexus can occur. When compression does occur in this area, the

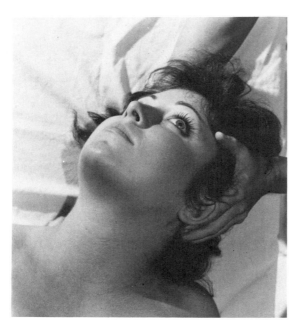

Fig. 11-19.   Vertebral artery testing.

patient has signs and symptoms similar to those of cervical dysfunction. Pain as well as associated paresthesia and muscle weakness can occur.

Compression can occur in three specific areas: the interscaleni triangle, the costoclavicular triangle, and the subcoracoid triangle. Adson's test, as described in many texts, is the test most commonly used to incriminate the thoracic outlet.[89,99,105] Reproduction of pain and a change in the radial pulse are considered positive signs of thoracic outlet involvement. In one study of asymptomatic persons, however, 82 percent had a diminished radial pulse.[106] With Adson's test, all three areas are compressed at one time, and a positive test does not help the therapist determine the exact structures at fault. Other authors describe three tests, one to incriminate each of the triangles.[98,107]

Another provocation test is that of the vertebral artery (Fig. 11-19). This test is important, especially if treatment is to be directed to the upper cervical spine. By performing this test, the therapist helps ensure that mobilization or stretching movements will not compromise the vertebral artery. During this test, the patient lies supine on the treatment table. The therapist cautiously bends the upper cervical spine backward and rotates the head to one side.[98] This position is held for approximately 30 seconds. The therapist then asks the patient whether any dizziness, nausea, tinnitus, or unusual sensations is experienced. The therapist also observes the patient's pupils for changes in constriction and dilation. The test is considered positive if any of these signs or symptoms occur. This test should then be repeated by rotating the head to the opposite side. Although this test is described late in the evaluation, it should be performed prior to any other subcranial testing maneuver. If signs and symptoms are positive, extreme care should be exercised during any further eval-

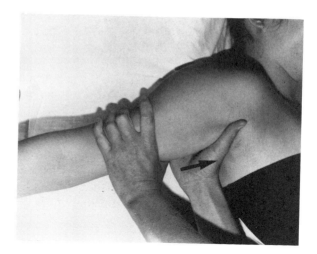

Fig. 11-20.   Shoulder locking maneuver.

uation and treatment of the cervical spine because a cerebral vascular accident (CVA) may occur.

To help rule out the shoulder as a major cause of the patient's symptoms, the shoulder locking maneuver can be used (Fig. 11-20). During this test, the therapist holds the patient's shoulder in abduction, extension, and slight medial rotation with one hand. With the other hand, the therapist imparts an anterior force to the patient's shoulder. Pain with this test signals the examiner to evaluate the shoulder girdle further.

NEUROLOGICAL EXAMINATION

The neurological examination consists of testing dermatomes, myotomes, and reflexes. The simple clinical testing of each area has its own difficulties with performance and interpretation. Dermatome evaluation involves using pin pricks to compare the patient's sensation side to side. This test relies heavily on the subjective response of the patient. Dermatome charts also vary from one text to another.[98] The patient may also experience some change in sensation even when no neurologic deficit exists. Travell documented changes in sensation in areas of referred pain from myofascial origin.[89] Total anesthesia in a dermatome is a true neurologic sign.[96] Hyperesthesia may also exist, as in trigeminal neuralgia.

Myotomes are then tested, and the strength of each muscle group is compared with that of the opposite side. When weakness is detected, the therapist must determine if the weakness is secondary to a neurological deficit or is secondary to pain or disuse. Generally, pain of a neurological origin is reflected in muscle weakness in only one or two muscle groups. If the weakness is diffuse, the therapist should not suspect a neurological deficit, but rather pain or disuse as the causative agent. Again, the reliability of this test depends on the patient to exert an equal amount of muscular effort bilaterally.

The reflex tests of the upper quarter are the biceps (C5), brachial radialis (C6), and triceps (C7). A diminished reflex may not exclusively indicate a neurological impingement. Mooney and Robertson showed changes in the lower quarter reflexes with injection of a local anesthetic into the corresponding lumbar facet joints.[96] All these tests should be documented and can be used as a mechanism to record change in the patient's status.

DENTAL EVALUATION OF THE UPPER QUARTER

The dentist can use an abbreviated form of evaluation of the upper quarter to help identify the patients to refer to physical therapy. The history is the chief portion of the examination that will help the dentist determine whether a physical therapy referral is necessary. If a patient complains of pain in the neck, shoulders, upper back, or down the arms, a physical therapy referral may be indicated. The dentist should ask the patient specifically if these areas are involved. If the dentist is not specific, patients may only describe their craniofacial pain since this is the area for which they are seeking the dental consultation. The first six questions in Table 11-8 are the most important questions for the dentist to ask the patient.

Next, observation of the patient's posture is important. The typical forward head posture should alert the dentist to possible musculoskeletal dysfunction in the upper quarter. To evaluate this further, the dentist can perform simple active ROM tests to the cervical spine and specific palpation tests (see Table 11–9).

The dentist should remember that this is only a screening examination and that some patients may have subtle findings that elude detection with this examination. If the patient does not respond as anticipated with the dental treatment, and if cervical spine dysfunction may be the reason, the dentist may still wish to refer the patient to a physical therapist for a more detailed evaluation.

OTHER CERVICAL SPINE PATHOLOGY

The physical therapist and dentist must both be alert to other pathology in the cervical spine that is not simply of a musculoskeletal-functional origin. They must also be aware of other medical problems of the patient that can affect or hinder their treatment. Patients with other pathology include: those involved in trauma in which a fracture may be suspected; those with upper extremity pain, sensory loss, and muscle weakness or atrophy in which the disc or nerve root may be involved; elderly patients especially women, who may have severe osteoporotic or spondylitic changes; patients who complain of dizziness when they look overhead, in whom a compromise of the vertebral artery may be suspected; and patients who have pain in the craniomandibular/ upper quarter area with few objective signs in this area and a strong profile for cardiac disease. All these patients must be referred to the appropriate physician for full medical management and/or clearing of their problem. After medical consultation, physical therapy and/or dental intervention may be appropriate. A medical consultation is also important when a patient does not respond as anticipated. Other less obvious medical problems may be hindering their progress.

Many other medical problems can affect the physical therapy treatment. These must be identified on an individual patient basis. Some of the more common problems include respiratory disease, allergies, poor vision or hearing, poor nutrition, and side effects of medications the patient may be taking. Respiratory problems or allergies that limit a patient's ability to be a nasal breather can significantly alter a patient's posture and use of cervical musculature. Mouth breathers tend to assume a more forward head posture (FHP) and to use their anterior cervical musculature to assist in respiration. A deficit in a patient's vision or hearing may cause compensation with stressful head and neck postures. Ill-fitting eyeglasses can significantly alter a patient's head/neck relationship. If a patient's eyeglasses tilt from one side to the other or slide down on the nose, the patient may unconsciously try to adjust the position of the head to compensate for this position of the glasses. This can keep the head and neck in a strained position for long periods of time. Moreover, people who wear bifocals often have to change their head/neck posture to see out both portions of the glass. Often these people tilt their heads backward to see through the lenses instead of lowering the reading material.

A patient with impaired hearing, especially unilaterally, may constantly maintain the head in a side-bent position toward the better side to get closer to the person speaking and improve the ability to hear.

The therapist should be aware of medication patients are taking and of their general nutritional status. Certain medications can hinder the effectiveness of certain modalities, especially TENS. This modality does not work well with diazepam, narcotics, and corticosteroids, and is enhanced with tryptophan and serotonin derivatives.[108] Some nutritional inadequacies can perpetuate muscle involvement.[89]

PHYSICAL THERAPY TREATMENT

The physical therapy treatment can be divided into three areas; modalities, hands-on manual techniques, and patient education. Modalities are discussed in the previous section of this chapter. This section covers hands-on-manual treatment and patient education. Treatment can be directed toward the muscle, joint, ligament, capsules and/or overall posture. The extent to which each structure is involved helps determine the emphasis and order of treatment.

Manual Techniques

Hands-on manual treatment includes various soft tissue stretching and massaging techniques as well as joint mobilization. This discussion is an overview and is not meant to be an exhaustive description of all possible techniques.

Joint manipulation is very helpful in decreasing pain and restoring mobility and proper posture to the cervical spine. Joint manipulation is a therapeutic maneuver applied to a joint that does not have normal movement to restore the joint's normal arthrokinematics.[109] Arthrokinematics refers to the intimate mechanics of the joint surfaces, such as their roll, spin, and slide movements.[110] There are various techniques and philosophies of joint manipulation. Three basic schools of thought exist.

Osteopathy and other disciplines including physical therapy have used manipulation to restore normal movement.[98] Other physical therapists, including the followers of Maitland[102] and Maigne[111] use manipulation to relieve pain. Chiropractic philosophy states that manipulation relieves nerve root pressure.[98] The techniques of joint manipulation are as varied as the philosophies. These techniques range from gentle oscillations to forceful thrusting maneuvers.

The physical therapy rationale for using joint manipulation has some basis in the scientific literature. Joint manipulation is used for its neurophysiologic effects of relieving pain or for its mechanical effects on connective tissue to restore normal movement.[109] Freeman and Wyke[112] showed that movement stimulates the various joint mechanoreceptors; in the gate control theory of Melzack and Wall,[113] this can inhibit pain. Mechanically, manipulation especially performed at end ranges can take the connective tissue into the plastic range of its stress–strain curve and assist in tissue elongation. Movement also helps in the alignment of the collagen fibers of the connective tissue[114,115] and thus helps normalize motion. There are a variety of joint manipulation techniques. Two specific techniques to promote the normal gliding of the facet joints are shown in Figures 11-21 and 11-22.

Another type of effective stretching to the cervical spine uses mechanical traction. The physical therapist must use caution when placing a patient with TMJ dysfunction in a conventional traction unit. Typical cervical traction units use head halters that pull through the mandible. This places a significant amount of pressure on the TMJs. Although this modality can be useful in treating the cervical spine, the benefit may be outweighed by the possibility of increasing TMJ dysfunction. Some possible solutions are to use manual traction, a head halter that pulls only through the occiput such as the Goodley polyaxial cervical traction system (E-Z-EM, 7 Portland Avenue, Westbury, NY 11590), or Saunder's cervical traction adaptation (Chattanooga, 101 Memorial Drive, Chattanooga, TN 37405) to the regular traction machines. If a conventional head halter is used, dental rolls should be placed between the back molars to minimize compressive forces on the TMJs.

In addition to the techniques directed toward the joint capsule and ligaments, the muscle must also be addressed. Soft tissue massage includes various effleurage, light stroking movements and pétrissage deeper kneading techniques to aid in muscle relaxation and elongation. Muscle stretching is also performed using passive as well as contraction–relaxation-type exercises as promoted by Knott and Voss.[116] These latter techniques use the principle of reciprocal inhibition. In the extremity joints, this type of active stretching is

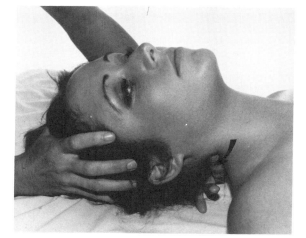

Fig. 11-21. This technique promotes posteroinferior gliding of the right facet joints.

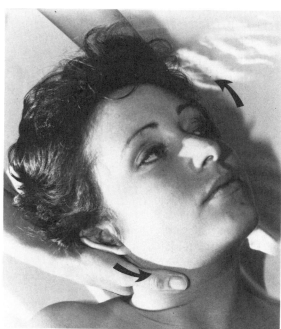

Fig. 11-22. This technique promotes anterosuperior gliding of right facet joints.

superior to passive stretching in achieving muscle elongation.[117,118] Strong resistive exercise in the cervical spine must be used judiciously, in acute cervical dysfunction because of the increased joint reaction forces created in the small facet joints with such exercise.

Other techniques include use of submaximal contractions to promote normal movement through various ROMs. Myofascial release techniques, first described in the osteopathic literature, are gaining increased popularity. These techniques try to balance the myofascial system through a mechanical and neuroreflexive approach.[119] Other schools of thought include those of Alexander[120], Feldenkreis[121] and craniosacral concepts[122] and techniques. Regardless of the approach, all the techniques are designed to normalize the patient's mobility, posture, muscle tone, strength, and coordination.

PATIENT EDUCATION

Education is the key to prevention. The patient needs to be educated as to the predisposing and precipitating factors that can aggravate TMJ/upper quarter dysfunction. These predisposing and perpetuating factors are the factors that the patient is responsible for controlling and may include poor postures, faulty work habits, poor stress management techniques, poor occlusion, and poor oral habits. These factors must be dealt with in the overall management of these patients. Physical therapy can help in most of these areas. The patient's education must extend into the home environment, and home instruction is a critical part of every physical therapy program. A home program enhances the patient's participation in the physical therapy treatment and also supplements treatment sessions. The home program can be divided into two areas: proper postures and home exercises.

Postures

The patient should be aware of three basic postures: standing, sitting, and lying postures. The components of proper standing posture have been described previously. Some patients may be able to attain proper posture simply through verbal guidance. Other patients may require physical therapy treatments to stretch, coordinate, and strengthen the various muscle groups and verbal guidance to achieve the proper posture. In one case study, various manual muscle stretching techniques, joint mobilization, active exercises, and a home program were used to help a patient achieve a more balanced posture.[123] Some verbal cues that can be used to assist the patient in achieving a better head–neck relationship are: "Tuck in the chin, keep the chest high, and tighten the abdominal muscles." The therapist must be aware of overdoers and help such patients to moderate attempts at achieving an improved posture.

Evaluation of the patient's posture in a sitting position is also important. Many people work sitting at their desks a good portion of their day. McKenzie observed that most people assume a slumped posture when sitting for any time. This posture increases backward bending of the cervical spine, increases upper thoracic kyphosis, and decreases lower lumbar lordosis.[95] The patient should be instructed to maintain the lumbar lordosis while sitting. This will help to maintain the proper positioning of the cervical and thoracic spine. Because most people assume a flexed position after sitting for a time, an external support such as a lumbar cushion to maintain the lumbar lordosis is invaluable.[124] The use of arm rests also helps relieve some of the stress on the shoulder girdle and upper trapezius muscles.

When a patient sits at a desk or other work surface, the work surface height can also influence sitting posture and stress on the upper quarter. The proper work height can be determined by evaluating the worker's shoulder position. The shoulders should be flexed approximately 25° and abducted 15 to 20°. This position minimizes the EMG activity of the trapezius, deltoids and erector spinae muscles.[125] Also, too low a work position increases the thoracic and lumbar kyphosis, whereas a high work surface causes abduction and elevation of the shoulder girdle. The ergonomics of the work environment is especially important for people who use computer terminals. One national survey reported that 56 percent of these workers complained daily of shoulder, neck, and back pain.[126]

The last posture to consider is the sleeping posture. The sleeping position is important in that it is probably the longest single postural activity a person undertakes. It is also the activity that persons may have the least control over, being in an altered state of consciousness. If the patient complains of an increase in pain on awakening in the morning, or of morning stiffness, the sleeping posture, pillow, and mattress must be examined. While one sleeps, the ideal posture is one that maintains the joints, ligaments, and muscles in a balanced neutral position. This can be most easily attained by sleeping in the supine position with a cervical pillow to support the cervical lordosis. Another pillow under the cervical pillow may be necessary, especially if the patient has a significant thoracic kyphosis. A pillow under the knees will help neutralize the lumbar lordotic curve. This may not be indicated in a person with an active lumbar disc condition. Sleeping side-lying, once again with the cervical pillow to support the neck and a pillow between the knees to keep the lumbar spine in a neutral position, is also an acceptable sleeping posture. Sleeping prone should be avoided because this position places the cervical spine in a rotated and extended position, which stresses the joints, muscles, and ligaments of the spine. The relative firmness of the mattress is a very individualized matter in regard to comfort. Generally, a firmer mattress will provide more support than will a soft or sagging mattress. Although no specific data have been recorded on the effectiveness of water beds, some patients find these beds very restful for sleeping. Water beds with a heating component may provide extra relaxation to the cervical, thoracic, and lumbar musculature.

Home Exercises

Specific self-mobilizing exercises are important to help the patient gain control over his musculoskeletal status. Many variations of exercises are helpful in this area. The major areas to focus on are: axial extension, upper trapezius, and levator scapula stretching; pectoralis major and minor stretching;

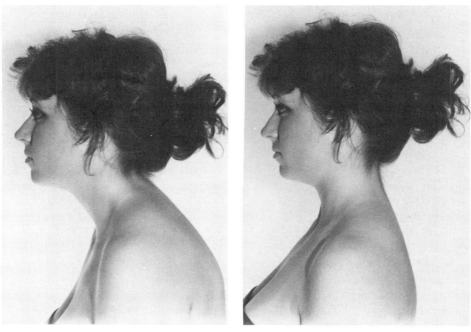

Fig. 11-23.   During axial extension, patient tucks in chin while keeping eyes level.

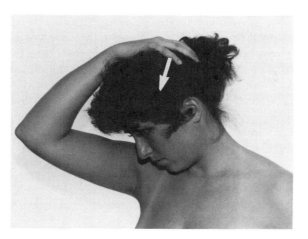

Fig. 11-24.   Upper trapezoid and levator scapula stretching.

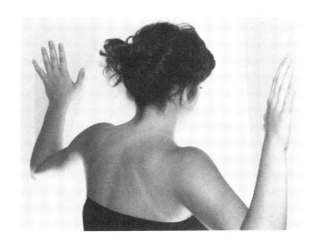

Fig. 11-25. Patient stands facing corner, keeping feet stationary, and then moves upper body into the corner, stretching the pectoralis muscle group.

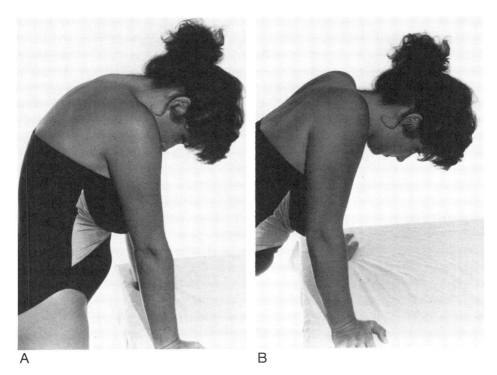

A   B

Fig. 11-26. Patient flexes and extends upper thoracic spine.

and retraction of the shoulder girdle, as well as upper thoracic movements. These exercises are shown in Figures 11-23 through 11-26.

Exercises should not be handed out on a piece of paper for the patient to read and follow. Although a written reminder or picture is helpful, a patient should not be expected to perform the exercise correctly and in a beneficial manner just by following a set of written instructions. The exercises must be personalized to each patient, taking into account the patient's dysfunction, body structure, and pain level. The therapist should observe the patient perform each exercise for maximal benefit.

PROBLEM ASSESSMENT AND
TREATMENT PLANNING

From the evaluation, the physical therapist tries to determine which anatomical structures are involved. With spinal pain, it is often difficult to determine the exact pathology. Cases have been documented in which patients have undergone discectomies without significant changes in their pain despite CT scan and myelogram documentations of this pathology. Likewise, conservative treatment methods have often been helpful in reducing the patient's symptoms and there has been no change on CT scans.[127] Even though a definite diagnosis may not be possible, the therapist can still determine a treatment approach based on objective signs and symptoms. These signs and symptoms must be assigned priority for each patient e.g., if pain is preventing a full evaluation, then rest, immobilization, or TENS may be the initial treatment of choice. Later, as the patient's pain subsides, a more thorough evaluation and a different treatment approach may be used; thus, the evaluation process is ongoing.

Prior to, during, and after each treatment session, the effects of the treatment are assessed through evaluation of one or two comparable signs. If no objective or subjective improvement is noted within three to four treatment sessions, the patient must be reevaluated and the treatment approach must be modified accordingly. From my clinical experience, most patients with upper quarter dysfunction realize some subjective and objective change within the first five to six treatment sessions over a 2- to 3-week period. If no change occurs in this time, the referring doctor is told. After discussion, we may decide to continue with treatment a little longer or to have the patient undertake a different course of treatment.

It is also my policy to communicate through written as well as verbal correspondence regarding each patient's evaluation findings, assessment, and treatment recommendations. This communication also includes anticipated goals and an expected time frame of treatment.

REFERENCES

Therapeutic Modalities

1. Mannheimer JS: TENS: uses and effectiveness. p. 73. In Michel TH (ed): Pain: International Perspectives in Physical Therapy. Churchill Livingstone, Edinburgh, 1985

2. Travell JG, Simons DG: Myofascial Pain and Dysfunction: The Trigger Point Manual. Williams & Wilkins, Baltimore, 1983

3. Mannheimer JS, Lampe GN: Differential evaluation for the determination of TENS effectiveness in specific pain syndromes, p. 63. In Mannheimer JS, Lampe GN (eds): Clinical Transcutaneous Electrical Nerve Stimulation. FA Davis, Philadelphia, 1984

4. Travell J: Temporomandibular joint pain referred from muscles of head and neck. J Prosthet Dent 10:745, 1980

5. Michlovitz SL: Biophysical principles of heating and superficial heating agents. p. 99. In Michlovitz SL (ed): Thermal Agents in Rehabilitation. FA Davis, Philadelphia, 1986

6. Scott BO: The effects of metal on shortwave field distribution. Ann Phys Med 1:238, 1953

7. Feucht BL, Richardson AW, Hines HM: Effects of implanted metals on tissue hyperthermia produced by microwaves. Arch Phys Med Rehabil 30:164, 1949

8. Kloth L: Shortwave and microwave diathermy. p. 208. In Michlovitz SL (ed): Thermal Agents in Rehabilitation. FA Davis, Philadelphia, 1986

9. Ziskin MC, Michlovitz SL: Therapeutic ultrasound. p. 141. In Michlovitz SL (ed): Thermal Agents in Rehabilitation. FA Davis, Philadelphia, 1986

10. Melzack R, Wall PD: Pain mechanisms: A new theory. Science 150:971, 1965

11. Warwick R, Williams PL: Gray's Anatomy, 35th Ed. WB Saunders, Philadelphia, 1973

12. Hassler R, Walker AE: Trigeminal Neuralgia. WB Saunders, Philadelphia, 1970

13. Gobel S: Principles of organization in the substantia gelatinosa layer of the spinal trigeminal nucleus. p. 165. In Bonica JJ, Albe-Fessard D (eds): Advances in Pain Research and Therapy. Raven Press, New York, 1976

14. Sessle BJ, Greenwood LF: Role of trigeminal nucleus caudalis in the modulation of trigeminal sensory and motor neuronal activities. p. 185. In Bonica JJ, Albe-Fessard D (eds): Advances in Pain Research and Therapy. Raven Press, New York, 1976

15. Rocabado M: Course Notes—Head, Neck and TMJ Dysfunction. Rocabado Institute for Craniomandibular and Vertebral Therapeutics, Tacoma, WA 1981

16. Kraus SL: Temporomandibular joint. p. 171. In Saunders HD (ed): Evaluation, Treatment and Prevention of Musculoskeletal Disorders. HD Saunders, Minneapolis, 1985

17. Kraus SL: Course Notes—Physical Therapy in Dentistry: Craniomandibular and Cervical Dysfunction. Clinical Education Associates, Atlanta, GA, 1985

18. Stillwell KG: Therapeutic heat. p. 233. In Krusen FH, Kottke FJ, Ellwood PM (eds): Handbook of Physical Medicine and Rehabilitation. WB Saunders, Philadelphia, 1965

19. Lehmann JF: Diathermy. p. 244. In Krusen FH, Kottke FJ, Ellwood PM (eds):

Handbook of Physical Medicine and Rehabilitation. WB Saunders, Philadelphia, 1965

20. Scott BO: The effects of metal on shortwave field distribution. Ann Phys Med 1:238, 1953

21. Feucht BL, Richardson AW, Hines HM: Effects of implanted metals on tissue hyperthermia produced by microwave. Arch Phys Med Rehabil 30:164, 1949

22. Gersten JW: Effect of metallic objects on temperature rises produced in tissues by ultrasound. A M J Phys Med 37:75, 1958

22a. Lehmann JF, Warren CG, Wallace JE, et al: Ultrasound: considerations for use in the presence of prosthetic joints. Arch Phys Med Rehabil 61:502, 1980

23. La Bar MM: Collagen tissue: Implications of its response to stress in vitro. Arch Phys Med Rehabil 43:461, 1962

24. Kramer JF: Ultrasound: evaluation of its mechanical and thermal effects. Arch Phys Med Rehabil 65:223, 1984

25. Gersten JW: Effect of ultrasound on tendon extensibility. Am J Phys Med 34:662, 1955

26. Lehmann JF, Masock AJ, Warren CG et al: Effect of therapeutic temperatures on tendon extensibility. Arch Phys Med Rehabil 51:481, 1970

27. Dyson M, Brookes M: Stimulation of bone repair by ultrasound (abstr). Ultrasound Med Biol 8:(suppl. 50), 50, 1982

28. Grieder A, Vinton PW, Cinotti WR, et al: An evaluation of ultrasonic therapy for temporomandibular joint dysfunction. Oral Surg 31:25, 1971

29. Lehmann JF, McMillan JA, Brunner GD, Blumberg JA: Comparative study of the efficiency of shortwave, microwave and ultrasonic diathermy in heating the hip joint. Arch Phys Med 40:510, 1959

30. Currier DP, Greathouse D, Swift T: Sensory nerve conduction: effect of ultrasound. Arch Phys Med Rehabil 59:181, 1978

31. Currier DP, Kramer JF: Sensory nerve conduction: heating effects of ultrasound and infrared. Physiother Can 34:241, 1982

32. Halle JS, Scoville CR, Greathouse DG: Ultrasound effect on the conduction latency of superficial radial nerve in man. Phys Ther 61:345, 1981

33. Antich TJ: Phonophoresis: the principles of the ultrasonic driving force and efficacy in treatment of common orthopaedic diagnoses. J Ortho Sports Phys Ther 4(2):99, 1982

34. Kahn J: Low Volt Technique. J Kahn, Syosset, NY, 1983

35. Sokoliu A: Destructive effect of ultrasound on ocular tissues. In Reid JM, Sikov MR: Interaction of Ultrasounnd and Biological Tissues. DHEW Pub (FDA) 73-8008, 1972

36. Bender LF, Janes JM, Herrick JF: Histologic studies following exposure of bone to ultrasound. Arch Phys Med Rehab 35:555, 1954

37. De Forest RE, Herrick JF, Janes JM: Effects of ultrasound on growing bone: an experimental study. Arch Phys Med Rehabil 34:21, 1953

38. Michlovitz SL: Cryotherapy: The use of cold as a therapeutic agent. p. 73. In Michlovitz SL (ed): Thermal Agents in Rehabilitation. FA Davis, Philadelphia, 1986

39. Knight KL: Cryotherapy: Theory, Technique and Physiology. Chattanooga Corp. Chattanooga, 1985

40. Lehmann JF, DeLateur BJ: Cryotherapy. p. 563. In Lehmann JF (ed) Therapeutic Heat and Cold. Williams & Wilkins, Baltimore, 1982

41. Lehmann JF, Delateur BJ: Therapeutic heat. p. 404. In Lehmann JF (ed): Therapeutic Heat and Cold, Williams & Wilkins, Baltimore, 1982
42. Buchtal F, Rosenfalck A: Evoked action potentials and conduction velocity in human sensory nerves. Brain Res 3:1, 1966
43. Mennel JM: The therapeutic use of cold. J Am Orthop Assoc 74:1146, 1975
44. Keatinge WR, Cannon P: Freezing point of human skin. Lancet 1:11, 1960
45. Kurland HD: Quick Headache Relief Without Drugs. William Morrow, New York, 1977
46. Mann F: Acupuncture: The Ancient Chinese Art of Healing and How it Works Scientifically. Vintage Books, New York, 1973
47. Austin M: Acupuncture Therapy. ASI Publishers, New York, 1972
48. Matsumoto T: Acupuncture for Physicians. Charles C Thomas Springfield, IL 1974
49. Cherney JV: Acupressure: Acupuncture Without Needles. Cornerstone Library, New York, 1974
50. Wolf SL: Neurophysiologic mechanisms in pain modulation. p. 41. In Mannheimer JS, Lampe GN (eds): Clinical Transcutaneous Electrical Nerve Stimulation. FA Davis, Philadelphia, 1984
51. Mannheimer JS: Clinical Transcutaneous Electrical Nerve Stimulation. FA Davis, Philadelphia, 1984
52. Duffin D: Acupuncture and acupressure. p. 122. In Michel TH (ed): Pain: International Perspectives in Physical Therapy. Churchill Livingstone, Edinburgh, 1985
53. Joachim G: Acupressure: a self-help technique for relieving headache pain. Can Nurse 38, 1984
54. Melzack R, Guite S, Gonshor A: Relief of dental pain by ice massage of the hand. Can Med Assoc J 122:189, 1980
55. Mannheimer JS, Lampe GN: Electrode placement sites and their relationship. p. 249. In Mannheimer JS, Lampe GN (eds): Clinical Transcutaneous Electrical Nerve Stimulation. FA Davis, Philadelphia, 1984
56. Melzack R: Prolonged relief of pain by brief, intense transcutaneous electrical stimulation. Pain 1:357, 1975
57. Peshek RJ: Electrical acupoint therapy for temporomandibular joint-myofacial pain. p. 340. In Morgan DH, House LR, Hall WP, Vamoas SJ (eds): Diseases of the Temporomandibular Apparatus. CV Mosby, St. Louis, 1982
58. Richardson PH, Vincent CA: The evaluation of therapeutic acupuncture: concepts and methods. Pain 24:1, 1986
59. Richardson PH, Vincent CA: Acupuncture for the treatment of pain: a review of evaluative research. Pain 24:15, 1986
60. Guillemin RT, Vargo T, Rossier J, et al: β-endorphin and adreno-corticotrophin are secreted concomitantly by the pituitary gland. Science 197:1367, 1977
61. Check WA: Old hormones reveal new surprises: complex connections link brain, pituitary. JAMA 243:499, 1980
62. Rees LH: Brain opiates and cortico-trophin-related peptides. J Coll Phys 2:130, 1981
63. Omura Y: Pain threshold measurement before and after acupuncture: controversial results of radiant heat method and electrical method and the roles of ACTH-like substances and endorphins. Acupuncture Electro Ther Res Int J 3:1, 1978
64. Binder SA: Applications of low and high voltage electrotherapeutic currents. p. 1. In Wolf SL (ed): Electrotherapy. Churchill Livingstone, Edinburgh, 1981

65. Lampe GN, Manheimer, JS: The patient and TENS. p. 219. In Mannheimer JS, Lampe GN (eds): Clinical Transcutaneous Electrical Nerve Stimulation. FA Davis, Philadelphia, 1984

66. Mannheimer JS, Lampe GN: Electrode placement techniques—the use of TENS during specific therapeutic procedures. p. 331. In Mannheimer JS, Lampe GN: Clinical Transcutaneous Electrical Nerve Stimulation. FA Davis, Philadelphia, 1984

67. Markovich SE: Pain in the head: a neurological appraisal. p. 125. In Gelb H (ed): Clinical Management of Head, Neck and TMJ Pain and Dysfunction. WB Saunders, Philadelphia, 1977

68. Quint H: Acupuncture. p. 335. In Morgan DH, House LR, Hall WP, Vamoas SJ (eds): Diseases of the Temporomandibular Apparatus. CV Mosby, St. Louis, 1982

69. Jankelson B. Radke JC: The myomonitor: its use and abuse II. Quintessence Int 3:7, 1978

70. Lampe GN, Mannheimer JS: Some limitations of TENS. p. 57. In Mannheimer JS, Lampe GN (eds): Clinical Transcutaneous Electrical Nerve Stimulation. FA Davis, Philadelphia, 1984

71. Kahn J: TMJ pain control. Whirlpool 5:14, 1982

72. Bertolucci LE: Introduction of anti-inflammatory drugs by iontophoresis: double blind study. J Orthop Sports Phys Ther 4:103, 1982

73. Harris PR: Iontophoresis: clinical research in musculoskeletal inflammatory conditions. J Ortho Sports Phys Ther 4:109, 1982

74. Scott DS, Lundeen TF: Myofascial pain involving the masticatory muscles: an experimental model. Pain 8:207, 1980

75. Carlsson SG, Gale En: Biofeedback in the treatment of long-term temporomandibular joint pain. Biofeedback Self Reg 2:161, 1977

76. Budzynski TH, Stoyva JM: An electro-myographic technique for teaching voluntary relaxation of the masseter muscle. J Dent Res 52:116, 1973

77. Dohrmann RJ, Laskin DM: An evaluation of electromyographic biofeedback in the treatment of myofascial pain—dysfunction syndrome. J Am Dent Assoc 96:656, 1978

78. Grossan M: Treatment of subjective tinnitus with biofeedback. Ear Nose Throat J 55:10, 1976

79. Principato JJ, Barwell DR: Biofeedback training and relaxation exercises for treatment of temporomandibular joint dysfunction. Otolaryngology 86:766, 1978

80. Dahlstrom L, Carlsson SG, Gale EN, Jansson TG: Clinical and electromyographic effects of biofeedback training in mandibular dysfunction. Biofeedback Self Reg 9:37, 1984

81. Scott DS, Gregg JM: Myofascial pain of the temporomandibular joint. A review of the behavioral-relaxation therapies. Pain 9:231, 1980

82. Abramson DI, Mitchell RE, Tuck S, et al: Changes in blood flow, oxygen uptake and tissue temperatures produced by the application of wet heat. Arch Phys Med Rehabil 42:305, 1961

83. Ottoson D, Ekblom A, Hansson P: Vibratory stimulation for the relief of pain of dental origin. Pain 10:37, 1981

84. Hansson P, Ekblom A: Transcutaneous electrical nerve stimulation (TENS) as compared to placebo TENS for the relief of acute oro-facial pain. Pain 15:157, 1983

85. Ekblom A, Hansson P: Extrasegmental transcutaneous electrical nerve stimulation

and mechanical vibratory stimulation as compared to placebo for the relief of acute oro-facial pain. Pain 23:223, 1985

86. Nordemar R, Thorner C: Treatment of acute cervical pain—a comparative group study. Pain 10:93, 1981
87. Kai HD: Relationship between the points of channels and the peripheral nerves. Acupuncture Electro Ther Res Int J 8:328, 1983
88. Mann F: Acupuncture points and meridians do not exist. Acupuncture Electro Ther Res Int J 8:329, 1983

Orthopedic Therapy

89. Travell JG, Simons DG: Myofascial Pain and Dysfunction: The Trigger Point Manual. Williams & Wilkins, Baltimore, 1983
90. Trott PH, Goss AN: Physiotherapy in diagnosis and treatment of the myofascial pain dysfunction syndrome. Int J Oral Surg 7:360, 1978
91. Lord Brain: Some unresolved problems of cervical spondylosis. Br Med J 1:771, 1963
92. Travell JG: Temporomandibular joint pain referred from muscles of the head and neck. J Prosthet Dent, 10:745, 1960
93. Edeling J: The true cervical headache. S Afr Med J 62:531, 1982
94. Griffiths RH: Report of the president's conference on the examination, diagnosis and management of temporomandibular disorders. J Am Dent Assoc 106:75, 1983
95. McKenzie RA. The Lumbar Spine—Mechanical Diagnosis and Therapy. Spinal Publications; Waikanea, New Zealand, 1981
96. Mooney V, Robertson J: The facet syndrome. Clin Orthop Rel Res 115:149, 1976
97. Kendall HO, Kendall FP, Wadsworth GE: Muscle Testing and Function. Williams & Wilkins, Baltimore, 1971
98. Paris SV: Course Notes—The Spine—Etiology and Treatment of Dysfunction Including Joint Manipulation, Institute Press, Atlanta, 1971
99. Hoppenfeld S: Physical Examination of the Spine and Extremities. Appleton-Century-Crofts, New York, 1976
100. Gonnella C, Paris SV, Kutner M: Reliability in evaluating passive intervetebral motion. Phys Ther 62:436, 1982
101. Cyriax J: Textbook of Orthopaedic Medicine. Bailliere Tindal, London, 1981
102. Maitland GD: Vertebral Manipulation. Butterworths, London, 1981
103. Stoddard A: Manual of Osteopathic Technique. Hutchenson Medical Publications, London, 1972
104. Johnston WL, Allan BR, Hendra JL, et al: Interexaminer study of palpation in detecting location of spinal segmental dysfunction. J Am Osteo Assoc 82:839, 1983
105. Lord JW, Rosati LB: Thoracic Outlet Syndromes. Clin Symp 23:3, 1971
106. Wright IS: The neurovascular syndrome produced by hyperabduction of the arm. Am Heart J 29:1, 1945
107. Smith KF: The thoracic outlet syndrome: a protocol of treatment. J Orthop Sports Phys Ther 1:89, 1979
108. Mannheimer JS: Clinical Transcutaneous Electrical Nerve Stimulation. FA Davis, Philadelphia, 1984
109. Paris SV: Mobilization of the spine. Phys Ther 59:988, 1979
110. Warwick R, Williams PL: Gray's Anatomy, 55th Br Ed. WB Saunders, Philadelphia, 1973

111. Maigne R: Orthopaedic Medicine. Charles C Thomas, Springfield, IL, 1972
112. Freeman MA, Wyke BD: Articular reflexes at the ankle joint: an electromyographic study of normal and abnormal influences of ankle joint mechanoreceptors upon reflex activity in the leg muscles. Br J Surg 54:990, 1965
113. Melzack R, Wall PD: Pain mechanisms: a new theory. Science 150:971, 1965
114. Akeson WH, Amiel D, Woo S: Immobility effects on synovial joints: the pathomechanics of joint contracture. Biorheology 17:95, 1980
115. Akeson WH, Amiel D, Mechanic GL, et al: Collogen crosslinking alterations in joint contractures: changes in reducible crosslinks in periarticular connective tissue collogen after nine weeks of immobilization. Connect Tissue Res 5:5, 1977
116. Knott M, Voss DE: Proprioceptive neuromuscular facilitation—patterns and techniques. Harper & Row, New York, 1968
117. Tanigawa MC: A comparison of hold-relax procedure and passive mobilization on increasing muscle length. Phys Ther 52:725, 1972
118. Wallin A, Ekblom B, Grahn R, et al: Improvement of muscle flexibility—a comparison of two techniques. Am J Sports Med 13:263, 1985
119. Ward RC: Course Notes—Tutorial on Level I Myofascial Release Techniques. Michigan State University, 1986
120. Barlow W: The Alexander Technique. Warner Books Ed. Alfred A. Knopf, New York, 1973
121. Feldenkreis M: Awareness Through Movement, Harper & Row, New York, 1977
122. Upledger JE, Vredervoogd JD: Craniosacral Therapy. Eastland Press, Chicago, 1983
123. Ayub E, Glasheen-Wray M, Kraus S: Head posture: a case study of the effects on the rest position of the mandible. J Orthop Sports Phys Ther 5:179, 1984
124. Knutsson B, Lindh K, Telhog H: Sitting an electromyographic and mechanical study. Acta Orthop Scand 37:415, 1966
125. Engdahl S: Specification for office furniture. p. 97. In Jonssor B (ed): Sitting Work Postures. National Board of Safety and Health, Sweden, 1978
126. Anonymous: VDT's—a new social disease, VIII. The Harvard Medical School Health Letter 5, April 1983
127. Natchev E: A Manual on Auto-Traction Treatment for Low Back Pain. Folksam Scientific Council, Stockholm, 1984

12 | Cervical Spine Influences on the Craniomandibular Region

Steven L. Kraus

A clinician's knowledge, experience, and expertise enhances his or her approach to the evaluation and treatment of patients and is applied to patients experiencing disorders of the craniomandibular region. Proper interpretations of signs and symptoms facilitate an appropriate treatment plan. A number of patients, however, continue to suffer various symptoms and dysfunctions of the craniomandibular region. The management of the craniomandibular region as it pertains to the occlusion, the TMJ, and associated muscles may be more complete if an evaluation and treatment of the cervical spine is included.

For the clinician to recognize the importance of the cervical spine and its role in the management of the craniomandibular disorders; two objectives must be addressed. The first objective is to review the mechanisms involved in the establishment of a head-neck posture. The second objective is to address the mechanisms by which the cervical spine influences mandibular movement and position.

ACHIEVEMENT OF A HEAD-NECK POSTURE

The mobility and positioning of the head–neck in humans is an interaction of numerous factors, factors we do not completely understand and have not yet recognized. Evolution, heredity, congenital, growth and development, and pathological factors influence the head-neck posture. Once musculoskeletal maturity is reached, other factors such as the aging process[1] and a decline in health[2] create changes in function and performance capabilities, contributing to a deterioration of head-neck posture. These factors are recognized as influencing, over the long term, the head–neck posture. Daily, the achievement, maintenance, and adaptability of a head-neck posture is dependent on two mechanisms: peripheral and central. These two mechanisms are the center of discussion of this section.

The peripheral and central mechanisms are paramount for adjusting and maintaining a head-neck posture. Achievement of a head-neck posture is within a physiological range. Within that physiological range, there may be great variability, although it will be minimal if peripheral and central mechanisms are functioning well. The head-neck posture is not static but instead is in dynamic equilibrium, constantly responding to environmental demands. Subsequent changes in head-neck posture due to these demands depends to a great degree on mobility within the cervical spine. I propose that when a person exceeds the physiological adaptive range of the cervical spine, adverse effects develop on the craniomandibular region.

Peripheral Mechanisms

Peripheral proprioceptive afferent information that relates specifically to achievement of a head-neck posture is divided into three systems. The three systems are the vestibular, ocular, and neck proprioceptive systems.

Vestibular System

The vestibular system is a sensory apparatus of the ear.[3] The ear may be subdivided into external, middle, and internal parts. The external and middle ears form the pathway for the transduction of sound energy into mechanical energy in the process of audition.[3] A part of the internal ear, the cochlea, acts as a sound analyzer and relays information to the brain. The remainder of the internal ear is the vestibular apparatus. The vestibular apparatus is contained within the temporal bone in a complex cavity known as the bony labyrinth. The vestibular apparatus is the sensory receptor detecting the position of the head and changes in the position of the head in space, thus serving as one of the major organs of equilibrium. The vestibular apparatus is composed of two groups of sensory receptors, the otoliths and semicircular ducts.[3]

There are two otolith organs, the utricle and the saccule. The sensory portion of the utricle (hair cells) is parallel to the ground when the head is upright. The saccule is just below the utricle. The sensory portion of the saccule (hair cell) is oriented approximately vertically in the upright human. The otolith organs with their spatial relationship to each other respond to alterations in head position in any direction.[4]

Each labyrinth has three semicircular ducts. The semicircular ducts are oriented in planes that are approximately at right angles to each other. One duct is nearly horizontal if the head is tilted forward 30°. The other two ducts are upright, the second being superior and the third posterior. When the head moves, the endolymph within the ducts causes distortion of the sensory hairs, which either increases or decreases the rate of afferent fiber firing. The afferent fibers from a given semicircular duct are most sensitive to movements in the plane of the duct (e.g., the most effective stimulus to the afferent fibers of the horizontal canals in humans is a rotation of the individual in a plane parallel to the ground when the head is tilted 30° forward. The function, then, of the semicircular ducts, is the detection of angular acceleration of the head.[3]

Once the afferent fibers from the vestibular system (otolith and semicircular ducts) have been stimulated, the impulses travel through the vestibular portion of cranial nerve VIII to the vestibular nuclei. The vestibular nuclei, in turn, send second-order axons to regions of the spinal cord, the cerebellum, the nuclei of the extrinsic eye muscles, the reticular formation, the contralateral vestibular complex, and the cerebral cortex. The bulk of the fibers reach the spinal cord and are in the vestibular spinal tract of the cord. The importance of this discussion is the close relationship of the vestibular system to the neck musculature.[5–7]

The vestibular spinal tract excites motor neurons on the ipsilateral side of the body. Some fibers reach the spinal cord through the medial longitudinal fasciculus (MLF). The descending fibers of the MLF appear to end within the upper cervical spinal cord. They appear to activate motor neurons participating in movements of the neck, perhaps in synergy with eye movements.[8] When balance is upset, the horizontal position of the head is first restored by vestibular action on the neck muscles.[9]

Ocular System

The function of certain eye proprioceptive mechanisms was described as early as 1785 by Thomas Reid.[10] Airapetyants et al, in 1957, investigated the role of the eyes and other specialized structures of proprioceptive significance in maintaining conditioned reflexes, demonstrating the ability of dogs to adjust their body equilibrium in space.[11] Edwards[12] and Travis[13] observed body-sway to be greater with eyes closed than with eyes opened.

During rapid head and eye coordinated voluntary movements in the alert animal, eye-neck muscles are synergistic.[14] Guitton et al, in 1980, demonstrated that neck EMG (biventer cervicis) discharges were affected by electrical stimulation of the superior colliculus,[15] which is located in the midbrain and receives fibers from the optic tract. The optic tract receives its fibers from the optic nerve, whose fibers originate in the retina.[16]

Wilson, et al showed that the splenius muscle of the cat responded to activation of ocular receptors that evoked head movements.[17] The results of Wilson's study confirm similar observations made by Vidal et al.[18] Electromyographic (EMG) activity of cervical muscles such as the obliquus capitis cranialis and caudalis and longissimus capitis is largely related to horizontal eye position in the orbit both during spontaneous eye movements and vestibular nystagmus.

The visual system, plays an important role not only in the perception of head position but also in the coordination of eye, head, and neck movement by influencing neck muscle activity.

Neck Proprioceptive System

The neck proprioceptive system consists of the muscle spindle and the tonic neck reflex (TNR). Recognition of the role played by muscle spindle receptors in providing abundant proprioceptive feedback cannot be overlooked.[19,20] The proprioceptive outflow from the muscle spindle is, however, a result of γ motor neuron activity, which is influenced greatly by the TNR.[21,22] Therefore I consider the TNR is the primary neck proprioceptor contributing to the achievement of a final head-neck posture.

The existence of the TNR and its role in reflexly orienting the limbs in relationship to the head-body angle was described by Magnus in 1912.[23] Magnus,[24] in his classic work, analyzed the postural reaction of the decerebrate quadrupeds when their heads were experimentally turned to an extreme right or left position. He found characteristic responses: (1) extension of the forelimb on the side toward which the head was turned, and (2) flexion of the opposite forelimb.

Localizing the origin of the TNR to a specific area and tissue began with Magnus and DeKleijn,[25] who had limited the receptive field for the TNR to the first three cervical segments of the spine. In their research, they showed that the decerebrate cat had TNR not labyrinthine in origin but due to activation to neck proprioceptors.

Not until 1951, did McCouch et al,[26] show that the TNR of the decerebrate labyrinthectomized cat was not abolished when the muscle mass of the neck was sectioned. The TNR was abolished only after the facet joints in the upper cervical spine were denervated, clearly demonstrating that the joint mechanoreceptors in the upper cervical spine are the origin of the TNR.

In 1921, Minkowski reported TNR could be elicited in the human fetus.[27] The TNR is a dominating characteristic of normal infancy in the first 3 months of life. The TNR, accordingly, has an ecology (the science of organisms are affected by the factors of their environments).[28] TNR subserves adaptations to the environment prior to birth as well as later.[28,29] The earliest reflex in the human embryo consists of contraction of the neck muscles elicited by light stroking of the perioral region at $7\frac{1}{2}$ weeks of menstrual age.[30] The TNR helps the fetus accomodate to the conformation of the uterine cavity. TNR may even facilitate the longitudinal presentation and orientation of the fetus at the entrance of the birth canal.[31] Postural attitudes assumed by the neonatal infant when suckled at the breast stem from the TNR.[31] Gesell[31] suggests that the TNR attitude promotes and directs visual fixation by the infant on the extended hand, leading to hand inspection, eye–hand coordination, prehensory approach, and eventually unidextrality. The TNR contributes to the organization of diagonal reflexes of prone locomotion, reduces the danger of suffocation to the infant and is well adapted to the acts of rejection and withdrawal.[31] Moreover, the TNR is related to an unlimited number of adult acts of skill, aggression, and extrication. The TNR always remains in reflex reserve and is subject to voluntary mobilization. Fukuda, described the ways in which any skilled athlete can use the posture of TNR for skilled motor coordination under unconscious control.[32]

The TNR is so basic that it is found in lower animals as well as in humans. The TNR is a natural but not a stereotyped reflex. TNR serves useful adjustments in the fetus as well as the infant in neonatal life. TNR is morphogenetically so fundamental that it has clinical value both as an index of maturity and as a symptom of neurologic abnormalities.[31]

Summary

The TNR influence plays a primary role in human ability to achieve a head-neck posture. Indeed, of the three peripheral systems discussed (vestibular, ocular, and neck proprioceptive systems), the TNR plays the major role in orienting an organism in its environment and maintenance of dynamic equilibrium.[33]

Although orientation of the head in space is the special role of the vestibular apparatus, there is, as Cohen says[34] "no conceivable way by which the semicircular canal or the otoliths can, by themselves, inform the brain of the angle formed by the head and the body." Orientation of the head to the body can only be achieved by the neck proprioceptive system. Information from the vestibular system indicating a position of the head in space would be inadequate without information from the neck proprioceptive system.

Regarding the visual system, vision affecting the cervical muscle activity has been discussed. De Kleijn[35] and others, however, described reflex effects of the neck proprioceptors on extraocular muscles of the eyes. Korovina[36] recorded the electrical activity of individual extraoccular muscles in response to combined vestibular and neck stimulation. Wapner et al[37] showed that the organism's ability to orient an environmental object was related to information from neck proprioceptors and that a vertical rod always appeared to rotate to the opposite side from the side on which an electrical stimulation of a neck muscle was induced. The influence of proprioceptive information from receptors in the neck on oculomotor control is well established.[38,39]

The preceding studies performed on animals and humans suggest the existence of ascending influences from neck proprioceptors on the vestibular and ocular systems. The neck proprioceptors play an important role in achieving and maintaining a dynamic equilibrium of head-neck posture to one's environment. Thus, adaptability of head-neck posture would seem to stem from the neck proprioceptive system with support coming from the vestibular and occular systems.

Symptoms related to neck proprioceptive system. The clinician must be alert to altered neck proprioceptive afferent activity contributing to unusual yet common symptoms. The origin of these symptoms may be of cervical spine dysfunction.

Some vestibular catastrophes such as vertigo and nystagmus can be caused solely by abnormalities related to neck proprioceptors.[33] Numerous studies[20,40–42] have shown that damage to deep cervical tissues, including neck muscles, produces a generalized ataxia, with symptoms of unbalance, disorientation and motor incoordination. Vertigo, ataxia, and nystagmus were induced in animals and humans by injecting local anesthetic into the neck.[43] The injections presumably interupted the flow of afferent information from neck muscles and joint receptors. Ataxia in humans was associated with a broad-based staggering gait, hypotonia of the ipsilateral arm and leg, and a strong sensation of ipsilateral falling or tilting.[43]

In addition to these previous symptoms, the clinician should be aware that the cervical spine is a source of local and or referred symptoms in areas of the neck, shoulders, and upper extremities. The clinician may not be aware, however, that the cervical spine is also a major source of referred symptoms to the head, face, and jaw.

The relation of the descending tract of the trigeminal nerve to the upper dorsal roots is of considerable physiological and clinical interest, particularly with reference to the mechanisms of hemicranial pain syndromes.[44] Neurons of the three divisions of cranial nerve V and cranial nerves VII, IX, and X share in the same neuron pool with neurons from the upper cervical spine segments C1, C2, and C3. This relationship of cranial and cervical neurons has been demonstrated in considerable detail.[44–46] The region shared by cranial nerves V, VII, IX, X and cervical nerves C1, C2, and C3 is called the subnucleus caudalis. The "pars spinalis" is the portion of the subnucleus caudalis that lies in the spinal cord.[47] The pars spinalis is characterized by its multiple cranial and cervical root inputs and by the pronounced anatomic convergence of these systems.[47] This convergence of the trigeminal and cervical root fibers on the same sensory neuron at high levels in the cervical spinal cord is an anatomic and physiologic basis for the referral of pain from cervical to trigeminal territories.[48]

Whenever a patient has symptoms related or believed to be related to the craniomandibular region, the cervical spine must be evaluated to rule out cervical spine dysfunction as a source of such symptoms. On many occasions I have seen inadequate results when treatments were administered to the craniomandibular region independent of treatment to the cervical spine or when such treatments were thought to help the cervical complaints.

Interaction of Neck Proprioceptors and Central Control Mechanisms in the Achievement of a Head-Neck Posture

In adults, peripheral afferent signals are very important for establishing programs for movement and posture.[49] The initiation and termination of movement and the subsequent maintenance of posture through the neck proprioceptive system is less well understood when the central control system's influences are considered. The mechanisms whereby central control centers (the brain) initiate movement through control of neck musculature have been studied.[50–53] One must ask whether maintenance of a head-neck posture is dependent on a readout of proprioceptive afferent information from the peripheral system or whether the head-neck posture is instead centrally programmed.

In contrast to the views of the importance of the peripheral system's influence on movement and head positioning, experimental evidence derived from deafferented animals[54] and humans[55] indicate that centrally initiated movements can be executed accurately without sensory feedback. These conclusions drawn from studies of deafferented animals may not apply to intact animals because postoperative training may have produced an adaptive rearrangement of motor preprogramming. Apparently, in intact humans, determining the final head position is an interaction between the peripheral system (TNR) and the central control system.[56,57]

The central control system compares feedback from the peripheral system to its own expected feedback which the central control system has acquired as an interaction between past and current proprioceptive experiences. Only when the expected feedback of the central control system matches the peripheral system's feedback does a certain head-neck posture exist. This designates a type of reverse action of one system's dependence on the other. This reverse action of interdependence is the concept of reafference, promoted by Nobel laureate Tinbergen.[58] This concept of reafference strongly indicates that at various levels of integration from single muscle units to complex behavior, the correct performance of many movements and positions is continuously checked by the central control centers.[59,60] Parts of this concept have been demonstrated in humans experimentally.[61] That a change in perceived position of the head without a physical deviation can influence eye posture indicates that the influence of neck proprioceptive afferents on the oculomotor nuclei must be centrally reinterpreted before affecting oculomotor motor control.

Factors Influencing Neck Proprioceptor Activity

Factors influencing the neck proprioceptors and thereby head-neck posture, can be broadly classified into two categories: trauma and misuse.

Trauma is essentially self-explanatory. Aberrant proprioceptive feedback from the neck proprioceptors occurs with macrotrauma such as whiplash injury or a blow to the neck. Not only does an altered head-neck position and movement occur due to the aberrant information but there are also various degrees of mechanical and physiological changes of the associated tissues. Symptoms such as those previously described would also be experienced by the patient.

Misuse (microtrauma), refers to positions and movements to which we subject our musculoskeletal system, that in turn become abusive to our neck proprioceptors. Examples of misuse are stomach sleeping, sitting on soft couches, and straining the cervical spine by lifting objects and carrying objects incorrectly, all of which conceivably place a stress on the tissues of our cervical spine.

Macrotrauma often results in pain and dysfunction; microtrauma does not initially result in pain, and the dysfunction is not as readily apparent. The intensity and duration of trauma is not the same between macro and micro injuries. Microtrauma usually occurs on numerous occasions, with minimal intensity, thus going unnoticed. The repetitive nature of the microtrauma could conceivably develop a significant amount of stress to the neck proprioceptors, resulting in aberrant afferent information. Microtrauma is usually not painful until tissues can no longer adapt to such prolonged stress. One would think that an individual would take subconscious/intuitive corrective action to avoid such prolonged abusive positions and movement patterns of the cervical spine. Self-correction of posture and movement often does not occur, owing to the individual's lack of cognitive awareness and reasoning as to what is wrong or right with posturing and movement of the head and neck. Environmental, occupational, and habitual influences daily force on us poor postural positions and movements. Such daily influences, plus the effects of gravity,[62] affect the use of our muscles in different postural positions throughout the day, continuously placing us in potential positions and movements of abuse.

Misuse of our posture and movement occurs slowly, usually in the absence of pain. The slowly developing afferent input from our peripheral system is interpreted by our central control system as being correct, when in fact, all is very wrong. The central control centers do not send out commands for corrective action; the result is a self-perpetuating cycle of improper positioning and movement of our head-neck.[58,59] A dilemma for persons who experiences "pain" for "no known reason" is the acceptance that their incorrect posture may be a preexisting, precipitating, or perpetuating cause to their cervical and craniomandibular symptoms. Postural correction for these persons should not be taken too lightly. Patients should not be told by the health professional that all they need to do is stand up straight. This would be as unacceptable as telling a person under a great deal of emotional stress: "All you need to do is learn to control your emotional stresses and everything will be fine." Rather, postural corrections can be achieved through a functional orthopedic approach offered by the physical therapist.

Factors Influencing the Central Control System

Kiernander[2] offers the following definition of posture, which reinforces that a part of posture is a psychosomatic affair: "[A] person's willingness and ability to maintain the relationship of different parts of the body which ensures their most efficient behavioral function and physiological functioning, both now and in the future.''

Posture may be a sum of a person's willingness and ability to maintain the best relationship of different parts of their body regardless of what other factors may be present.

Studies of postural movement (body sway) during normal standing reveal that body movement is significantly influenced by the mental state.[63] In patients with psychosomatic disorders or anxiety reactions, a specific fluxation in postural movement was observed.

Several texts have addressed, the ways in which one's attitude and feelings are expressed through posture.[64-66] The central control system's influence now applies a new meaning to the word misuse, which acquires a psychosomatic connotation. Misuse may be a result of modern living conditions of a culturally determined stress, interreacting with the individual's own psychological makeup, which (more or less) will determine how the individual responds to the environmental stressors. Poor posture may result from a feeling that the person is not quite up to facing the monotonous work ahead for the day; one's posture may be very different if one has a meaningful and immediately satisfying occupation. The education of children has changed almost beyond recognition into an extremely demanding training, creating additional psychosomatic stresses to posture at an early age. Psychologically, poor posture may result from how we respond to auditory and visual input of the daily news reports, a request by an employer that we perform duties outside our range of ability, and financial comparison between ourselves and our peers. All these ongoing stressors would appear to place the central control system in a favorable state to misuse one's achievement of a head-neck posture. Our abilities to adapt may allow us to accommodate to such stressors until our physiological adaptive range has been exceeded, but then it is often too late. Recognizing environmental stressors is a key to decreasing misuse of our musculoskeletal system. Environmental pressure is a very difficult area to cope with and manage.[67]

Because stress is with us at all times, is there a consistent way that our head-neck posture responds to stress? Stimuli such as anxiety (giving a speech), fear (losing a job), the startle reaction (facing heavy traffic while driving to and from work) are with us daily to varying degrees. Active postural changes in response to stress often occur so slowly that we do not actively see these changes; instead, we see usually the result of the changes. A patient's slow active response to daily stressful stimuli such as anxiety, fear, and the startle reaction may be easily seen through an objective experiment that studied the ''startled'' pattern.[68-70] During an EMG study of subject's head-neck muscle tension and the postural image, the subjects acquired a comfortable postural position and then, without their having any knowledge of what was to occur, a door was slammed. The results consistently showed that:

> The head, though keeping the same angle with the horizon, has been trust forward and down, and an "attitude" has been imposed to the body in

which the knees are flexed, the arms extended, the shoulders raised and the chest flattened. The character of the response which is completely left in a second is similar to what is seen in aging and in abnormal postures of disease.[70]

Other experiments have demonstrated predictable responses of head-neck position in humans subjected to stress. This suggests that the TNR operates preeminently when unsurmountable stress is imposed. Head-neck postural responses were recorded when subjects were placed in a stressful environment of performing heavy resistive exercises of the extremities. The resulting head-neck posture assumed appeared to be a facilatory physiological adaptation.[71] When subjects were asked to resist bilateral wrist extension, there was an associated straightening of the vertebral column with dorsiflexion of the head. If unilateral wrist extension was resisted, there was still dorsiflexion of the head, but with rotation of the head to the same side of wrist extension. Resisting bilateral wrist flexion resulted in a strong ventroflexion of the head.[72] The movement patterns induced appear so regularly under standardized conditions that they suggest that the TNR may play a fundamental role in the integration of the autonomous component of purposive motor acts.[73] Daily, we habitually place ourselves in a working environment in which our central control system is asking that a repetitive task be performed (typing, hairdressing, art, dentistry, etc.) in which our extremity actions are facilitated by our TNR.

In summary, when the neck proprioceptors and central control systems have "failed" to achieve and maintain a person's upright postural position, the most common altered head-neck posture seen clinically is the "forward head posture" (FHP). The FHP may occur following macrotrauma and or microtrauma. Influences stemming from the central control system on head-neck posture appear to work through the TNR. The central control system responds to environmental stress (fear, anxiety, the startle reaction) or stress that stems from having to perform a repetitive, tedious, and monotonous task with our extremities. Such environmental stress results in overuse and abuse of our cervical spine. These attitudinal TNRs in themselves do not fatigue.[74] Not only should the clinician be aware of muscle hyperactivity occurring in the masticatory region in response to stress but also of muscle hyperactivity occurring in the cervical spine in response to stress. Later in this chapter, the mechanisms that allow the TNR to cause jaw muscle hyperactivity directly are discussed.

The resulting FHP leads to a decrease in the person's physiological adaptive range. When such an adaptive range has been exceeded, numerous symptoms of the cervical spine may develop. Unless the clinician is aware of the impact that the cervical spine has on contributing to various symptoms, the patient may not receive the appropriate therapy to the cervical spine. Abuse to the cervical spine often has an insidious onset, with such symptoms frequently aggravated by emotional stress. The word stress covers not only emotions, but also physical stress. If physical stress is decreased, the person can often manage environmental–emotional stress better.

Therapy must not only deal directly with the cervical spine dysfunction

(FHP) but also with central control influences. Treatments offered to the cervical spine dysfunction, consisting of manual techniques and modalities, are the first choice. Improving the patients' awareness of their environment through patient education and the application of rhythmic, mobility, coordinating, cognitive awareness exercises performed often throughout the day will improve central control influences.

CERVICAL SPINE INFLUENCES ON MANDIBULAR POSITION AND MOVEMENT

To enhance the reader's awareness of the various clinical conclusions that will be established pertaining to the cervical spine influencing the craniomandibular region, a brief review of head-neck positioning associated with craniofacial morphology is addressed. Clinicians must consider possible relationship between head-neck position and mandibular position in the very early postnatal years.

Head-Neck Positioning and Craniofacial Morphology

Clinical observations indicate that most patients experiencing TMJ dysfunction have an underdeveloped (retrognathic) mandible.[75] This does not imply, however, that a cause and effect relationship exists between an underdeveloped mandible and TMJ dysfunction. Many patients who have a retrognathic mandible and then developed TMJ dysfunction often have orthodontics and/or orthognathic surgery performed in the stabilizing stage of their treatment.

Much interest has resulted in investigation of the causes of mandibular retrognathism. Such studies have centered on the debate between the genetic hypothesis and the environmental hypothesis. Observations of current trends, both in research and clinical studies reveal a strong interest in the influences of environment or function on the orofacial complex.[76] The environmental position does not deny the role of genetic factors in development. Moss summarizes; ". . . the intrinsic factors in skeletal tissue cells provide only the possibility of an appropriate response to an extrinsic stimulus."[77] Available data from many fields and from many workers make it more reasonable to suggest that postnatal environmental factors primarily regulate skeletal form and function.[76-79]

During orofacial growth, the mandible as a whole is passively and literally lowered in space,[77] down and forward.[80] Mandibular growth occurs as the volume of functional oral spaces increases with age. Such spaces are surrounded by muscles and connective tissues. Because the mandible originates, grows, and exists completely embedded within the oral facial space, enlargement of these spaces allows such mandibular growth to occur.[77]

In the search for an environmental factor(s) that influences the oral facial space and therefore the down and forward growth pattern of the mandible, the possible role of head posture has received little attention. A relationship between head posture and craniofacial morphology was suggested in 1926 by Schwartz,[81] who attributed the development of a class II malocclusion to hyperextension of the head relative to the cervical column during sleep. Experimentally, the presence of a relationship between craniofacial morphology and posture has been supported by the demonstration of craniofacial morphologic changes in animals following artificially induced changes in body positions.[82,83] Within the last 10 years, studies have evaluated variations in head position and its relationship with craniofacial morphology, resulting in several interesting findings. Solow and Tallgren[84,85] showed statistical associations between head posture to craniofacial and dentoalveolar morphology. A consistent pattern of association emerged. On the average, *extension of the head relative to the cervical column (such extension occurring at the craniocervical segment) was noted in association with mandibular retrusion development.* Additional findings associated with an extended head posture are; large anterior (long face) and small posterior facial heights, small anteroposterior craniofacial dimensions, large inclination of the mandible relative to the anterior cranial base and to the palatal plane, a large cranial base angle, and a small nasopharyngeal space. Conversely, those who had flexion of the head relative to the cervical column showed the opposite traits. These findings of Solow and Tallgren were supported by Posnick,[86] and Thomas,[87] and similar findings were made by Opdebeek et al.,[88] Marcotte,[89] and Treuenfels.[90]

The resulting forces on the developing mandible created by the extension of head-on-neck posture appears to be a retrusive force on mandibular development.[78] In theory, an extension of the head posture would involve a passive stretching of the facial soft-tissue layer draping the face and neck.[91] Such soft-tissue restraints on the facial skeleton and dentition consists of the lips, skin, and fascia, continuing into the investing fascia of the neck and superficial musculature.[92] Conversely, a release of tension by the soft tissue and muscles by establishing an anterior position of the head in relation to the cervical column may allow the mandible to develop as it should in a down and forward position.

Because a statistical association exists between extension of the head on the neck and craniofacial and dentoalveolar morphology[84,85] the question is; what functional factor(s) contribute to the extended head–neck posture? Physiological functions such as respiration, swallowing, and speech are dependent on maintenance of a sufficient nasopharyngeal space and may be related to the craniocervical posture.[84]

Of the physiological functions in which the orofacial complex participates, respiration is the most essential, being vital for survival. To remain viable, one must be able to accommodate. Such accommodation to facilitate respiration is the variation in muscle behavior controlling the position of the mandible, lips, tongue, and cranium in relationship to the cervical spine.[76] Experimentally induced interruption of nasal respiration in humans resulted in a progressive extension of the head, reaching a peak at about 1 to 1½ hours after introduction of the stimulus.[93] Removal of the nasal obstruction allowed the preexisting

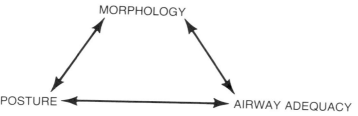

Fig. 12-1.   Simplified theoretical model for developmental relationships between craniofacial morphology, craniocervical posture, and airway adequacy. In principle, each factor may be the site of a primary affliction triggering cycle. (Solow B, Siersbaek-Nielsen S: Airway adequacy, head posture, and craniofacial morphology: Am J Orthod 86:214, 1984.)

respiratory pattern to resume, resulting in a return of head posture to baseline values.

Complete nasal obstruction in humans is rare, and total oral respiration, although possible in humans, is the exception rather than the rule. Total oral respiration is both uncomfortable and difficult to sustain.[76] Is it possible then for a minimal to moderate airway resistance to contribute to craniofacial morphology and the associated postural changes that occur? Is it possible for postural changes to occur (extension of the head on the neck) with normal airway resistance and still have a high correlation to craniofacial morphology (mandibular retrusion)?[94]

A theoretical model for developmental relationships between craniofacial morphology, craniocervical posture, and airway adequacy is illustrated in Fig. 12-1. In principle, each factor may be the site of a primary affliction triggering the cycle. A common denominator among the three factors (morphology, posture, and airway adequacy) may be altered muscle activity. Vig[76] suggests that minimal muscle activity of the orofacial, pharyngeal, and craniocervical complex should be present simply to resist the force of gravity. If altered muscle activity were present, Vig[76] indicates:

> [s]uch a heightened state-of-tone beyond the minimum electrical activity of a true resting posture, would provide a long-acting, low-level biophysical stimulus for a morphogenetic effect to occur.

In summary, a high correlation exists between an extended head-neck posture (FHP) and the development of the mandible into a retrognathic posture. Evidence today supports the contention that a growth-coordinating mechanism relates mandibular development to craniocervical angulation.[94] Thus, craniocervical postural changes may be the primary factor in the cycle of events leading to craniofacial and dentoalveolar morphology. Early treatment of functional postural abnormalities may in theory retard or reverse craniofacial and dentoalveolar morphologic changes.

Treatment of the oral-masticatory region today begins at such an early age for cosmetic, dysfunctional, symptomatic, and/or preventive reasons that neuromuscular influences stemming from the cervical spine must be considered if results are to be complete and functional. Until more research is done, clinicians who treat airway and craniomandibular disorders in the growing child must realize the profound influences a primary craniocervical dysfunction may have on the short- and long-term success and choice of treatment. I am in agreement with the concept of Schwartz: "... the development of the jaw will be permanently influenced by the position of the head if it is habitually or forcibly kept in one certain position."[95] Such a concept is not meant to be misunderstood as a solution pertaining to the etiology of craniomandibular disorders. The objective is to indicate another possible influence affecting jaw morphology and the craniomandibular region (occlusion, TMJ and associated muscles).

In adults whose mandible is advanced by orthognathic surgery, the head-neck posture should be considered. Relapses in orthognathic surgery have been related to resistance caused by the suprahyoid musculature as one possible factor.[96,97] Resistance of the suprahyoid musculature may result from an extended head-neck posture in postnatal years and or be secondary to an acquired FHP in later years. I suggest that an extended head-neck posture may, theoretically, be a factor to consider in orthognathic cases in which mandibular relapse was believed to occur secondary to suprahyoid resistance.

Cervical Spine Influences On the Upright Postural Position of the Mandible in Adults

Functional movements of the mandible occur during talking, mastication, swallowing, yawning, coughing, and licking of the lips. During these functional movements, tooth-to-tooth contacts may occur. When functional movements of the mandible cease, the teeth are apart and the mandible is considered to be in the "rest position." Such a rest position has been extensively explored, defined, and redefined during the past 50 years. The persistent interest in a postural jaw position has been inspired by the hypothesis stated by Sherrington[98]: "[P]osture is the basis of movement and all movement begins and ends with posture."

The rest position of the mandible varies from one person to another as well as within the same person not only from day to day but from moment to moment. Identifiable yet imprecise, the mandibular rest position is a position to which reference is made as a basic datum in many procedures in clinical dentistry. Dentistry often uses this mandibular rest position as a guide to determine vertical dimension of occlusion (VDO) for diagnostic and therapeutic purposes in edentulous as well as dentulous patients.[99–101] The rest position of the mandible is the position where all noncontact and masticatory movements of the mandible start and end.[102,103] According to Thompson, in cases involving extensive restorative procedures or orthodontics, classification of malocclusion should be based on the mandibular rest position and not on the occlusion of the teeth.[104]

The rest position of the mandible has several names, such as the clinical rest position, tonic rest position, and rest relation. Use of the term rest implies a state of equilibrium, quiet, or repose. A rest position of the mandible is said to exist when there is a space, referred to as the freeway space, between the upper teeth and the lower teeth.[104] The average freeway space is 3 mm between the tips of the anterior central upper and lower incisors.[105] The freeway space is variously called interocclusal distance, interocclusal clearance, interocclusal gap, or interocclusal rest space.[106] Numerous subtle factors can influence the rest position of the mandible even if a freeway space exists. Anatomical factors (i.e., the weight and number of teeth), physiological factors (i.e., tongue positioning and breathing), and pathological factors (i.e., ridge resorption under dentures) may all influence the rest position of the mandible.[106,107] Other influences such as age, drugs, and emotions have been suggested as influencing the rest position of the mandible.[108]

Dentistry continues to devise means of scientifically evaluating the rest position of the mandible other than clinical judgment.[100] Conventional methods such as swallowing, phonetics, esthetics, and the physiological approach are still being used today.[109] Electromyography (EMG) with or without biofeedback, myomonitor/kinesiograph,[110] and cephalometric analysis[111] have all been used to varying degrees. Judgment and clinical trial is still the common choice of the clinician when determining the "clinical" rest position of the mandible.[101]

A concern has developed over the use of the word rest; it is a misnomer according to Edwards (1955).[112] Edwards indicated that not all muscle fibers are at rest; rather, some of them are in tonic contraction. Kawamura and Fujimoto[113] found, as have others, spontaneous motor activity in masticatory muscles in the clinical rest position and concluded: ". . . it is not logical to decide the resting position of the mandible as the condition in which the jaw closing muscles are in complete electrical silence". These findings have led to the conclusion that there is more than one rest position of the mandible.[114]

Mandibular rest positions other than the clinical rest position that have been investigated are called the transcutaneous electrical stimulation (TES) and the EMG rest position.

The TES is often applied by the myomonitor.[115] The myomonitor rest position is suggested to be achieved by induction of an electrical current into the preauricular areas of the face to induce relaxation of the muscles of mastication and facial expression.[116] The rationale of TES by using the myomonitor hinges on several debatable issues. One central issue is whether stimulation of the motor branches of cranial nerves V and VII at the preauricular areas bilaterally actually occurs with use of surface electrodes[116] or is the stimulus that results in direct depolarization of the muscle membrane of the masseter muscle fibers.[117] The myomonitor is suggested for a variety of uses (e.g., production of a muscularly oriented maxillomandibular registration, diagnosis, and occlusal adjustment).[116] On the contrary, other studies[118,119] suggest that the myomonitor does not produce group function of the closing muscles, and does not result in a reproducible or uniqued mandibular position. This method of acquiring a rest position for diagnostic purposes should be examined more closely before such use is applied clinically.

Various studies[120-123] investigated the EMG rest position of the mandible. The various muscles studied are the masseter, anterotemporal, posterotemporal, and the anterior digastric muscles. The mandibular EMG rest position, which has an average freeway space of 11 mm, was never found at or near the clinical rest position, which has an average freeway space of 3 mm.[123] Diagnostically and therapeutically, encouraging a freeway space of 11 mm or increasing the vertical dimension of occlusion by 8 mm to achieve the mean clinical freeway space of 3 mm would not be realistic or functional.

Therefore, judgment and clinical trial is still the preferred method to establish a rest position of the mandible. Regardless of the method/technique used to determine the rest position, the influence of head-neck posture must be considered a major factor. I believe that the head-neck posture has a significant influence on the mandibular rest position.

When head-neck influences are considered, the term rest, should no longer be used to describe the mandibular position at rest. Numerous studies show the mandibular muscles not to be at rest when the mandible is in the clinical rest position.[113,124-127] Even though a "term" does not influence a "technique," the word or phrase used may influence a clinician's thinking regarding the significance of other variables that must be considered. A more appropriate term to use for the rest position of the mandible is "the upright postural position of the mandible (UPPM)," as suggested by Rugh and Drago in 1981.[122] The emphasis on phrases such as "head upright,"[104,128] "patient at ease in the upright position,"[106] "patient relaxing comfortable in the upright position,"[129] "patient resting comfortably in the upright position"[130] existed prior to the suggestions of Rugh and Drago. These past definitions seem to place emphasis on the existence of an upright postural position for achievement of the "ideal" mandibular position with teeth apart.

The UPPM is defined in nonclinical words such as: upright, resting, relaxing, and at ease. Clinical definitions are often obscure and quite variable as indicated by the use of other terms such as, centric relation (CR), centric occlusion, and centric position. For the clinician to know whether the patient has met the criteria of the previous definitions would be difficult to determine scientifically. I suggest that if the mandibular position is related to the upright head-neck posture, such a relationship places an emphasis on the need to evaluate and treat the cervical spine to achieve the appropriate UPPM. Emphasis must be placed on the dynamics and posturing of the mandible/cervical spine and the functional interrelationships between the two.

Mechanisms Influencing Upright Postural Position of the Mandible

Muscle tone. One of the generally accepted mechanisms in controlling the UPPM is the continuous state of tonic muscle activity occurring in the mandibular elevator muscles, namely the masseter, temporalis, and the medial pterygoids. This tonic activity is similar to the original concept of muscle tone in antigravity muscles elsewhere in the body.

Muller in 1838 designated tone to be "the slight contractile tension characteristic of normal skeletal muscle when at rest."[131] Tone in a muscle results from the number, size, and frequency of firing of the active motor units in the muscles.[132,133] The motor unit consists of the anterior horn cell, the cell's axon, and all the muscle fibers innervated by the axon.[134] The anterior horn cell's activity, and thus the motor unit activity, is influenced by the peripheral and central control systems. Under normal circumstances, the number and activity of the motor units of the mandibular elevators should be minimal if the ideal UPPM is to be achieved.

The prevailing tone (tension) at any moment of any skeletal muscle is, however, the collective sum of two additional factors[135,136]; (1) the static elastic properties of the connective tissue components of the muscles (the fascial sheaths, intermuscular septa, and tendons); and (2) the static elastic properties of the fibrillary muscle portein molecular aggregates (myosin and actin) within the individual muscle fibers. In normal circumstances, factors 1 and 2 cannot be modified directly by the nervous system. Primary pathological conditions such as muscle fibrosis or collagen diseases can affect factor 1. Old age, malnutrition, and muscle atrophy can affect factor 2. Clinically, in the absence of such pathological conditions, factors 1 and 2 provide a background of static tension to the tone provided by the motor unit activity.

Tissue elasticity tone. Tissue elasticity tone refers to the elastic tissue properties of connective tissues outside the epimysium, the connective tissue sheath surrounding each muscle. The elastic components within each muscle (factors 1 and 2 previously described) also contribute to this tissue elasticity tone. Therefore, the UPPM is influenced by ". . . the tissue elastic properties of the associated tissues, especially muscles."[137]

Tissue elasticity tone is present in the mandibular elevator muscles, the suprahyoid and infrahyoid muscles, and associated connective tissues. Several studies have demonstrated tissue elastic qualities influencing mandibular positioning and movement. One study showed that slow closure of the mandible from a fully opened position toward occlusion occurred without any change in muscle activity of the jaw-closing muscles.[138] Another study showed that closing from a fully opened position was controlled by the elastic qualities of the diagastric muscles.[139] In studies involving chewing, elastic recoil of the elevator muscles has been suggested as being important in the first part of the chewing stroke.[140] The UPPM has been suggested as being an equilibrium position that can be independent of muscle activity.[137]

For the most ideal UPPM to exist, neuromuscular and soft tissue harmony of the muscles and the associated connective tissue of the mandible must exist.

Head-Neck Posture Influencing Tissue Elasticity and Muscle Tone

Originally the UPPM was believed to be stable throughout life.[104] Subsequent studies have shown the UPPM to vary according to the occlusion,[141] loss of teeth,[142] insertion of dentures,[143] environmental changes,[144] and a host of other factors previously mentioned, ranging from age to temperature changes to use of drugs. All the above factors must be recognized and controlled when feasible. I believe that head-neck posture will have the most immediate and long-lasting effect on the UPPM. This belief seems to shared in part by other researchers.[102,145-148]

Postural changes of the head-neck in the sagittal plane influencing the mandible in the sagittal plane are discussed in this chapter. Other dimensional changes occurring with mandibular and cervical spine postures are not intentionally ignored. An understanding of a three-dimensional concept of the ways in which the UPPM is affected by the cervical spine is desirable. Patients do manifest varying degrees of head-neck postures that are either rotated or side-bent or a combination of both. Our state of scientific and clinical knowledge is just beginning to encompass an understanding of changes of the cervical spine in the sagittal plane relevant to the UPPM. To this end, the reader is cautioned regarding conclusions drawn for clinical applications.

Postural changes of flexion and extension in the sagittal plane affecting the UPPM are analyzed first. Extension will be considered to occur in the upper cervical spine (occiput and the first three cervical segments), although extension does occur in the lower cervical spine segments; however, we are not considering full ROM in order to draw certain conclusions. Extension is synonymous with dorsiflexion, posterior rotation of the occiput on atlas, and backward bending. Flexion also is to be considered as occurring in the upper cervical spine. Flexion is synonymous with ventroflexion, anterior rotation of the occiput on the atlas, and forward bending.

Extension and Flexion Influencing Tissue Elasticity

Extension. When the chin is taken away from the chest during extension, an increase in tension occurs in the suprahyoid and infrahyoid musculature, resulting in depression and retrusion of the mandible.[137,148,149] Subsequently an increase in the freeway space results. (Fig. 12-2)

Flexion. Flexion produces a decrease in the freeway space.[137,148] and results in a decrease in the tissue elastic forces, thereby allowing the mandible to posture itself upward and forward.

Extension and Flexion Influencing Muscle Activity

The tonic neck reflex (TNR), as discussed earlier in this chapter, plays a key role in the achievement of a head–neck posture. The TNR has a significant influence on jaw muscle activity, especially those muscles innervated by cranial nerve V.[150] The trigeminal mesencephalic nucleus in the superior colliculus is believed to be necessary for the TNR to influence jaw muscle activity.[151,152] Trigemino-neck reflexes have been demonstrated to occur through motor neurons located in the subnucleus caudalis and probably in the dorsal horn of the upper cervical spine.[153] A closely organized neurophysiological reflex relationship appears to exist between TNR activity and trigeminal reflex activity.

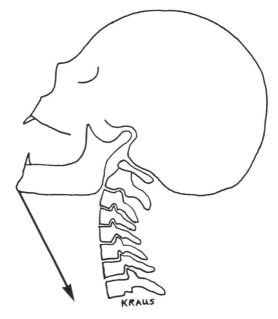

Fig. 12-.2 Tissue elastic force results in depression and retrusion on mandible during extension of head and on neck.

In one study, electric stimulation was applied to the central end of the cut first cervical nerve, and EMG activity was recorded from the masticatory muscles.[152] In the same study,[152] EMG responses were abolished after the first three cervical nerves were cut. The effect the TNR has on jaw muscle activity is appreciated by observing animals biting on a hard object such as a bone or a nut between the right molars. The animal turns its head to the left and tilts it to the right. The head position causes an increased masticatory muscle tone and a shift of the mandible to the working side.[152] The animal is then prepared for a powerful bite with the right molars by facilatation through the TNR. Several independent studies have investigated head position influencing jaw muscle activity; the following consistent pattern emerges.

Extension. Extension produces an increase in jaw muscle activity in the temporalis, masseter, and anterior digastric muscles.[152] A second study of the same muscles showed a major increase in activity in the temporalis muscles, a moderate increase in activity in the masseter muscles, and no increase in activity in the digastric muscles.[154] An investigation that recorded only masseter and anterior digastric muscle activity showed a marked increase in the masseter and a decrease in the anterior digastric muscle.[150] The results from these studies infer that extension causes an increase in temporalis and masseter muscle activity, producing a force of elevation and retrusion on the mandible (Fig. 12-3). A decrease in the freeway space results.[149]

Flexion. The previous studies reveal that flexion causes a general decrease in jaw muscle activity, especially in the temporalis and masseter muscles. Anterior digastric activity consistently increased with head flexion. Such activity of the anterior digastric may stabilize the hyoid bone primarily. The resulting

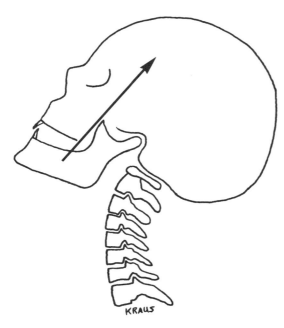

Fig. 12-3. Muscle activity force results in elevation and retrusion on mandible during extension of head on neck.

forces on the mandible, with the head postured in flexion, is apparently minimal depression and retrusion.

The forces acting on the mandible during head flexion or extension may be summarized as follows.

Head extension → Tissue elasticity → Depression and retrusion
Head extension → Muscle activity → Elevation and retrusion
Head Flexion → Tissue elasticity → Elevation and protrusion
Head Flexion → Muscle activity → Depression and Retrusion.

The previous discussion shows that extension and flexion of the head on the neck influence mandibular tissue elasticity and muscle activity tone. The degree of gravitational influence on the tissues of the mandible must also be considered. The position of the head in the earth's gravitional field, in going from the upright to the supine position, also influences tissue elasticity and muscle activity tone about the mandible.[132,155] A patient lying supine with the head extended or flexed further alters the soft tissue and muscle activity forces on the mandible.

The influence of the forward head posture on the management of the position and movement of the mandible is discussed next.

Forward Head Posture Influencing Mandibular Position and Movement in Adults

A common sign of cervical spine dysfunction is a FHP. The FHP as described by Kendall et al.[156] is an increased thoracic kyphosis and cervical hyperextension (backward bending) with the eyes kept level. *Cervical hyper-*

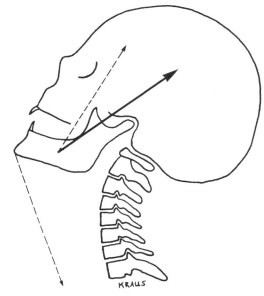

Fig. 12-4. When head is extended on neck, a force of elevation and retrusion maybe occurring on mandible. Trajectory of mandibular closure and initial occlusal contacts are posterior to maximum intercuspated position.

extension occurs in the upper cervical spine. A flattening or decrease in cervical lordosis occurs in the lower cervical spine. Spinal variations undoubtedly occur within the FHP from person to person. The main emphasis is on the head being forward of the vertical reference line. The correct vertical reference line as described by Kendall[157] should pass through the tip of the shoulder and the lobe of the ear. When the head is forward, the chin is up, keeping the eyes level and placing the occiput and the upper cervical spine segments, in extension.

Cervical spine dysfunction is recognizable by signs other than the FHP. A thorough musculoskeletal evaluation (see Chapter 11) will determine if a forward head posture is significant.

Forward Head Posture Influencing Mandibular Positioning

In summary, there is a high association between a retrognathic mandible and an extended head posture during growth and development.[84,85] An extended head-neck posture suggests that retrusion force is exerted on the mandible during growth. Second, the soft tissue (Fig. 12-2) and muscle activity (Fig. 12-3) forces independently influencing mandibular position when the head is held in extension relative to the neck was discussed. When a person's head is held in extension on the neck, the resulting forces on the mandible may result in a force of elevation and retrusion, as shown in Figure 12-4. Third, a study[158] demonstrated that as normal subjects assumed different degrees of a FHP, a significant decrease in the freeway space resulted, as measured by the kinesiograph. Such a decrease in the freeway space indicates that an elevation force

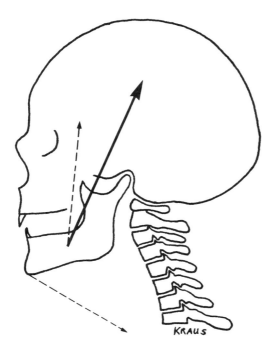

Fig. 12-5. In forward head posture, it is proposed that a force of elevation and retrusion is occurring on mandible. Trajectory of mandibular closure and initial occlusal contacts are posterior to maximum intercuspated position.

is exerted on the mandible. Fourth, other studies[159–162] have demonstrated the effects of a natural head posture and of a forward head posture on mandibular positioning.

I propose that in adults who have acquired a FHP, the resulting force on the mandible is elevation and retrusion, as shown in Figure 12-5. This concept evolved not only from clinical observations but by the previously presented supportive material.

Individual variations must be recognized as to the degree of cervical spine dysfunction. Cervical spine dysfunction refers to the FHP and altered mobility of the cervical spine. Varying degrees of soft tissue and muscle activity secondary to cervical spine dysfunction will cause variability in the UPPM. Skeptics suggest that such variations in the UPPM in response to head–neck changes occur constantly and should be expected. Therefore, how important is the influence of head-neck posture on the UPPM to the craniomandibular region? Unlike the person who has good position and movement of the head-neck area, persons with cervical spine dysfunction associated with an improper UPPM clinically have far less adaptability. Cervical spine dysfunction often has existed for many months to years, decreasing the person's physiological adaptive range. Cervical spine dysfunction causing an improper UPPM both in positioning and mobility may result in various craniomandibular dysfunctions with emphasis on muscle activity. Clinically, I observe that cervical spine dysfunction contributes to less tolerance by the person who is receiving treatment(s) to the craniomandibular region (occlusion, TMJ, muscles). A lack of patient's response to treatments of the craniomandibular region often leads to incorrect conclusions if cervical spine influences are not recognized.

A clinical example demonstrating how a patient's adaptibility is decreased due to cervical spine dysfunction is the patient's adverse response to a change in the VDO. VDO is the distance designated from the base of the nose to the base of the chin when the teeth are in maximum intercuspation.[101] The freeway space is the space between the UPPM and VDO. Freeway space is physiologically necessary to allow the muscles of the oral–masticatory system to relax.[141] Freeway space that is infringed on (by increasing VDO) may cause disturbances in the oral–masticatory system.[141]

Contrary to the belief that an increase in VDO is hazardous, a study by Carlsson et al.[163] indicated that most patients adapt to changes in vertical dimension and that the determination of the height of occlusion might not be a critical procedure as has often been stated. As is the case in most studies dealing with functional occlusion, no mention was made of the state of function of the cervical spine. If cervical spine dysfunction existed in this previous study, I would anticipate that for the following reasons the change in VDO may not have been tolerated as easily by the subjects.

Dentistry can influence VDO in many ways. Intraoral applicances used to treat muscle imbalances and/or TMJ dysfunctions always cover some of the occlusal surfaces. The new VDO that results from application of the intraoral appliance will increase the VDO or, if an insufficient vertical existed, may establish a correct VDO. Regardless of the extent of the preexisting VDO, every appliance alters the VDO.

In the example of an anterior repositioning appliance, which is often used to stabilize disc–condyle dislocations, the VDO and anterior mandibular position are often overcorrected positions. The patient's oral–masticatory system may not be able to tolerate such a change in VDO. An increase in the VDO in the presence of an already decreased freeway space secondary to a FHP (Fig. 12-5) may have an adverse affect. The result may be an increase in signs and symptoms such as bruxism, headaches, and neck pain, as I have observed.

I propose that a change in VDO changes the relationship of the head on the neck. Several studies support the view that the head is maintained by synergistic activity of the anterior head-neck and posterior head-neck muscles, as documented by EMG.[164,165] Studies have shown a close correlation between trigeminal inputs and neck muscle activity,[166,167] suggesting that some degree of synergy exists between these two areas. Neural communication also has been shown to exist between the trigemino-neck reflex and the jaw-opening reflex.[168] Research documents[120,123] that as VDO is increased, minimum EMG activity of mandibular muscles is recorded in a resting range of approximately 11 mm. In 30 male students whose bite (VDO) was opened 8 mm, Daly et al.[169] demonstrated that 90 percent of the subjects had an extension of the head on the neck after 1 hour. This finding is sequential to the observation of Vig et al.[93] In our study,[161] increased VDO caused a tendency for the head to rise, as measured by lateral cephalometric radiographs.

From the previous information, a cycle of events may occur. As VDO is altered (increased), supramandibular muscle activity is decreased. Increasing the VDO may result in decrease in posterior neck muscle activity owing to the synergistic activity and neural organization of the trigemino-neck reflex. As VDO increases, the head is placed in an extended position, thereby influencing

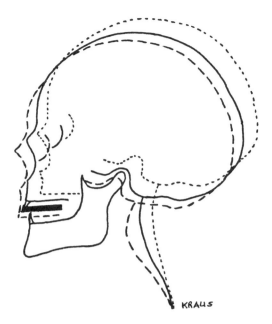

Fig. 12-6. Possible adaptive responses of head-neck posture to a change in vertical dimension of occlusion (VDO). Regardless of change in head posture, peripheral mechanisms (vestibular, ocular, neck proprioceptive systems) will maintain the eyes in horizontal plane. Preexisting forward head posture prior to any change in VDO (solid line); change in head-neck posture to a more upright posture in response to a change in VDO (dotted line); change in head-neck posture to a more forward head posture in response to a change in VDO (dashed line).

the TNR. When head balance is upset, the horizontal position of the head is first restored by vestibular action on the neck muscles.[9] From such an extended position, the TNR, in conjunction with the ocular and vestibular systems, will attempt to bring the eyes level. The eyes may be brought level by *the head adjusting to a more upright position* or by *the head adjusting to a greater FHP.* (Fig. 12-6) How the head-neck posture responds to such a change in VDO will be, I believe, dependent on the degree of cervical spine dysfunction and/or how much the VDO is increased.

Dentists should be aware that the head-neck may not be able to adapt to even a minimum change in VDO if cervical spine dysfunction exists.

In the example of using an anterior repositioning appliance for an anterior disc dislocation that reduces, the beginning vertical and anterior components to mandibular position (placing the mandible into a down and forward position) is often an overcorrected position. This mandibular position is necessary to "recapture" the disc but may also encourage an appropriate head-neck positioning that is responding to the change in VDO. Symptoms related to both the TMJ and cervical spine may then be diminished significantly. The dentist may then progress to a "CR" appliance, which often places the mandible in a less vertical and anterior horizontal position as compared with the original anterior repositioning appliance. This change in vertical of the appliance may then alter the head-neck posture again, with a recurrence of symptoms. Such a recurrence of symptoms is related to the cervical spine and not to the TMJ disorder. Symptoms may not recur if the associated cervical spine dysfunction is treated before and/or during the application of the anterior repositioning appliance. Treatment of the FHP to a more upright posture allows the mandible to posture

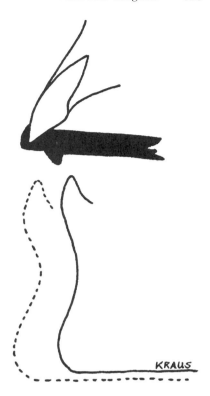

Fig. 12-7. An anterior reposition-ing appliance influences mandible to posture itself down and forward and to close in a trajectory of closure more anteriorly (dashed line); Forward head posture influences mandible to posture itself up and back and to close in a trajectory of closure more posteriorly (solid line).

I prefer that the occlusion or appliance be adjusted in the patient's given head-neck posture in the sitting or standing position. As the patient's cervical spine posture is managed by physical therapy, additional adjustments on the appliance may be necessary.

When an intraoral appliance is used to control for muscle hyperactivity secondary to a malocclusion and/or head-neck posture, the guidelines for use and design of the appliance given in Chapter 5 should be followed. Such an appliance controls for occlusal influences while allowing cervical spine postural corrections to occur.

An intraoral appliance can affect the trajectory of habitual mandibular opening and closing movements.[188] The head-neck posture can affect the trajectory of habitual mandibular opening and closing movements. What can be visualized as occurring is a battle over the UPPM and the trajectory of jaw closure. The battle is between the head-neck posture and the appliance/occlusion. A clear example of this battle over the UPPM and the trajectory of jaw closure can be observed clinically with an anterior repositioning appliance. The anterior repositioning appliance places the mandible in an overcorrected position, namely a down and forward position, influencing the patient to posture the mandible further forward and to close in an anterior trajectory of closure. The FHP influences the mandible to posture itself in an elevated and retruded position and thus to take a trajectory of closure more posteriorly (Fig. 12-7). The use of an anterior repositioning appliance with cervical spine dysfunction may result in an increase in muscular symptoms related to the cervical spine and craniomandibular areas. Classically, this occurs in the patient with an anterior disc dislocation that reduces with associated muscular symptoms. Once the anterior repositioning appliance is in place, the patient may no longer experience clicking and popping, but muscular symptoms may either fail to improve or get worse.

Postural treatment before and/or during use of an anterior repositioning appliance may allow better patient acceptance of the appliances and relief of symptoms. Correction of the FHP (cervical spine dysfunction) through physical therapy allows the mandible to posture itself in a down and forward position, which is a position similar to that encouraged by an anterior repositioning appliance.

In summary, the degree of postural change, occlusion, and patients' individual adaptive capacity and psychological profile play key roles in contributing to muscle and joint symptoms. Ways in which head-neck position/mobility affects the UPPM and trajectory of jaw closure have been suggested. Clinical examples that I have frequently observed have been cited. The clinician must consider each person individually. In some persons, the cervical spine dysfunction may play a primary role; in others, it may have a secondary role. The clinician must learn to recognize an individual's needs and wants in order to direct the person toward the most appropriate treatment(s). Members of the physical therapy and dental professions, working together, play a significant role in the management of the craniomandibular complex. This chapter has emphasized the role of the cervical spine. In conclusion, Mohl states[145]:

> It therefore seems reasonable to consider that at least some of the dysfunctional problems involving the masticatory system could be in some way related to the adaptive requirements imposed by chronic or acute postural demands.

REFERENCES

1. Shock P: Current concepts of the aging process. JAMA 175:108, 1961
2. Kiernander B: Discussion on postural re-education—a critical examination of methods. Proc R Soc Med Phys Med 49:667, 1956
3. Willis WD Jr, Grossman RG: Medical Neurobiology. 2nd Ed. CV Mosby, St. Louis, 1977
4. Peterson B: Distribution of neural responses to tilting within vestibular nuclei of the cat. J Neurophysiol 33:750, 1970
5. Wilson V, Maeda M: Connections between semicircular canals and neck motoneurons in the cat. J Neurophysiol 37:346, 1974
6. Akaike T, Fanardjian V, Ito M, et al; Electrophysiological analysis of the vestibulospinal reflex pathway of rabbit. Exp Brain Res 17:497, 1973
7. Wilson V, Yoshida M: Monosynaptic inhibition of neck motoneurons by the medical vestibular nucleus. Exp Brain Res 9:365, 1969

8. Suzuki J, Cohen B: Head, eye, body and limb movements from semicircular canal nerves. Exp Neurol 10:393, 1964

9. Roberts TDM: Neurophysiology of Postural Mechanisms. Butterworths, London, 1967

10. Reid T: An inquiry into the human mind on the principles of common sense. Sect. 22. In Hamilton W (ed): The Works of Thomas Reid. Edinburgh, Maclachlan, Stewart, London, 1846

11. Airapetyants E, Kislyakov V, Lobanav L, et al: The role of the motor analysor in the compensatory function of the cerebral cortex. Physiol Bohemoslov 6:297, 1957

12. Edwards A: Body sway and vision. J Exp Psychol 36:526, 1946

13. Travis R: An experimental analysis of dynamic and static equilibrium. J Exp Psychol 35:216, 1945

14. Outerbridge JS, Melvill J: Reflex vestibular control of head movements in man. Aerospace Med 42:935, 1971

15. Guitton D, Crommelinck M, Roucoux A: Stimulation of the superior colliculus in the alert cat. Exp Brain Res 39:63, 1980

16. Everett NB: Functional Neuroanatomy. 6th ed. Lea & Febiger, Philadelphia, 1971

17. Wilson V, Precht W, Dieringer N: Responses of different compartments of cats splenius muscle to optokinetic stimulation. Exp Brain Res 50:153, 1983

18. Vidal P, Roucoux A, Berthoz A: Horizontal eye position-related activity in neck muscles of the alert cat. Exp Brain Res 46:448, 1982

19. Goodwin GM, McCloskey DI, Matthew PBC: The persistence of appreciable kinesthesia after paralysing joint afferents but preserving muscle afferents. Brain Res 37:326, 1972

20. Manzoni D, Pompeiano D, Stampacchia G: Tonic cervical influences on posture and reflex movements. Arch Ital Biol 117(2):81, 1979.

21. Wyke B: Neurology of the cervical spinal joints. Physiotherapy 65:72, 1979

22. Wyke B: Articular neurology—a review. Physiotherapy 58:94, 1972

23. Magnus R: Some results of studies in the physiology of posture. Lancet 2:531, 1926

24. Magnus R: Animal Posture, Croonian Lecture. Proc R Soc B 98:339,1925

25. Magnus R, DeKleijn A: Die Abhangigkeit des Tonus der Extremitatenmuskeln von der Kopfstellung. Pflugers Arch Physiol 145:455, 1912

26. McCouch G, Deering I, Ling T: Location of receptors for tonic neck reflexes. J Neurophysiol 14:191, 1951

27. Minkowski M: Sur les mouvements, les reflexes et les reactions musculaires du foetus humain de 2 a 5 mois et leur relations avec le systeme nerveux foetal. Rev Neurol 37:1105, 1921

28. Gesell A, Thompson H: Infant Behavior: Its Genesis and Growth. McGraw-Hill, New York, 1934

29. Gesell A, et al: The tonic neck reflex (TNR) in the human infant. From the photographic library of the Value Clinic of Child Development, 1938

30. Humphrey, T: Spinal tract of the trigeminal nerve in human embryos between 7.5 weeks of menstrual age and its relation to early fetal activities. J Comp Neurol 97:143, 1952

31. Gesell A: The tonic neck reflex in the human infant. J Pediatr 13:455, 1938

32. Fukuda T: Studies on human dynamic postures from the viewpoint of postural reflexes. Acta Otolarayngol (Stockholm), suppl., 161:1, 1961

33. Igarashi M, Watanabe T, Maxian P: Role of neck propriocepters for the maintenance of dynamic bodily equilibrium in the squirrel monkey. Laryngoscope 79:1713, 1969
34. Cohen L: Role of eye and neck proprioceptive mechanisms in body orientation and motor coordination. J Neurophysiol 24:1, 1961
35. DeKleijn A: Action reflexes du labyrinthe et du con sur les muscles de l'oeil. Arch Neerl Physiol 2:643, 1918
36. Korovina M: Electrical changes in the various eye muscles produced by impulses from the vestibular apparatus and from the neck muscles in animals of different ages. Fiziol Zh Mose 45:32, 1959
37. Wapner S, Werner H, Chandler K: Experiments on sensory-tonic field theory of perception. J Exp Psychol 42:351, 1951
38. Kleijn, de A: Tonische Labyrinth und Halsreflexe auf die Augen. Arch Ges Physiol 186:84, 1921
39. Meyer DL, Schott D, Buttner U, Schaefer KP: Influence of head position on excitation patterns of oculomotor neurons during nystagmus. Programs and abstracts, Society for Neuroscience, Abstract 456, Fourth Annual Meeting 1974
40. Cope S, Ryan GMS: Cervical and otolith vertigo. J Laryngol 73:113, 1959
41. Gray LP: Extralabyrinthine vertigo due to cervical muscle lesions. J Laryngol 70:352, 1956
42. Weeks VD, Travell J: Postural vertigo due to trigger areas in the sternocleidomastoid muscle. J Pediatr 47:315, 1955
43. De Jong PTVM De Jong JMBV, Cohen B, Jongkees LBW: Ataxia and nystagmus induced by injection of local anesthetics in the neck. Ann Neurol 1:240, 1977
44. Kerr FWL: Structural relation of the trigeminal spinal tract to upper cervical roots and the solitary nucleus in the cat. Exp Neurol 4:134, 1961
45. Kerr FWL: Facial, vagal and glossopharyngeal nerves in the cat: afferent connections. Arch Neurol 6:264, 1962
46. Kerr FWL: The divisional organization of afferent fibres of the trigeminal nerve. Brain 86:721, 1963
47. Bell WE: Orofacial pains Differential Diagnosis. 2 Ed. Year Book Medical, Chicago, 1980
48. Kerr WLF, Olafson RA: Trigeminal and cervical volleys—convergence on single units in the spinal gray at C1 and C2. Arch Neurol 5:171, 1961
49. Paillard J: Proprioception musculaire et sens de la position. Arch Ital Biol 111:451, 1973
50. DeLong M: Activity of pallidal neurons during movement. J Neurophysiol 34:414, 1971
51. Evarts E: Representation of movements and muscles by pyramidal tract neurons of the precentral motor cortex. p. 215. In Yahr M, Purpura D (eds): Neurophysiological Basis of Normal and Abnormal Motor Activities. Raven Press, New York, 1967
52. Thack W: Discharge of Purkinje and cerebellar nuclear neurons during rapidly alternating arm movements in the monkey. J Neurophysiol 31:785, 1968
53. Coulter JD, Bowker SP, Wise EA, et al: Cortical, tectal and medullary descending pathways to the cervical spinal cord. p. 263. In Granit R, Pompeiano O (eds): Reflex control of posture and movement. Elsevier/North-Holland Biomedical Press, Amsterdam, 1979
54. Taub E, Goldberg I, Taub P: Deafferentation in monkeys pointing at a target without visual feedback. Exp Neurol 46:178, 1975

55. Lashley K: The accuracy of movement in the absence of excitation from the moving organ. Am J Physiol 43:169, 1917

56. Gibbs C: The continuous regulation of skilled response by kinesthetic feedback. Br J Phychol 45:24, 1954

57. Eccles J, Sabah N, Schmidt R, et al: Modes of operation of the cerebellum in the dynamic loop control of movement. Brain Res 41:73, 1972

58. Tinbergen N: Ethology and stress diseases. Science 185:20, 1974 (Lecture delivered in Stockholm, Sweden, by Dr. Tinbergen on 12 December 1973 when he received the Nobel Prize for Physiology or Medicine and was published with the permission of the Nobel Foundation.)

59. Holst E, Mittelstaedt H: Das Reafferenzprinzip. Naturwissenschaften 37:464, 1950

60. Tinbergen N: Functional ethology and the human sciences. Proc R Soc Lond (B) 182:385, 1972

61. Teixeira R, Lackner J: Influence of apparent head position on optokinetic nystagmus and eye posture. Exp Brain Res 24:435, 1976

62. Hellebrandt F, Riddle K, Larsen E, et al: Gravitational influences on postural alignment. Physiother Rev 22:143, 1942

63. Sugano H, Takeya T: Measurement of body movement and its clinical application. Jpn J Physiol 20:296, 1970

64. Kurtz R, Prestera H: The Body Reveals. Harper & Row, San Francisco, 1984

65. Lowen A: The Language of the Body. Collier Books, New York, 1971

66. Lowen A: Depression and the Body. Coward, McCann and Geoghegan, New York, 1972

67. Tinbergen N: Functional ethology and the human sciences. Proc R Soc London (B) 182:385, 1972

68. Jones F, Hanson J, Miller J, et al: Neck muscle tension and the postural image. Ergonomics 4:133, 1961

69. Jones F, Hanson J, Miller J, et al: Quantitative analysis of abnormal movement: the sit-to-stand pattern. Am J Phys Med 42:208, 1963

70. Jones F, Hanson J, Gray F: Startle as a paradigm of malposture. Percept Mot Skills 19:21, 1964

71. Walshe F: On certain tonic or postural reflexes in hemiplegia with special reference to the so-called "associated movements." Brain 46:1, 1923

72. Hellebrandt F, Houtz S, Krikorian A: Influence of bimanual exercise on unilateral work capacity. J Appl Physiol 2:446, 1950

73. Hellebrandt F, Houtz S, Partridge M, et al: Tonic neck reflexes in exercises of stress in man. Am J Phys Med 35:144, 1956

74. Magnus R: Animal posture. Proc R Soc London (B) 98:339, 1925

75. Dibbets JM, vander Weele LT, Uildriks AK: Symptoms of TMJ dysfunction: indicators of growth patterns? J Pedod 9:265, 1985

76. Vig PS: Respiratory mode and morphological types: some thoughts and preliminary conclusions. p. 233. In McNamara J: Nasorespiratory Function and Craniofacial Growth, Monogram No. 9. Craniofacial Growth Series. Center for Human Growth and Development, The University of Michigan, Ann Arbor, MI, 1979

77. Moss ML: A functional cranial analysis of centric relation. Dent Clin North Am 19:431, 1975

78. Solow B, Kreiborg S: Soft-tissue stretching: a possible control factor in craniofacial morphogenesis. Scand J Dent Res 85:505, 1977

79. Moss ML: An introduction to the neurobiology of oro-facial growth. Acta Biotheoret 22:236, 1972

80. Massler M., Schour I: Atlas of the mouth in health and disease. 2nd Ed. Am Dental Assoc Chicago Ill. 1958
81. Schwartz AM: Kopfhaltung und Kiefer. Z Stomatol 24:669, 1926
82. Lisowski FP, Stelt A, Vis JH: Upright posture: an experimental investigation. Acta FRN Univ Comen 5:127, 1961
83. Moss ML: Rotation of the otic capsule in bipedal rats. Am J Phys Anthrop 19:301, 1961
84. Solow B, Tallgren A: Head posture and craniofacial morphology. Am J Phys Anthrop 44:417, 1976
85. Solow B, Tallgren A: Dentoalveolar morphology in relation to craniocervical posture. Angle Orthod 47:157, 1977
86. Posnick B: Craniovertical angulation and morphogenic variables in children: a cephalometric study. M.S. Thesis, University of North Carolina, 1978
87. Thomas BP: Craniocervical angulation and morphologic variables in children: a cephalometric study. M.S. Thesis, University of North Carolina, 1978
88. Opdebeek H, Bell WH, Eisenfeld J, Mishelevich D: Comparative study between the SFS and LFS rotation as a possible morphogenetic mechanism. Am J Orthod 74:509, 1978
89. Marcotte MR: Head posture and dentofacial proportions. Angle Orthod 51:208, 1981
90. von Treuenfels H: Die Relation der Atlasposition bei prognather und progener Kieferanomalie. Fortschr Kieferorthop 42:482, 1981
91. Solow B, Greve E: Craniocervical Angulation and Nasal Respiratory Resistance pp. 87. In McNamera J.: Naso-respiratory Function and Craniofacial Growth. Monograph Number 9, Craniofacial Growth Series, Center for Human Growth and Development, The University of Michigan, Ann Arbor, Michigan 1979
92. Archer SY, Vig PS: Effects of head position on intraoral pressures in class I and Class II adults. Am J Orthod 87:311, 1985
93. Vig PS, Showfety KJ, Phillips C: Experimental manipulation of head posture. Am J Orthod 77:258, 1980
94. Solow B, Siersbaek-Nielsen S, Greve E: Airway adequacy, head posture, and craniofacial morphology. Am J Orthodontics 86:214, 1984
95. Schwartz AM: Positions of the head and malrelations of the jaws. Int J Orthodontic Oral Surg Radiogr 14:56, 1928
96. Schendel SA, Epker BN: Results after mandibular advancement surgery: an analysis of 87 cases. J Oral Surg 38:265, 1980
97. Proffit WR, Bell WH: Openbite p. 1075. In Bell WH, Proffit WR, White RP (eds): Surgical Correction of Dentofacial Deformities. WB Saunders , Philadelphia, 1980
98. Sherrington CS: Reflexes elicitable from the pinna vibrassae and jaws of cats. J Physiol 51:404, 1917
99. Krajicek DD, Jones PM, Radzyminski SF, et al: Clinical and electromyographic study of mandibular rest position. J Prosthet Dent 11:826, 1961
100. Turrell AJ: Clinical assessment of vertical dimension. J Prosthet Dent 28:238, 1972
101. Weinberg LA: Vertical dimension: a research and clinical analysis. J Prosthet Dent 47:290, 1982
102. Preiskel HW: Some observations on the postural position of the mandible. J Prosthet Dent 15:625, 1965
103. Kazis H, Kazis AJ: Complete Mouth Rehabilitation. Henry Kimpton, London, 1956.
104. Thompson JR: The rest position of the mandible and its significance to dental science. J Am Dent Assoc 33:151, 1946

105. Beyron HL: Characteristics of functionally optimal occlusion and principles of occlusal rehabilitation. J Am Dent Assoc 48:648, 1954
106. Atwood DA: A review of the fundamentals on rest position and vertical dimension. Int Dent J 9:6, 1959
107. Murphy WM: Rest position of the mandible. J Prosthet Dent 17:329, 1967
108. Landa JS: Integration of structure and function of the temporomandibular joint. NY J Dent 24:290, 1954
109. Fieldman S, Leupold RJ, Staling LM: Rest vertical dimension determined by electromyography with biofeedback as compared to conventional methods. J Prosthet Dent 84:216, 1978
110. George JP, Boone ME: A clinical study of rest position using the kinesiograph and myomonitor. J Prosthet Dent 41:456, 1979
111. Basler FL, Douglas JR, Moulton RS: Cephalometric analysis of the vertical dimension of occlusion. J Prosthet Dent 11:831, 1961
112. Edwards LF: Some anatomic facts and fancies. J Prosthet Dent 5:825, 1955
113. Kawamura Y, Fujimoto J: Some physiologic considerations on measuring rest position of the mandible. Med J Osaka Univ 8:247, 1957
114. Wessberg GA, Epker GN, Elliott AC: Comparison of mandibular rest positions induced by phonetics, transcutaneous electrical stimulation, and masticatory electromyography. J Prosthet Dent 49:100, 1983
115. Jankelson B, Swain CW: Physiological aspects of masticatory muscle stimulation: the myo-monitor. Quintessence Int 3:57, 1972
116. Jankelson BJ, Sparks S, Crane PF: Neural conduction of the myo-monitor stimulus: a quantitative analysis. J Prosthet Dent 34:245, 1975
117. Bessette RW, Quinlivan JT: Electromyographic evaluation of the myo-monitor. J Prosthet Dent 30:19, 1973
118. Remien JC, Major MA: Myo-monitor centric: an evaluation. J Prosthet Dent 31:137, 1974
119. Bessette RW, Quinlivan JT: Electromyographic evaluation of the myo-monitor. J Prosthet Dent 30:19, 1973
120. Manns A, Miralles R, Guerrero F: The changes in electric activity of the postural muscles of the mandible upon varying the vertical dimension. J Prosthet Dent 45:438, 1981
121. Rugh J. D., Drago C. J., Barghi N: Comparison of electromyographic and phonetic measurements of vertical rest position (abstr No. 899). J Dent Res 58 (special issue A): 316, 1979
122. Rugh JD, Drago CJ: Vertical dimension: a study of clinical rest position and jaw muscle activity. J Prosthet Dent 45:670, 1981
123. Garnick J, Ramfjord SP: Rest position. An electromyographic and clinical investigation. J Prosthet Dent 12:895, 1962
124. Miralles R, Manns A, Guerrero F: Study of EMG postural activity in mandibular muscles at different body positions. Physiology 8:122, 1980
125. Latif A: An electromyographic study of the temporalis muscles in normal persons during selected positions and movements of the mandible. Am J Orthod 43:577, 1957
126. Carlsoo S: Nervous coordination and mechanical function of the mandibular elevators. An electromyographic study of the activity and an anatomic analysis of the mechanics of the muscles. Acta Odontol Scand, 10:suppl. 11:1, 1952
127. MacDougall JDB, Andrew BL: An electromyographic study of the temporalis and masseter muscles. J Anat 87:37, 1953

128. The Academy of Denture Prosthetics. Glossary of Prosthodontic Terms, 1st Ed. J Prosthet Dent 6:25, 1956
129. The Academy of Denture Prosthetics, Glossary of Prosthodontic Terms. 2nd. Ed. J Pros Dent, 10:30, 1960
130. The Academy of Denture Prosthetics, Glossary of Prosthodontic Terms. 4th ed. CV Mosby, St. Louis, 1977
131. Sherrington CS: Medical and Biological Research Dedicated to Sir William Osler, Vol. 1, Hoeber, New York, 1919
132. Wyke BD: Neuromuscular mechanisms influencing mandibular posture: a neurologist's review of current concepts. J Dentistry 2:111, 1972
133. Guyton AC: Textbook of Medical Physiology. 4th Ed. WB Saunders, Philadelphia, 1971
134. Goodgold J, Eberstein A: Electrodiagnosis of Neuromuscular Diseases. Williams and Wilkins, Baltimore, 1972
135. Basmajian JV: Muscles Alive. Their Functions Revealed by Electromyography. 2nd Ed. Williams & Wilkins, Baltimore, 1967
136. Granit R: The Basis of Motor Control. Academic Press, New York, 1970
137. Yemm R: The mandibular rest position: The roles of tissue elasticity and muscle activity. J DASA, 30:203, 1975
138. Yemm R, Berry DC: Passive control in mandibular rest position. J Dent Res 22:30, 1969
139. Carlsoo S: An electromyographic study of the activity of certain suprahyoid muscles, and of reciprocal innervation of the mandible. Acta Anat 26:81, 1956
140. Ahlgren J: The mechanisms of mastication. A quantitative cinematographic and electromyographic study of masticatory movements in children, with special reference to occlusion of the teeth. Acta Odontol Scand, suppl. 24:72, 1966
141. Ramfjord SP, Ash MM Jr: Occlusion. 2nd Ed. WB Saunders, Philadelphia, 1971
142. Atwood DA: A cephalometric study of the clinical rest position of the mandible. Part I: The variability of the clinical rest position following the removal of occlusal contacts, J Prosthet Dent 6:504, 1956
143. Carlsson, GE, Ericson S: Postural face height in full denture wearers. A longitudinal x-ray cephalometric study. Acta Odontol Scand 25:145, 1967
144. Yemm R: Irrelevant muscle activity: Dent Pract 91:51, 1968
145. Mohl DN: The role of head posture in mandibular function. p. 97. In Solberg WK, Clark G (eds): Abnormal Jaw Mechanics Diagnosis and Treatment, Quintessence, Chicago, 1984
146. Posselt U: Studies on the mobility of the human mandible. Acta Odontol Scand 10:1, 1952
147. Brill N, Lammie GA, Osborne J, et al: Mandibular positions and mandibular movements. Br Dent J 106:391, 1959
148. Dombrady L: Investigation into the transient instability of the rest position. J Prosthet Dent 16:479, 1966
149. Mohamed sE, Christensen LV: Mandibular reference positions. J Oral Rehabil 12:355, 1985
150. Bratzlavsky M, Vander Eecken H: Postural reflexes in cranial muscles in man. Acta Neurol Belg 77:5, 1977
151. Kerr FWL: Central relationships of trigeminal and cervical primary afferents in the spinal cord and medulla. Brain Res 43:561, 1972
152. Funakoshi M, Amano N: Effects of the tonic neck reflex on the jaw muscles of the rat. J Dent Res 52:668, 1973

153. Sumino R, Nozaki S, Katoh M: Trigemino-neck reflex. p. 81. In Kawamura Y, Dubner R: Oral-Facial Sensory and Motor Functions. Quintessence, Tokyo, 1981

154. Funakoshi M, Fujita N, Takehana S: Relations between occlusal interference and jaw muscle activities in response to changes in head position. J Dent Res 55:684, 1976

155. Lund P, Nishiyama T, Moller E: Postural activity in the muscles of mastication with the subject upright, inclined, and supine. Scand J Dent Res 78:417, 1970

156. Kendall HO, Kendall FP, Boynton DA: Posture and Pain. Robert E. Krieger, Huntington, NY, 1952

157. Kendall FP, McCreary EK: Muscles: Testing & Function. 3rd Ed. Williams & Wilkins, Baltimore, 1983

158. Goldstein DF, Kraus SL, Williams WB, et al: Influence of cervical posture on mandibular movement. J Prosthet Dent 52:421, 1984

159. Darling DW, Kraus SL, Glasheen-Wray MB: Relationship of head posture and the rest position of the mandible. J Prosthet Dent 52:111, 1984

160. Milidonis MK, Kraus SL, Segal RL, et al: Suprahyoid muscle activity in response to changes in anterior/posterior head posture. Am J Orthod (submitted for publication)

161. Root GR, Kraus SL, Razook SJ, et al: Effect of an intraoral appliance on head and neck posture. J Prosthet Dent 58:90, 1987

162. Ayub E, Glasheen-Wray MB, Kraus SL: Head posture: a case study on the effects on the rest position of the mandible. J Orthop Sports Phys Ther 5:179, 1984

163. Carlsson GE, Ingervall B, Gulumser K: Effect of increasing vertical dimension on the masticatory system in subjects with natural teeth. J Prosthet Dent 41:284, 1979

164. Halbert R: Electromyographic study of head position. J Can Dent Assoc 24:11, 1958

165. Davis PL: Electromyographic study of superficial neck muscles in mandibular function. J Dent Res 58:537, 1979

166. Green JD, Groot GD, Sutin J: Trigemino-bulbar reflex pathways. Am J Physiol 189:384, 1957

167. Manni E, Palmier G, Marini R, et al: Trigeminal influences on extensor muscles of the neck. Exp Neurol 47:330, 1975

168. Sumino R, Nozaki S: Trigemino-neck reflex: its peripheral and central organization. p. 365 In Anderson DJ, Matthews B (eds): Pain in the Trigeminal Region. Elsevier/North-Holland Biomedical Press, Amsterdam-New York, 1977

169. Daly PD, Preston CB, Evans WG: Postural response of the head to bite opening in adult males. Am J Orthod 82:157, 1982

170. Ramfjord SP: Bruxism, a clinical and electromyographic study. J Am Dent Assoc 62:21, 1961

171. Krough-Poulsen WB, Olsson A: Management of the occlusion of the teeth. p. 236 In Schwartz L, Chayes CM (eds) Facial Pain and Mandibular Dysfunction: WB Saunders, Philadelphia 1968.

172. Posselt U: The temporomandibular joint syndrome and occlusion. J Prosthet Dent 25:432, 1971

173. Lowenstein WR, Rathkamp R: A study on the pressoreceptive sensibility of the tooth. J Dent Res 34:287, 1955

174. Matthews B: Mastication, p. 199. In Lavelle CLB (ed): Applied Physiology of the Mouth. John Wright and Sons, Bristol, England 1975

175. Yemm BDS: Neurophysiologic studies of temporomandibular joint dysfunction. Oral Sc Rev 7:31, 1976

176. Weinberg LA: Temporomandibular dysfunctional profile: a patient-orientated approach J Prosthet Dent 32:312, 1974

177. Newton AV: Predisposing causes for temporomandibular joint dysfunction J Prosthet Dent 22:647, 1969

178. Rugh JD, Solberg WK: Psychological implications in temporomandibular pain and dysfunction. Oral Sci Rev 7:3, 1976

179. Mohl N: Head posture and its role in occlusion. New York State Dental Journal 42:17, 1976

180. McLean LF: Gravitational influences on the afferent and efferent components of mandibular reflexes. Ph.D. dissertation, Thomas Jefferson University of Philadelphia, 1973

181. Watt DM: Gnathosonics—a study of sounds produced by the masticatory mechanism. J Prosthet Dent 16:73, 1966

182. Eberle WR: A study of centric relation as recorded in a supine position. J Am Dent Assoc 42:15, 1951

183. McLean LW, Brenman HS, Friedman MGF: Effects of changing body position on dental occlusion. J Dent Res 52:1041, 1973

184. Brenman HS, Amsterdam M: Postural effects on occlusion. Dent Prog 4:43, 1963

185. Pruzansky S: The application of electromyography to dental research. J Am Dent Assoc 44:49, 1952

186. Jarabak JR: An electromyographic analysis of muscular and temporomandibular joint disturbances due to imbalances in occlusion. Angle Orthod 26(3):170, 1956

187. Perry HT: Functional electromyography of the temporal and masseter muscles in class II, division I malocclusion and excellent occlusion. Angle Orthod 26:49, 1955

188. Maruyama T, Nishio K, Kotani M, Miyauchi S: The effect of changing the maxillomandibular relationship by a bite plane on the habitual mandibular opening and closing movement. J Oral Rehabil 11:455, 1984

Index

Page numbers followed by *f* indicate figures; those followed by *t* indicate tables.